Introduction to
Statistical
Mediation Analysis

Multivariate Applications

Sponsored by the Society of Multivariate Experimental Psychology, the goal of this series is to apply complex statistical methods to significant social or behavioral issues, in such a way so as to be accessible to a nontechnical-oriented readership (e.g., nonmethodological researchers, teachers, students, government personnel, practitioners, and other professionals). Applications from a variety of disciplines such as psychology, public health, sociology, education, and business are welcome. Books can be single- or multiple-authored or edited volumes that (1) demonstrate the application of a variety of multivariate methods to a single, major major area of research; (2) describe a multivariate procedure or framework that could be applied to a number of research areas; or (3) present a variety of perspectives on a controversial topic of interest to applied multivariate researchers.

There are currently 12 books in the series:

- *What if there were no significance tests?* co-edited by Lisa L. Harlow, Stanley A. Mulaik, and James H. Steiger (1997).
- *Structural Equation Modeling with LISREL, PRELIS, and SIMPLIS: Basic Concepts, Applications, and Programming* written by Barbara M. Byrne (1998).
- *Multivariate Applications in Substance Use Research: New Methods for New Questions*, co-edited by Jennifer S. Rose, Laurie Chassin, Clark C. Presson, and Steven J. Sherman (2000).
- *Item Response Theory for Psychologists*, co-authored by Susan E. Emberston and Steven P. Reise (2000).
- *Structural Equation Modeling with AMOS: Basic Concepts, Applications, and Programming*, written by Barbara M. Byrne (2001).
- *Conducting Meta-Analysis Using SAS*, written by Winfred Arthur, Jr., Winston Bennett, Jr., and Allen I. Huffcutt (2001).
- *Modeling Intraindividual Variability with Repeated Measures Data: Methods and Applications*, co-edited by D. S. Moskowitz and Scott L. Hershberger (2002).
- *Multilevel Modeling: Methodological Advances, Issues, and Applications*, co-edited by Steven P. Reise and Naihua Duan (2003).
- *The Essence of Multivariate Thinking: Basic Themes and Methods*, written by Lisa Harlow (2005).
- *Contemporary Psychometrics:* A Festschrift for Roderick P. McDonald, co-edited by Albert Maydeu-Olivares and John J. McArdle (2005).
- *Structural Equation Modeling with EQS: Basic Concepts, Applications, and Programming, Second Edition*, written by Barbara M. Byrne (2006).
- *Introduction to Statistical Mediation Analysis*, written by David P. MacKinnon (2008).

Anyone wishing to submit a book proposal should send the following; (1) author/title; (2) timeline including completion date; (3) brief overview of the book's focus, including table of contents, and ideally a sample chapter (or more); (4) a brief description competing publications; and (5) targeted audiences.

For more information, please contact the series editor, Lisa Harlow, at Department of Psychology, University of Rhode Island, 10 Chafee Road, Suite 8, Kingston, RI 02881-0808; Phone (401) 874-4242; Fax (401) 874-5562; or e-mail LHarlow@uri.edu. Information may also be obtained from members of the advisory board: Leona Aiken (Arizona State University), Gwyneth Boodoo (Educational Testing Services), Barbara M. Byrne (University of Ottawa), Patrick Curran (University of North Carolina), Scott E. Maxwell (University of Notre Dame), David Rindskopf (City University of New York), Liora Schmelkin (Hofstra University), and Stephen West (Arizona State University).

Introduction to
Statistical
Mediation Analysis

David P. MacKinnon

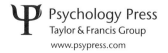

Psychology Press
Taylor & Francis Group
www.psypress.com

Lawrence Erlbaum Associates
Taylor & Francis Group
270 Madison Avenue
New York, NY 10016

Lawrence Erlbaum Associates
Taylor & Francis Group
27 Church Road
Hove, East Sussex BN3 2FA

Printed in the United States of America on acid-free paper
10 9 8 7 6

International Standard Book Number-13: 978-0-8058-6429-8 (Softcover) 978-0-8058-3974-6 (Hardcover)

Library of Congress Cataloging-in-Publication Data

MacKinnon, David Peter, 1957-
  Introduction to statistical mediation analysis / by David P. MacKinnon.
    p. cm.
  Includes bibliographical references and index.
  ISBN-13: 978-0-8058-6429-8 (soft cover)
  ISBN-10: 0-8058-6429-6 (soft cover)
  ISBN-13: 978-0-8058-3974-6 (hard cover)
  ISBN-10: 0-8058-3974-7 (hard cover)
  1. Mediation (Statistics) I. Title.

QA278.2.M29 2008
519.5'36--dc22   2007011793

Visit the Taylor & Francis Web site at
http://www.taylorandfrancis.com

and the LEA and Psychology Press Web site at
http://www.psypress.com

Contents

Preface

The main reason I became interested in mediation analysis was its potential for improving public health by helping to identify how to prevent problem behavior and promote healthy behavior. Mediation is also fundamental to many substantive areas, especially psychology (i.e., health, social, clinical, developmental, and cognitive) and the social and medical sciences. The idea of mediation is a simple one—that a third variable transmits the effect of one variable to another. Although the idea is simple, the scientific investigation of these variables is more complex than might be expected. I can't imagine tiring of the intriguing conceptual and statistical aspects of assessing whether a variable is intermediate between two other variables. There is much remaining work to be done in the area of mediation analysis. I view this book as a way to combine information on mediation analysis from a variety of disciplines in one place.

The goal of this book is to provide a comprehensive introduction to statistical, methodological, and conceptual aspects of mediation analysis. Throughout the book, substantive applications of mediation methods are described for a wide variety of research areas, from biology to sociology. In particular, readers will find applications in the development and evaluation of prevention and treatment programs in many fields as well as applications in epidemiology, social psychology, developmental psychology, and other areas. The book covers the single mediator model in detail before discussing extensions to advanced statistical methods including multilevel mediation models and longitudinal mediation models. The reader will notice the complexity involved even in the simplest single mediator model and remember these issues as the models become more complex. The goal is to prepare the reader for applying mediation analysis to a research program including estimation of effects, consideration of assumptions, and understanding of the limitations of the methodology.

There are four parts to the book. Part I, consisting of chapters 1 and 2, covers definitions, history, and applications for the mediation model. The purpose of this section is to provide an overview of the research questions the mediation model can answer. In Part II, consisting of chapters 3,

4, and 5, the conceptual model described in the first part of the book is quantified in the estimation of mediation in single and multiple mediator models. This part of the book describes the estimation of mediation effects including assumptions of the methods, statistical tests, and construction of confidence limits for the mediated effect. The methods described in this section serve as the foundation for the rest of the book. In Part III, consisting of chapters 6 to 12, advanced mediation models including mediation in path analysis, longitudinal mediation models, mediation with multilevel data, mediation for categorical variables, and mediation in the context of moderation are described. In Part IV, consisting of chapters 13, 14, and 15, general issues in the investigation of mediation including causal inference for mediation models, additional approaches to identifying mediating variables, and future directions are discussed. The importance of developing a program of research investigating mediational hypotheses is emphasized.

This book is intended to be an introduction to statistical mediation analysis. In general, the book assumes some exposure to a graduate level research methods or statistics course, although persons without this preparation will find many of the chapters useful. The entire book is designed so that a person with some exposure to graduate research methods and statistics could master the material in each chapter with sufficient time and determination. The primary audiences for this book are advanced undergraduate students, graduate students, and researchers from many substantive areas. I expect that there will be two general types of readers of this book. The first type will consist of persons skilled in a substantive area but less experienced with statistical methods. Persons designing prevention or treatment programs based on the mediation model would fall in this group. Researchers planning a study in which mediating mechanisms are investigated also fall in this group. For this group, it will be important to start with Chapters 1 and 2 even though some of this material may be familiar to substantive readers. Chapters 3 and 5 provide the general introduction to statistical methods for the mediator model. Once chapters 1 through 5 are understood, substantive researchers will have an easier time discussing mediation analysis with fellow researchers and the person conducting the statistical analysis. Chapters 6, 7, and 8 generally assume at least 1 year of graduate level research methods. Chapters 1 to 8 provide a general introduction to statistical mediation analysis. The remaining chapters describe special topics in mediation analysis. Chapter 13 is important because it summarizes the limits of what can be concluded from a mediation analysis. Chapter 14 describes additional approaches to investigating mediation including experimental designs for a program of research. Chapter 15 provides an overview of mediation analysis along with guidelines for conducting a mediation analysis.

The second type of reader is sophisticated statistically but without much exposure to mediation analysis. These persons may be interested in mediation in multilevel models (Chapter 9) or mediation with a binary outcome (Chapter 11) and already have some background in statistical methods. Chapters 1 and 2 provide a general background for the mediation model. The rest of the book is written so that statistically sophisticated persons may be able to focus on their particular area of interest. Future directions for statistical development are described in chapter 15.

There are several aspects of the book that should enhance learning. At the beginning of each chapter there is an overview of what is covered in the chapter. The summary at the end of each chapter provides links with subsequent chapters. Worked examples are provided in the text to make the topics in the book more concrete. Exercises at the end of each chapter solidify and extend topics covered in the chapter. Answers to the odd numbered questions are given in appendix A. The CD accompanying this book contains computer programs and output that are described in the book. The methods described in the book are illustrated with SAS and SPSS general computer programs and covariance structure analysis software including LISREL, EQS, Mplus, and CALIS. The CD also includes instructions for downloading a program to compute the most accurate confidence limits for the mediated effect based on the distribution of the product. A program to simulate the mediation model is also included on the CD.

Last, a word about notation: I have tried to keep notation consistent with existing literature on mediation in psychology with relations represented by a, b, c, and c' in the single mediator model. In Chapter 6, when model specification with matrix formulas are introduced, coefficient matrices are specified consistent with existing literature on structural equation modeling. Similarly, the multilevel mediation model chapter uses notation consistent with the research literature on multilevel analysis. However, whenever possible I have attempted to keep the simple notation for the single mediator model widely used in psychology even in more complicated models. As a result, in some places regular letters are used to represent relations in a mediation model and in other places Greek letters are used to represent relations in a mediation model. The cost of this is some ambiguity regarding coefficients representing relations, but the benefit is that the simpler single mediator notation is most widely used in social sciences research literature. Appendix B contains information on notation used in the book.

Acknowledgments

I sincerely acknowledge the support of the National Institute on Drug Abuse (DA09757) for my research on mediation analysis. Several data sets in this book were obtained as part of the Adolescents Training and Learning to Avoid Steroids study funded by the National Institute on Drug Abuse (DA07356).

Many former and current graduate students have provided feedback and contributed to this book on mediation analysis. In particular, I would like thank Chondra Lockwood, Jeewon Cheong, Jennifer Krull, Antonio Morgan-Lopez, Jason Williams, Ghulam Warsi, Marcia Taborga, Amanda Fairchild, Matt Fritz, Oi-Man Kwok, Myeongsun Yoon, Aaron Taylor, Krista Ranby, Davood Tofighi, Jeanne Hoffman, Felix Thoemmes, Vanessa Ohlrich, and Ehri Ryu. Matt Fritz and Amanda Fairchild also completed the computer programs and output in the CD that accompanies this book.

I also thank Andy Johnson, Craig Enders, Peter Killeen, Kristopher Preacher, Jenn Tein, Morris Okun, Michael Hecht, Irwin Sandler, Manuel Barrera, Nancy Eisenberg, Booil Jo, Michael Sobel, Diane Elliot, and Esther Moe for many helpful comments and edits. The book benefited from discussion with Dave Kenny, John Graham, Bill Hansen, Leona Aiken, Sanford Braver, Roger Millsap, Kim Johnson, Alex Zautra, Linda Luecken, Nancy Hay, Bill Fabricius, Helena Kraemer, and Linn Goldberg. I thank Hendricks Brown, Bengt Muthen, Wei Wang, George Howe, Dan Feaster, Lee Van Horn and other members of the Prevention Science Methodology Group (MH40859) for their feedback and comments on mediation topics. Mary Ann Pentz and Jim Dwyer provided sound advice and clear thinking when I first started investigating mediation.

I thank Lisa Harlow, the editor of this series, Patrick Curran, and Steve West for their extensive and challenging comments on many chapters in the book. I especially thank Ellen Laing and also Kristen Judd and Camden Bay for help preparing the manuscript. I thank Kim, Lea, and Ross for their support and patience as I wrote this book. I thank Pete, Al, and Will for inspiration.

Many people have helped me with this book. Remaining errors in this book are mine. If you have comments or improvements to the book, I would appreciate hearing from you.

1

Introduction

> "From the best statistics which I could get on the Isthmus, I found that the French lost yearly by death from yellow fever about one-third of their white force. . . . During the fall of 1905 yellow fever rapidly decreased, and by November, the last case of this disease had occurred in Panama. This fact quieted alarm on the Isthmus, and gave the sanitary officials great prestige. Not only among the now large body of Canal employees, but also among the native population living on the Isthmus."
>
> **—William Crawford Gorgas (1915, pp. 149, 156)**

1.1 Overview

This book addresses the question of how and why two things are related. How do knowledge and beliefs lead to behavior? Why does poverty lead to juvenile delinquency? How do tobacco prevention programs reduce tobacco use? How does psychotherapy reduce depression? These questions are addressed by considering variables that explain how or why two things are related. These variables are called mediating variables or mediators. More formally, a mediating variable is intermediate in the causal sequence relating an independent variable to a dependent variable. That is, the independent variable causes the mediating variable which then causes the dependent variable. *Webster's New World Dictionary of the American Language* (Guralnik, 1970, p. 881) defines mediate as "(1) to be in an intermediate position or location. (2) to be an intermediary or conciliator between persons or sides." and mediated as "(1) intermediate or intervening. (2) dependent on, acting by or connected through some intervening agency; related indirectly." The notion of a mediating variable in this book differs from the more common conception of a mediator as a person who negotiates between two parties. Mediation between two parties by a person is not described in this book. Methods to investigate variables that explain how or why two variables are related are the focus of this book.

Questions relating to mediating processes are central to basic and applied research in many fields. Here are a few mediational hypotheses: attitudes cause intentions, that then cause behavior; exposure to contagious bacteria causes infection that then causes disease; and exposure to information causes learning that causes behavior based on that learning. Many other examples are described throughout this book, and you can probably think of several right now. The purpose of this book is to describe methods to investigate such mediating variables.

Chapter 1 introduces the notion of a mediating variable in scientific research and defines several concepts used throughout the book. Two mediation examples are described. The first example, one of the most common examples of mediation, originated in the study of how an organism mediates the relation of a stimulus to a response (Woodworth, 1928). The substantial impact of this stimulus to organism to response (S–O–R) approach in psychology is described. The second mediation example is the description of the control of yellow fever during the building of the Panama Canal in the early 1900s. The same mediation approach is now widely used in health promotion and disease prevention. After these examples, several concepts are defined and a brief history of the mediating variable is given.

1.2 Stimulus–Organism–Response Model: A Mediation Theory

The stimulus–response (S–R) formulation dominated 20th century psychology (Hebb, 1966), and its influence continues today. In the S–R formulation of behavior, behavior is a response to stimuli. In a lower organism such as an insect, neural and muscular physiological mechanisms translate a stimulus to behavior. In higher organisms, mental processes in addition to physiological mechanisms translate a stimulus into behavior. Woodworth (1928) outlined a stimulus–organism–response (S–O–R) model for explaining how the organism mediates the relationship between the stimulus and response by postulating different mediating mechanisms operating in the organism. Mediating mechanisms are what determines how an organism responds to a stimulus. For example, a stimulus may trigger a memory mechanism that identifies the stimulus as a threat that leads to an avoidance response, or a stimulus may trigger an attraction process that leads to a physiological response such as pupil dilation and an approach response.

The S–R formulation was first applied in studies of learning, primarily with animals. In these experiments, animals learned how to avoid an electric shock or how to find food in a maze. Experimental manipulations elucidated many aspects of learning such as the ideal reward schedule to maintain behavior and how unrewarded behaviors decrease. Researchers theorized about the processes occurring between when a stimulus is given and a response is made. In an American Psychological Association presidential address devoted to describing why rats turn the way they do in mazes, Tolman (1938) proposed that mental processes such as demand, appetite, and biases translate stimuli into response. Tolman (1935) was also the first to use the term intervening variable for these mediating processes coming between the stimulus and response. In contrast to Tolman's mental processes, Hull (1937) postulated more materialistic variables such as habit strength and drive as mediating the relation of stimulus to response. In his view, learning consisted of organization and reorganization of reinforced drives. For both views, mathematical functions determined how the stimulus affected the intervening variables and how the intervening variables affected the response.

Two examples further demonstrate the S–O–R model. Suppose that you are given two numbers 16 and 18 and are asked to respond with their product. The two numbers, 16 and 18, are the stimulus and your answer is the response. The mediating process is the thinking and other activities done in the time between when you were given the stimulus and when you made your response. Another example is from a study of learning in monkeys by Tinklepaugh (1928). The monkeys were allowed to view the experimenter put food such as lettuce in one of two cups out of the monkey's reach. A screen was put up and after a delay the monkey was allowed to retrieve the food from one of the cups. In one experiment, the experimenter put lettuce in a cup that the monkey took and ate after a delay. In another experiment, the monkey saw the experimenter put a banana, the monkey's favorite food, in one cup, but after the screen was put up, the experimenter replaced the banana with lettuce. When the screen was removed and the monkey picked up the lettuce, the monkey showed surprise and would not eat the lettuce, and some monkeys "turned toward observers present in the room and shrieked at them in apparent anger" (Tinklepaugh, 1928, p. 224). This study suggested that the stimulus of showing the food initiated expectancy in the monkey that then affected how the monkey responded to the food. The expectancy was the mediating or intervening variable.

The S–O–R model illustrates that the mediational process can be complicated. First, the mediating process is generally unobservable. If each link in the S–O–R model is studied, then some way to measure the mediating process is required. For the S–O–R model, examples of measuring mediators are electroencephalography, pupil dilation, galvanic skin response, and self-reports. Second, the mediating process may operate at different levels. Mediating processes contain physiological changes that translate the stimulus to the response and mental processes. Within the physiological domain, there are neuronal, sensory, and muscular mediational processes, even for simple S–R relations. Mediating mechanisms may be present outside the organism as well, such as group and community level processes (e.g., the socioeconomic status of a neighborhood may affect social cohesion that affects crime rates). Third, the mediating process can be the sum of a variety of mediating processes happening simultaneously or in sequence. Fourth, the chain of mediation may be extensive, for example, a sequence of sensory, neuronal, and muscular activity. In the S–R formulation, molar mediation approaches that focused on the major variables were preferred to molecular processes involved in detailed chains (Hull, 1943, p. 19). Decisions about the level of detail investigated in a mediational chain are required for any mediation analysis.

The S–O–R model is an example of the more general black box model, in which the black box refers to unobservable mechanisms by which an input affects an output (Weed, 1998). The variables in the black box are mediating variables and the mechanisms hypothesized in the black box are mediating mechanisms. The S–O–R and black box models provide the framework for mediation analysis. The black box model applies to many areas of science. Early in history, atomic mechanisms were hypothesized for the observable processes of chemical reactions. These atomic chemical reactions are unobserved and must be inferred from the results of experiments. In these experiments, chemicals are the input to the black box and chemicals are the output from the black box. Experiments by John Dalton and Antoine Lavoisier demonstrating that mass was conserved and proportions of original elements were identical after chemical reactions led to the conclusion that matter was composed of atoms (Brown, LeMay, & Bursten, 2000). Atomic reactions are what transform the chemical input to the chemical output. Scientific developments such as the electron microscope have improved the ability to view and measure these processes, and this has led to even more unobservable hypotheses such as subatomic particles. Gregor Mendel hypothesized that particles or genes were the mechanisms for his studies of inheritance in pea plants (Campbell, Reece, Taylor, & Simon, 2006). Genetic theory describes how parent traits, the input to the black box, lead to offspring traits, the output from the black box. With the discovery of deoxyribonucleic acid (DNA) and now the measurement of the human, rat, and fruit fly genome, direct measurement of the previously unobserved genetic mechanisms is possible. The genetic and atomic theory examples illustrate how theory is used to understand unobservable inner mechanisms in the black box. These examples also demonstrate how science progresses by measuring previously unobserved mediating mechanisms. In fact, investigation of mediating variables may be considered a measurement problem, for which progress occurs with more accurate measurement of the mediating process.

1.3 Yellow Fever and the Panama Canal: An Applied Mediation Example

The control of yellow fever during the building of the Panama Canal provides an early example of an intervention designed to change mediators to change an outcome variable. The French attempt to build the Panama Canal during 1889 to 1898 was stopped by yellow fever—a disease that killed or incapacitated so many workers that continuous work on the project was impossible. But the Panama Canal had to be built, as the trip around Cape Horn at the bottom of South America was too long and dangerous. Because the Panama Canal was vital to the interests of the United States, it followed that the United States would take up the task to build the canal. Recognizing the health as well as the engineering challenges to build the canal, Dr. William Gorgas was selected to lead the public health attack on yellow fever and malaria (Gorgas, 1915).

Two major theories for the cause of yellow fever were present at this time (Gorgas, 1915). The first theory held that person-to-person contact was the main cause of disease transmission. These arguments flowed naturally from the findings that anthrax and other diseases were spread by contact with sick individuals or their body fluids. This theory suggested that yellow fever could be battled by improving sanitation and quarantining infected persons. A second theory was that mosquitos carried malaria and yellow fever. Here the reduction of human exposure to mosquitos was the critical component to prevent yellow fever.

Convinced that malaria and yellow fever were transmitted by mosquitos, Dr. Gorgas set out with a comprehensive plan to reduce human exposure to mosquitos (Gorgas, 1915). The purpose of these activities was to reduce the number of mosquitos under the theory that fewer mosquitos led to fewer human bites, consequently fewer disease cases, and ultimately fewer deaths due to malaria and yellow fever. Such a multiple cause model was elegant but also unwieldy with many opportunities for failure. For example, if mosquitos were not the carrier of disease, no effect would be observed. If the species of mosquito that carried disease was not reduced, then the prevention activity would fail even if many mosquitos were killed.

To reduce human exposure to mosquitos, the number of animals that eat mosquitos was increased, drainage canals were built, and plumbing was introduced wherever possible to reduce the amount of standing water ideal for mosquito breeding. Sleeping quarters were screened to keep out mosquitos. The result of these interventions, based on the theory that mosquitos caused the diseases, was a significant reduction in malaria and yellow fever cases. Consequently, the Canal was built, at least partly, because of prevention activity based on a hypothesized causal connection based on theory, a target of the intervention or mediating variable (human exposure to mosquitos), and components to change the mediating variable. These results led to subsequent research identifying the viruses responsible for the diseases. Many disease prevention and health promotion activities are of this type in which theory is used to identify important mediators and activities are designed to change those mediators. This mediation model links the intervention activities to changes in mediators to changes in an outcome variable.

1.4 Two-Variable Effects

The translation of mediation concepts to statistical methods begins with the simplest form of a relation between two variables. Much of statistics focuses on the association of one variable, X, with another variable, Y. Often a distinction is made between the independent variable, X, and the dependent variable, Y, to identify the direction of the hypothesized relationship between the variables. Effects in which one variable causes another variable are called asymmetric effects to specify that one variable is the cause of another variable (Rosenberg, 1968). A symmetric relation is one in which both X and Y cause each other. By restricting the discussion to two variables and assuming no other variable affects the relation between X and Y, there are four possibilities: X and Y are unrelated, X causes Y, Y causes X, or X causes Y and Y causes X at the same time, a reciprocal relation. Much research and theory are based on statistics from this two-variable system of relations. The correlation coefficient, regression coefficient, odds ratio, and the difference in the mean between two groups (where X represents assignment to the groups) are examples of quantitative measures from a two-variable system. Even in a two-variable system, it can be very difficult or impossible to identify causal relations because these relations are inferred from observed data.

1.5 Three-Variable Effects

The addition of a third variable to the interpretation of the relation between an independent and dependent variable increases the number and complexity of the possible relations among the three variables. It is still possible that X causes Y or Y causes X, but there are many additional possibilities. Assuming asymmetric effects, now the third variable, Z, can be in any order of causal direction with X and Y, e.g., X to Z to Y, Z to X to Y, X to Y to Z, as well as other possibilities as described later. Reciprocal relations are also possible between any two variables and among all three variables. Given the number and complexity of the possible relations among these variables, there are several generally accepted descriptions of conceptual relations among three variables. These descriptions form a general way to understand effects in even more complicated systems of relations.

Confounder. One possibility is that the relation between X and Y changes when Z is considered because Z causes both X and Y, leading to an observed relationship between X and Y that may be considered causal if Z is not included in the analysis (see Greenland & Morgenstern, 2001, for comprehensive discussion of confounding). Such a Z variable is a confounder of the effect and it may decrease or increase the relation between X and Y. *A confounder is defined as a variable that changes the relation between an independent and dependent variable because it is related to both the independent and the dependent variable.* Meinert (1986, p. 285) defined a confounder as "a variable related to two variables of interest that falsely obscures or accentuates the relation between them." In many research studies, an effect is said to be adjusted for a confounder, which means that the reported relationship between X and Y has been adjusted for the confounder effect of Z. It is important to note that a third variable, Z, may actually increase the relation between X and Y, in which case Z is a suppressor variable. A suppressor variable is one in which the original relation between two variables increases in magnitude when a third variable is adjusted for in an analysis (Conger, 1974; MacKinnon, Krull, & Lockwood, 2000). It is also possible that a relation between X and Y actually is reversed when a third variable is included in the analysis, which is a distorter variable (Rosenberg, 1968). A distorter variable is a variable that changes a relation between two variables such that when it is included in an analysis a relation emerges between previously unrelated variables or the direction of relation between two variables reverses in sign.

Covariate. Another possibility is that the third variable, Z, is another predictor of Y such that both X and Z predict Y. In this case, the additional predictor, Z, will make the prediction of Y more accurate because it explains variability in the Y variable. If there is no relation between X and Z, the addition of the third variable, Z, to the analysis will not change the relation between X and Y. These types of variables have been called covariates or predictors. *A covariate is a variable related to the dependent variable that typically has a minimal relation to the independent variable.* Covariates may also be related to both the dependent and independent variables. Typically, a confounder differs from a covariate in that a confounder is also related to X and Y but in a way that consideration of the confounder changes the relation between X and Y.

Mediator. A more complicated relation may be present such that the third variable is intermediate in the causal chain relating X and Y such that X causes Z and Z causes Y. This type of relationship is called mediation, and the Z variable is called a mediator or mediating variable (M). A mediating (M) variable is intermediate in the causal path from an independent variable to a dependent variable. A mediating variable represents asymmetric relations among variables. *In a mediation model, the independent variable causes the mediator which then causes the dependent variable.* Baron and Kenny (1986, p. 1173), defined mediation as "the generative mechanism through which the focal independent variable is able to influence the dependent variable of interest." In Last's (1988) medical dictionary, a mediator is defined as "a variable that occurs in a causal pathway from an independent variable to a dependent variable. It causes variation in the dependent variable and itself is caused to vary by the independent variable." So a mediator (M) is a variable that transmits the effect of an independent variable on a dependent variable. Mediation also implies a temporal relation with X occurring before M and M occurring before Y. These mediating variables and methods to test for them are the focus of this book.

Another widely used definition of a mediator has led to some confusion because both a confounder and a mediator satisfy the definition, "In general, a given variable may be said to function as a mediator to the extent that it accounts for the relation between the predictor and the criterion" (Baron & Kenny, 1986, p. 1176). Both the confounder and the mediator account for the relationship between X and Y. A confounder explains the relation because it is related to both X and Y, but not as part of a causal mediation process. The mediator explains the relation between X and Y because it transmits the effect of X on Y through the mediator Z. Several other definitions of a mediating variable also include this ambiguity regarding a confounding and mediating variable. For example, Hoyle and Smith (1994, p. 437) stated "The question that gives rise to mediational hypotheses can be stated, How or why does X affect Y or, more specifically, Can the effect of X on Y be attributed to Z?" A confounder or a mediator will satisfy this definition as either explains how or why an effect occurs. Mediation explains the effect by the causal sequence from the independent variable to the mediator to the dependent variable. The confounder effect also explains the relation because a confounder is related to both the independent and the dependent variable.

Some references identify a mediator as not necessarily in the causal sequence between the independent and dependent variable and only require that the independent variable influences the mediator and the mediator influences the dependent variable (Holmbeck, 1997, p. 600). This view has led to confusion regarding the meaning of mediation and, as a result, in this book, a mediator is intermediate in the causal sequence between the independent variable and the dependent variable. It is true that other variables may explain a relation between an independent and dependent variable, but these other variables may serve as confounders of the relation and explain the relation in that manner. It does not explain the relation in terms of a mediation model.

Further misunderstanding has arisen because some mediation tests require that there is a significant relation between the independent and the dependent variable for mediation to exist. Although these effects may be rare, it is possible that there is a significant mediational process, even if there is not a significant overall relation between the independent variable and the dependent variable (Collins, Graham, & Flaherty, 1998; MacKinnon et al., 2000; Shrout & Bolger, 2002). If there is not a significant relation of an independent variable with a dependent variable and the indirect effect is statistically significant, Holmbeck (1997) concludes that there is an indirect effect but not a mediated effect. The idea is that if there is not a significant relation between two variables then it does not make sense to talk about mediation, but it does make sense to talk about indirect effects. As described in Holmbeck (1997, p. 603), "findings suggest that the mediator does not (and cannot) significantly 'account' for the predictor–criterion relationship (because there was not a significant relation between the predictor and the criterion in the first place)." Even if there is not a significant relation between the independent variable and the dependent variable, mediation can exist. This pattern may occur because the test of the mediated effect has more statistical power than the test of the overall relation of X on Y in some situations. It is easy to simulate data with a pattern such that the overall relation between X and Y is not statistically significant, but there is a significant mediation effect. One substantive example of this pattern of effects is the small relation between age and typing proficiency, which is explained by the opposing mediational processes whereby age increases reaction time reducing typing proficiency and age increases cognitive typing skills improving typing proficiency (Salthouse, 1984). In this case, the mediating variables reveal important mediation relations as described in Rosenberg (1968, chapter 4) in his discussion of distorter variables.

Mediating variables are often called intervening or intermediate variables to clearly indicate their role as coming between an independent and a dependent variable. Mediating variables have also been called process variables (Judd & Kenny, 1981b) referring to their function as variables that describe the process by which an independent variable affects a dependent variable. In the medical literature, mediating variables are sometimes called surrogate or intermediate endpoints because these variables represent proximal measures of a distal outcome (Prentice, 1989).

Different names are also used for the sequence of variables in a mediational process. Kenny, Kashy, and Bolger (1998) described the three variables as initial to mediator to outcome variables. James and Brett (1984) referred to the antecedent to mediating to consequent variables to clearly define the time sequence of a mediational process. Shipley (2000) described a mediator that transmits the effect of a causal ancestor on its descendant. In the medical literature, program exposure to intermediate endpoint to ultimate endpoint is used (Freedman, Graubard, & Schatzkin, 1992). Another common nomenclature distinguishes between proximal and distal measures, where mediators are typically the proximal measures and the distal measures are outcome measures. The purpose of different variable names is to be precise about the nature of the variables studied. In this book, the variables will be described as the independent variable, mediator, and dependent variable because of the simplicity and the general applicability of these terms. Technically, there will be cases in which the independent variable is not strictly independent of other variables as the independent variable in a randomized study, for example. The independent variable will refer to the first variable in the mediational sequence.

Researchers often make the distinction between a mechanism and a mediator. The mechanism is described as the true causal process by which two variables are related in contrast to a mediator or mediating variable, which is the measure used to investigate the mechanism. This distinction is the same as the difference between a hypothetical mediating mechanism and intervening variable made by MacCorquodale and Meehl (1948). Inference regarding mediation must be based on sample data. In many cases, it will not be possible to fully distinguish between mediation and other third-variable effects, and additional information such as theory will be required to build a case for mediation. As clearly stated by McCullagh and Nelder (1989, p. 8), all models are generally wrong in some way and, "we must recognize that eternal truth is not within our grasp." Inference regarding a true mediating mechanism is most likely to emerge based on a body of research evidence rather than one study.

Moderator. A third variable may also change the relation between the independent variable and the dependent variable because it moderates the relation between the two variables. Baron and Kenny (1986, p. 1174) defined a moderator as "a qualitative (e.g., sex, race, class) or quantitative (e.g., level of reward) variable that affects the direction and/or strength of the relation between an independent or predictor variable and a dependent or criterion variable." Sharma, Durand, and Gur-Arie (1981, p. 291) define a moderator as a variable that "systematically modifies either the form and/or strength of the relationship between a predictor and a criterion variable." In fact, Sharma et al. (1981) described three different types of moderators depending on the correlation between the moderator variable and X and Y, and whether there is a statistically significant interaction between the moderator and the X variable. Moderators are variables that interact such that the relation between X and Y is different at different levels of the moderator variable. *A moderator is a variable that changes the sign or strength of the effect of an independent variable on a dependent variable.* It is typically (but not always) an interaction such that the effect of an independent variable on a dependent variable depends on the level of the moderator variable. Here the relation between X and Y changes at different values of the third variable. Moderator variables have also been called effect modifiers or effect measure modifiers given that the effect is modified by the levels of the third variable (Rothman & Greenland, 1998). Effect modification is the term most often used in the medical literature. Information on the investigation of moderator or interaction variables is described in Aiken and West (1991). More detailed information regarding moderator variables and types of models that have both moderator and mediator effects are described in chapter 10.

1.6 Mediators and Moderators

In addition to the Baron and Kenny (1986) landmark article, interesting discussions of the distinction between mediating and moderating variables have been described for nursing (Bennett, 2000), industrial and organizational psychology (James & Brett, 1984), child psychotherapy (Kazdin & Nock, 2003), clinical psychology (Holmbeck, 1997), psychoneuroimmunology (Stone, 1992), and programs for children (Petrosino, 2000). More recently a series of comments and discussion on mediators and moderators appeared in the *Journal of Consumer Psychology*, Volume 10, 2001 (Ambler, 2001; Heath, 2001; Lehmann, 2001). There are many valid, useful definitions of mediators and moderators in the literature. For example, Kraemer, Stice, Kazdin, Offord, and Kupfer (2001) specified mediators as variables that change over time after an intervention and moderators as variables that are measured before an intervention. More detailed definitions of confounding and confounders are also available (Greenland & Morgenstern, 2001). To clarify the discussion in this book, the definitions in italics in this chapter will be used throughout this book.

For the most part, the relative priority of investigating moderators versus mediators depends on the research question of interest. However, as stated by Stone (1992, p. 14), "Perhaps it is in some sense flashier to focus solely on mediators, because they address more central hypothesized linkages." Generally, mediators are more interesting because they address the mechanisms by which an effect occurs, whereas moderators provide information on when effects are present. Once a moderator effect is found, mediation analysis is often used to explain the source of the ef the case of experimental manipulations, in which an effect is present for one group but not another, a subsequent study may investigate mediational process in the group for which the manipulation was successful. In another respect, the failure of a mediating process in a subgroup defined by a moderator may imply that the mediation theory is limited and needs revision. The ideal theory applies across subgroups and situations. There are also situations in which moderation is consistent with a mediated effect. In an exercise promotion study, for example, it is not likely that an intervention can improve exercise habits of persons who are already high on a mediator such as belief that exercise is important. As a result, there will be a moderator effect whereby program effects are only observed for persons low on beliefs about exercise at baseline.

1.7 Four or More Variable Effects

The number of possible relations among variables increases rapidly as the number of variables increases. An example of a four-variable effect is described in chapter 10, where a mediational process differs across levels of a moderator. Another more common example of a four-variable effect is a four-way interaction in analysis of variance. Perhaps as knowledge in a field progresses, more complicated effects will be hypothesized and tested. A more common way to deal with this complexity is to identify third-variable effects in more complicated models.

Given the many possible relations among four or more variables, how should a researcher proceed? Theory and prior research provide the clearest motivation for reducing the number of realistic relations. Pilot and exploratory analysis further clarify the relations suitable for further study. Randomized experimental designs provide a way to localize the effect of one or more variables. In general, programs of research based on theory, prior research, qualitative methods, longitudinal studies, and experimental designs are necessary to investigate mediational processes.

1.8 Some Historical Background for Mediation Analysis

This section describes several major historical issues that provide the background for modern approaches to identify mediating variables. An attempt has been made to describe the issues in chronological order but this is difficult because the issues overlap in content and when they were first discussed.

Cause. At approximately age 3, persons begin to interpret their world in terms of processes by which one thing leads to another (Shultz, 1982). These young persons can generate and answer questions about how two things are related, including whether one thing causes another. It is not surprising that the identification of how and why things are related has played a central role in how humans view their environment because once real causal sequences are identified, they are likely to be present in new situations. As summarized by Shultz (1982, p. 1), ". . . the concept of causation is just as indispensable to human understanding as are the concepts of object, space, time, quantity, and logic."

The first written historical examples of questions similar to mediation begin in the 3rd century BC, with Aristotle's identification of material, formal, efficient, and final causes. The efficient cause refers to how a thing comes about and is most similar to the investigation of mediation. The research literature on causality is voluminous so only a few examples related to mediation and research to investigate mediational processes are presented here. In general, the literature focuses on a causal relation between one cause and one effect. Hume (1748) argued that observers are not capable of identifying causes but are capable of observing the regularity of events and may consider one thing as a cause of another under certain conditions consisting of spatial/temporal contiguity (two events occur close in time and space), temporal succession (one event always precedes another), and constant conjunction (whenever one event is observed, the other event is also observed). In this framework, observed events form the basis for inferring mediation. Another view of causality argues that the causes of effects can be found and that is what humans do well (Kant, 1965/1781). Mill (1843) introduced the notion of covariation as being indicative of a causal relation and advocated experimentation to identify causes. Similarly, Suppes (1970) emphasized covariation as a manifestation of a causal relation and suggested tests of whether additional variables reflecting alternative causes remove the covariation. Popper (1959) argued that causes can never be proven, but that data can be viewed as consistent or inconsistent with a cause. Further, Popper argued that the best research strategy is to focus on testing whether hypothesized causal relations are false so that false causal hypotheses are rejected. In this way science advances by systematic testing and refutation of causal hypotheses.

Wright's path analysis. Modern approaches to quantifying mediating mechanisms began with Sewall Wright's (Wolfle, 1999; Wright, 1920, 1921) methods for the path analysis of systems of relations among variables that included mediating processes as an important component. Wright used this system of equations for the relations among variables to quantify the hereditary and environmental influences on the color patterns of piebald guinea pigs. Wright's method, called path analysis, defined a model in terms of mathematical equations and displayed the model visually in a path diagram, in which variables were represented with symbols and causal relations between variables with arrows to indicate the direction of the relation. Path analysis provided a way to specify the causal relations among many variables and generated coefficients reflecting the size of the relation between variables. Path analysis generated quantitative estimates of the coefficients including mediated effects based on observed correlations among variables. Wright showed that the path coefficient for a mediating process was the product of all the path coefficients in a chain of mediation. The same quantification of mediation as a product of coefficients is described later in this book starting in chapter 3.

As with many new statistical methods, path analysis was developed to extract the maximum amount of information from data. In this case, the data were from the U.S. Department of Agriculture's extensive studies on breeding guinea pigs. Wright wrote several papers (Wright, 1920, 1921) on the quantitative analysis of the guinea pig data, which was an ideal application of path analysis methods because of clear genetic hypotheses and linear relations between parent and offspring variables. Wright used the methods to partition the variance in guinea pig breeding into heredity and environment.

Niles (1922, 1923) provided an important criticism of Wright's path analysis. The criticisms by Niles are the same criticisms of path analysis and mediation methods that are voiced today. Niles criticized Wright on several accounts, of which three are most relevant here. First, Niles stated that correlation and causation are the same thing so it was senseless to contrast them, an idea popularized by Pearson in his classic book, *The Grammar of Science* (Pearson, 1911). Pearson (1911) argued that correlation was a broad category with causation at its limit (Pearl, 2000) because all things are associated. The difficulty was the assessment of how closely things are associated, for which Pearson proposed the correlation coefficient.

Niles' second criticism was that it was impossible to specify a correct system of the action of causes. In Wright's most important response to Niles' criticisms, Wright (1923, p. 240) stated an argument used to defend path analysis approaches to this day, "the combination of knowledge of correlations with knowledge of causal relations, to obtain certain results, is a different thing from the deduction of causal relations from correlations implied by Niles' statement. Prior knowledge of the causal relations is assumed as a prerequisite in the former case." Wright (1923, p. 241) further divided the application of theory into three cases, "(1) where the causal relations among the variables may be considered as known, (2) where enough is known to warrant an hypothesis or alternative hypothesis, and (3) where even an hypothesis does not seem justified." In case 1, he argued that knowledge of causation and correlation justifies the modeling. In case 2, he noted that models can be compared with new data. He suggested that perhaps nothing could be done for case 3 because there is nothing to combine with knowledge of the correlations.

Wright agreed with Niles' third criticism that the chain of causation must be cut off at some point, but argued that this was true of all scientific research. In particular, Niles noted Pearson's idea that the causes of any individual thing can widen out in an unmanageable way. Wright argued that a portion of the unmanageable number of causes can be studied by isolating a portion of the system and investigating causation in this more limited system. Wright (1923, p. 250) stated, "In subtracting the total cause of one event from another there is an enormous cancellation of common factors." This discussion of the chain of causation is the ubiquitous issue of molar versus molecular mediation where molecular or micromediation refers to the specification of causal pathways in minute detail, and molar mediation specifies causal pathways with more general variables that reflect aggregated micromediational pathways. It is often only possible to study mediation at a molar level because of the unfeasible level of detail for measurement of micromediation.

In summary, Wright argued that path analysis was not a method to infer causation, it was a method to quantify already supposed causal relations. The attempt to quantify causal relations required an initial set of causal sequences that was deduced from all available information including theory, prior correlations, and results of prior experiments. These causal relations were then quantified using path analysis. Wright (1923) also gave a clear outline of path analysis including definitions of coefficients and applications of the method to study causal relations.

Many of these same criticisms and responses have been repeated in modern discussions of structural equation modeling of covariance and correlation matrices, which includes path analysis as a special case (Cliff, 1983; Ling, 1982; MacCallum, Wegener, Uchino, & Fabrigar, 1993). Most criticisms relate to the case for which there is insufficient information to specify causal relations and the usefulness of applying the model is unclear. Others would argue that even in this case, specifying a model could be used to explore relations that will be tested in a subsequent study. Overall, these criticisms focus on the additional information that must be brought to bear on any research problem, rather than inferring relations based on correlations or associations (Berk, 1991; Blalock, 1991; Freedman, 1991).

Conceptualizations of mediation. During the 1950s, several important conceptualizations of mediation were developed in psychology, agriculture, and social science. As described earlier, one of the first substantive examples of a mediation hypothesis in modern research comes from the S–O–R (Woodworth, 1928) ideas of classic psychology. Later a distinction between theoretical mediating variables and intervening variables was made by MacCorquodale and Meehl (1948) and also Ginsberg (1954), where theoretical mediating processes were hypothetical constructs and intervening variables were the measures of those hypothetical constructs. This distinction between the theoretical nature of a mediating process and the variables used to measure that process is important for applications of mediation analysis. A similar distinction was made between molar mediation, whereby more general variables are investigated, in comparison with molecular or micromediation where each variable in the chain of mediation is investigated. Rozeboom (1956) described a mediation model in terms of functional relations, whereby the mediator is a function of the independent variable and the dependent variable is a function of the mediator. In this model, for mediation to exist, the relation between the independent variable and the dependent variable and the mediator and the dependent variable must not be independent. Mediation as functional relations has been the basis of subsequent conditional probability definitions of mediation (Freedman & Schatzkin, 1992).

Another line of related research began with Fisher's (1934) development of analysis of covariance as a means to adjust the results of analysis of variance for an additional variable called a covariate. A covariate can reduce unexplained variability and clarify the true effects of an experimental manipulation. Original applications of analysis of covariance were in agricultural studies in which, for example, the effects of an experimental manipulation on crop yield in plots of land were adjusted for covariates such as variation in soil quality among the plots. A covariate is also called a concomitant variable because in some situations it was not sensible to remove the effects of the additional variable by covariance analysis (Cochran, 1957; Smith, 1957). For the case of mediation, the concomitant variable and the dependent variable are affected by the experimental manipulation. For example, fumigation reduces the number of eelworms, which increases oat yield because eelworms reduce oat yield (Cochran, 1957). The number of eelworms in a volume of soil is a mediating variable. The true effect of fumigation of farmland is not obtained by removing the effect on eelworms from the effect of fumigation on oat yield because changes in the number of eelworms are affected by fumigation. This conceptualization of mediation in terms of a concomitant variable affected by the independent variable forms the basis of several important modern contributions to mediation analysis based on the meaning and function of concomitant variables (Rosenbaum, 1984; Rubin, 2004).

Another historical precedent for mediation analysis is the elaboration method developed by Paul Lazarsfeld (1955) and colleagues (Kendall & Lazarsfeld, 1950). The elaboration method adds variables into statistical analysis to see how an original relation between two variables changes. The elaboration model was developed to formalize the analysis of contingency table data from the research of Stouffer, Suchman, DeVinney, Star, and Williams (1949) on American soldiers during World War II. Stouffer and colleagues added variables to the statistical analysis to understand the meaning of observed relations between two variables. For example, based on elaboration analysis, Stouffer and colleagues demonstrated that the relation of soldier morale was primarily a function of soldiers' feelings of deprivation relative to other soldiers around them rather than to soldiers in other locations. Lazarsfeld and colleagues formalized the methodology involved in elaboration, based on how the addition of a third variable affects the relation between two variables. If the addition of a third variable does not appreciably change the original relation, it is called replication, so the third variable is a covariate as discussed earlier. If the addition of a third variable changes the observed relation because the third variable is related to the two original variables but does not intervene between them, it is called explanation, and the third variable is the same as a confounder. Interpretation corresponds to a third variable that changes an observed relation because it comes between the independent and dependent variable and is interpreted as an intervening or mediating variable. Specification refers to a third variable that specifies when and at what levels of the third variable a relation is observed or not observed, corresponding to a moderator variable. A primary aspect of elaboration is the identification of the time ordering of variables based on theory and prior research, necessary to identify the independent, intervening, and dependent variables. Rosenberg (1968) further developed the elaboration method including the notion of a distorter variable that may make a relation emerge and may reverse the sign of an original relation. The elaboration method is widely used in the social sciences.

Structural equation models. The next important events in the quantification of mediating processes occurred when sociologists and economists developed models for sets of causal relations (Blalock, 1971; Duncan, 1966; Goldberger, 1972; Simon, 1954). Simon (1954) clarified the assumptions for the relations in three variable models. Duncan (1966) applied the path analysis methods described by Wright to examine models including mediated effects in sociology. Here one of the primary research topics was the effects of parental characteristics on child characteristics, such as the effects of parent socioeconomic status (SES) on child SES mediated by child education. Sociology has continued to be an active area of application of mediation models as well as an important area of statistical development and application for new methods. Because there are often many variables in sociological theory, there are often many mediators.

The modeling tradition started by Wright and rediscovered by Duncan and Blalock was made more general with the development of covariance structure modeling including the Jöreskog (1970, 1973) Keesling (1972)

Wiley (1973) or the JKW covariance structure model (Bentler, 1980). The LISREL (Jöreskog & Sörbom, 2001) program for the JKW approach was developed and has received widespread application. The Bentler–Weeks formulation (Bentler & Weeks, 1982) that required half as many matrices as the JKW approach was included in the EQS program (Bentler, 1997). Covariance structure models combine traditions. The path analysis multiple equation tradition, started by Wright and extended to sociology and economics, was combined with the psychometrics tradition with its focus on measurement. These models, which are also called structural equation models, combine a measurement structure from factor analysis (Mulaik, 1972) with the path analytical framework by specifying latent, unobserved, constructs formed by separating true and error variance in observed measures. In this way, covariance structure models distinguish between the measurement model for observed measures of a construct and the structural model for the relations among the constructs. These covariance structure analysis models improve the accuracy of the estimation of mediated effects in a model that includes both methods to assess mediation and also methods to model measurement error in the analysis. The use of maximum likelihood estimation for covariance structure models allows for a statistical test of how close the predictions of the model are to the actual data (Shipley, 2000).

The estimation of each of the mediated effects in structural equation and path analysis models is called effect decomposition to identify the fact that there is a separation of effects in terms of direct effects and mediated effects (Alwin & Hauser, 1975). According to Duncan, effect decomposition in path analysis is important because "it makes explicit both the direct effects and indirect effects of causal variables on dependent variables" (Duncan, Featherman, & Duncan, 1972, p. 23). General methods to decompose effects into direct and indirect effects for covariance structure models were derived (Alwin & Hauser, 1975; Graff & Schmidt, 1982). Sobel (1982) derived the standard error of these direct and indirect effects and shortly thereafter several covariance structure analysis programs included these standard errors as part of their output. These standard errors are used to compute confidence intervals for indirect effects.

There has been consistent development of statistical methods for covariance structure modeling such as methods for non-normal data (Browne, 1984), ordinal or limited variables (Muthén, 1984), alternative specifications of the models (Bentler & Weeks, 1982; McArdle & McDonald, 1984), and growth curve models (Rogosa, 1988). Statistical software, such as EQS (Bentler, 1997), Mx (Neale, Boker, Xie, & Maes, 2002), & LISREL (Jöreskog & Sörbom, 2001), Mplus (Muthén & Muthén, 2004), AMOS (Arbuckle & Wothke, 1999), and CALIS (SAS, 1989) has simplified the estimation of these models. Recent developments include the description and comparison of different tests of mediation (MacKinnon, Lockwood, Hoffman, West, & Sheets, 2002) and the estimation of mediated effects for continuous and categorical outcomes using single sample and resampling methods (Bollen & Stine, 1990).

Mediation in prevention and treatment research. Starting in the 1970s, researchers in several fields noticed the usefulness of the mediation model in treatment and prevention research. Susser (1973) clarified the different types of variables present in epidemiological studies including the mediating variable notion for health program development. During the late 1980s, the distinction between molar and molecular mediation arose in the medical and epidemiological literature on intermediate or surrogate endpoints (Prentice, 1989). Here the mediation model was used to identify mediating variables called surrogate or intermediate endpoints that serve as early indicators of later disease. These surrogate endpoints are important because treatment effects on these variables are easier to study than treatment effects on disease, which may be of low frequency and require a long time to occur.

The Judd and Kenny article (1981a) and book (1981b) described the use of the mediation model in experimental health promotion and disease prevention programs and marked the beginning of applying theoretical mediating mechanisms to the development and evaluation of prevention programs from a social science perspective. Baron and Kenny (1986) provided a major treatment of mediating variables in the social sciences and included methods to examine their effects. These articles are now widely cited in the research literature and have led to incorporation of mediation analysis in psychological research. MacKinnon and Dwyer (1993) outlined the application of mediation analysis in prevention research and evaluated several statistical aspects of assessing mediation.

Modern causal inference. Recent developments related to assessing mediation center around situations in which it is possible to make definitive statements about whether a variable is truly intermediate in a causal sequence (Frangakis & Rubin, 2002; Holland, 1988a; Pearl, 2000; Rubin, 1974, 2004). This research continues to formalize the work of Simon (1954) and Wright (1921, 1934). Here the assumptions required for identifying mediation are laid out and discussed. In general, these models demonstrate that identifying true mediation is difficult. The models suggest that the only true way to identify causality is with randomized experiments because only with this design is it possible to rule out alternative explanations of results. In several of these models, if a variable cannot be manipulated, such as sex or race, then it is not reasonable to consider causal relations. Furthermore, for the case of a mediating variable, true causal relations are only possible in specific circumstances related to counterfactual situations in addition to random assignment (Frangakis & Rubin, 2002). This pessimistic view of identifying mediating variables is challenged by causal approaches developed as part of artificial intelligence research. This work grew out of the need to train machines to identify causal mediating processes necessary for proper operation. Often the computer must make a decision based on incomplete information. In many cases, the machine does not have the luxury of deciding that a task is impossible, but must make a decision.

The general notion of these causal inference approaches is that X is related to Y through a mediating variable M such that X would not affect Y if it had no effect on M. More on these philosophical notions of causation can be found in Holland (1986) and Pearl (2000, especially the epilogue) and also in chapter 13. The general causal approach of this book is that all relevant research can shed light on the accuracy of a mediational hypotheses, but some research designs lead to more defensible conclusions. In general, true causal relations cannot be known exactly, but observed manifestations of mediational theory can be repeatedly tested, thereby generating a body of research to bolster a mediational hypothesis. Mediation results from one study inform the predictions for the next, more detailed, study in the same or different research context. Furthermore, the identification of mediational processes is a multifaceted approach that involves substantive skill and theory, results across substantive areas, and careful research design.

1.9 Summary

The purpose of this chapter was to introduce the notion of a mediating variable and to define several concepts. The major applications of mediation in terms of identifying the mechanisms in the black box exemplified by the S–O–R research and mediation in prevention were described. The mediating variable and related variables (confounder, concomitant, covariate, distorter, and moderator) were defined and the history of the mediating variable was briefly summarized. More information about specific applications of the mediation model is included in chapter 2.

1.10 Exercises

1.1. Look up the words *mediator, mediating,* and *mediate* in the Oxford English Dictionary (OED). The OED is usually available on-line as part of university library systems. Briefly describe some of the meanings of these words and the first use of the words.

1.2. Describe possible mediators to be targeted if the transmission of yellow fever was through person-to-person contact.

1.3. Describe two examples of S–O–R models. Describe two examples of mediation in prevention.

1.4. Chapter 1 focused on two- and three-variable systems. Describe several effects in a four-variable system. Why is the four-variable system so complicated?

1.5. Given the number of possible types of effects in four or more-variable systems, when is it sensible to consider these more complicated models?

1.6. Use a literature search program such as the Web of Knowledge (http://www.isiwebofknowledge.com) and search for the keywords, *moderators* and *mediators*. How many articles did you find and from how many different fields? Search for the word *mediator* and count the number of articles listed for this keyword.

1.7. For each of the following examples describe whether the variable is a mediator, moderator, or confounder.
   a. The age effect is removed from the relation between stress and health.
   b. Effect of dissonance on a court decision depends on whether the court case was a harassment or product liability case.
   c. Physical fitness affects feelings of athletic competence, which then affects body image.
   d. The relation between stress and health symptoms is compared across ages.

1.8. Here are two examples described in Simon (1954) for the measurements of three variables in groups of people. Identify each variable as an independent variable, mediator, confounder, or dependent variable.
   a. The percentage of persons that are married, average pounds of candy consumed per month, and average age.
   b. The percentage of female employees who are married, average number of absences each week per employee, and number of hours of housework completed each week per employee.

1.9. In a classic psychological study, Horst (1941) observed that the coefficient relating mechanical ability and pilot performance increased when verbal ability was added to the regression equation. Is verbal ability a confounder or a mediator? Why? Is verbal ability a suppressor?

1.10. In a hypothetical example, McFatter (1979) described relations among worker intelligence, boredom, and errors on an assembly line task. More intelligent workers make fewer errors but are also more likely to be bored. Is boredom a confounder or a mediator? Describe how the relations among these variables may indicate suppression.

1.11. Rosenberg (1968) described a real data example showing a positive relation between being married and rate of suicide; that is, married persons had a higher rate of suicide. He gives evidence that age was a distorter variable of this relation. Explain how holding age constant could reverse the positive relation between marital status and rate of suicide.

1.12. Section 1.5 describes situations in which the overall relation between two variables is not statistically significant, but there is significant mediation. Describe one real or hypothetical substantive example of how this could occur.

2

Applications of the Mediation Model

"In the absence of a concern for such mediating or intervening mechanisms, one ends up with facts, but with incomplete understanding."

—Morris Rosenberg, 1968, p. 63

2.1 Overview

Chapter 2 describes applications of the mediation model, thereby providing a substantive context for the statistical topics in the following chapters. Examples outlined in this chapter are used throughout the book and are chosen to reflect disparate fields to illustrate the widespread utility of the mediation model. Important methodological developments for mediation analysis in each research area are briefly mentioned. As an example of studies designed on the basis of hypothesized mediating mechanisms, program development is described as a guide for designers of health promotion and disease prevention programs. The focus of this chapter is substantive application rather than quantitative methods, which are the focus of the rest of the book.

2.2 Mediation for Explanation and Mediation for Design

There are two main uses of mediating variables in research studies. Once a relation between an independent and dependent variable is established, researchers often try to explain why or how the two variables are related. In this context, the purpose of mediation analysis is to investigate the processes underlying the observed relation between an independent variable and dependent variable. There are many examples of this purpose of mediation analysis, which is most common in psychology, sociology, and related fields. This approach to assessing mediation stems from the elaboration model whereby additional variables are analyzed to understand an observed relation (Lazarsfeld, 1955).

A second approach to mediation attempts to select mediating variables beforehand that are causally related to the dependent variable, rather than explaining an observed relation between two variables. Once these mediating mechanisms are identified, a manipulation is designed to change the selected mediating variables. If the assumption that the mediating variables are causally related to the outcome is correct, then a manipulation that changes the mediating variables will change the dependent variable. Studies using a mediation for design approach have increased because of the usefulness of this approach for applied research.

Both mediation for explanation and mediation for design approaches are used in the study of the same research topics. Often mediation results from explanation studies are used in subsequent mediation by design studies. Mediation for explanation is more common in basic research to explain an observed relation between an independent and dependent variable. Mediation for design is often a primary characteristic of applied experimental studies. The main difference between these two types of studies is when mediation is considered in the research process, either planned before the study to change a dependent variable or conducted after an effect is observed to understand how or why the effect occurred. Mediation for design research focuses on designing actions to solve a problem. Mediation for explanation attempts to explain how or why there is an observed relation between two variables.

2.3 *Social Psychology*

Mediation studies are common in social psychological research. In many psychological studies mediation is investigated with a randomized experimental design, but there is no attempt to measure the mediating process. In these studies, participants are randomly assigned to receive different experimental conditions, and differences in means in the conditions are either consistent or inconsistent with a mediation theory. For example, cognitive dissonance is a social psychological theory which explains that persons make decisions at least in part to reduce internal discomfort or dissonance. Sherman and Gorkin (1980) studied dissonance by randomly assigning participants to either solve a brainteaser that invoked feelings of sexism or a brainteaser not related to sex roles. After the brainteaser, participants judged a legal case that involved sex discrimination. After exposure to the brainteaser, participants with feminist beliefs were more likely to make feminist judgments about the discrimination case if they failed the sexism brainteaser than participants with feminist beliefs who did not fail the brainteaser. It was hypothesized that failure to solve the sex role brainteaser induced discomfort regarding feelings of sexism and the discomfort led to stronger judgments in favor of the sex discrimination case.

Although these results were taken as evidence of a cognitive dissonance mediation relation, the mediation relation was not investigated in a statistical analysis. Experimental studies will always be critically important for the study of mediation but more information may be extracted from a research study if measures of the mediating process are incorporated in the analysis. If measures of the mediator are obtained, more links in the mediated relation can be studied.

Taylor and Fiske (1981) described how mediation analysis is typically conducted in social psychological research when mediating variables are measured by testing the experimental effect on the dependent variable and the mediator. If the experimental effects on the mediator and the dependent variable are both statistically significant, then the experimental manipulation changed the dependent variable, and the mediator was changed as expected. Taylor and Fiske (1981) demonstrated that this method of testing mediation is incomplete because the association between the mediator and the dependent variable is not tested in this framework. An important aspect of mediation is that the mediator is related to the dependent variable. It is possible for the experimental effects on the mediator and the dependent variable to be statistically significant, when the relation between the mediator and the dependent variable is zero.

In a later article, Fiske, Kenny, and Taylor (1982) applied structural equation modeling to test the relation between the mediator and the dependent variable in addition to the test of the experimental effect on the mediator and the dependent variable. This research is one of the first applications of mediation analysis in an experimental research design. The researchers examined the psychological phenomenon whereby directing a person's attention to stimuli in a social situation makes the person attribute more importance to that stimuli. Participants in the study viewed two persons talking together. Attention to specific stimuli, called salience, was manipulated by instructing participants to watch one of the two persons. After viewing the two persons talking together, participants rated the influence of each person in the conversation and also recalled the characteristics of each person. The researchers were interested in the characteristics of the persons that mediated the relation between salience (attention to one person) and ratings of influence. There was evidence that salience increased positive visual recall and positive visual recall was related to influence, consistent with the mediation hypothesis.

Harris and Rosenthal (1985) described potential mediational processes for how expectancies about a person's behavior lead to actual changes in behavior. The origin of this research was a study of rat maze learning. Rosenthal and Fode (1963) had psychology students teach maze learning to rats that were either maze-dull or maze-bright, when, in fact, the labels were randomly assigned to the rats. Despite the random assignment of labels, after 1 week rats labeled maze-bright were better at running the maze than maze-dull rats. The results were described as a self-fulfilling prophecy—the expectancy introduced by the label led to actual performance changes. A teacher expectancy effect on children's learning was also reported such that children randomly labeled as bright had greater achievement than other children (Rosenthal, 1987). Harris and Rosenthal (1985) investigated the mediational processes that may explain the expectancy effect in a meta-analysis of 86 expectancy effect studies. For example, a teacher may devote more attention to a student whom the teacher expects to perform well, and this increase in attention to the student increases the student's subsequent performance. The expectancy effect remains somewhat controversial (Rosenthal, 1987; Wineburg, 1987) and is an active area of research. Mediation of the expectancy effect is an example used in chapter 6.

Another mediational hypothesis is the extent to which intentions mediate the relationship between attitudes and behavior (Fishbein & Ajzen, 1975). Alternatively, others have suggested that behavior changes intentions (Bem, 1972). Bentler and Speckart (1979, 1981) found that, in general, attitudes affect behavior, but there was evidence of reversed patterns for some of the behaviors studied. In a related study, Smith (1982) investigated the relations among the social cognition variables of beliefs, attributions, and evaluations. The article had the classic substantive focus of research examining how an individual's responses to achievement are mediated by attributions (Weiner, Russell, & Lerman, 1979) and how attitudes about objects are mediated by beliefs about the objects (Fishbein & Ajzen, 1975). The methods of the study allowed for estimation of reciprocal paths among the measures; that is, beliefs cause attributions and attributions cause beliefs. One of the challenges in many research areas is that measures are reciprocally related, such that symmetric relations exist between variables. For example, the mediator may cause the dependent variable and the dependent variable may cause the mediator. Smith (1982) proposed an ingenious method to investigate these types of relations and quantify these reciprocal paths using an experimental methodology. Smith also described the many assumptions required for accurate estimation of reciprocal relations. As expected, there was evidence for substantial reciprocal relations among beliefs, attributions, and evaluations.

The seminal Baron and Kenny (1986) article describing mediation and moderator analysis in psychology was published in the *Journal of Personality and Social Psychology*. This article is now widely cited and contains guidelines for mediation and moderation analysis. A set of criteria widely used for establishing mediation was described.

2.4 Industrial Psychology

Several topics in industrial psychology involve mediation (James & Brett, 1984). The first topic is how job perceptions mediate the effect of work environments on worker productivity and employment. Aspects of the work environment include reward systems, management styles, and workgroup composition. For example, one model proposes that goals predict effort that then predicts performance (Hall & Foster, 1977). A second mediation topic is the extent to which the environment affects intentions that then affect worker retention. Third is attribution in leadership whereby subordinate performance evaluations by a leader are mediated by the leader's perceptions about the attributions of the causes of the subordinate's performance. Billings and Wroten (1978) summarize the usefulness of path analysis including mediation in industrial psychology. Importantly, industrial psychology articles often describe assumptions underlying the application of the mediation model including decisions about the time ordering of variables, linear relations, and measurement error (see James, Mulaik, & Brett, 1982).

In James and Brett's (1984) article on mediation, they highlight the assumptions of the mediation and moderation model with an example of how effort and ability attributions mediate the relation between performance feedback and intended persistence in the future among workers. The moderator variable was the self-esteem of the worker; for example, persons with high self-esteem given poor performance feedback attributed it to lack of effort and intended to work harder. More recently, Prussia and Kinicki (1996) examined the mediation of performance feedback on group effectiveness with potential mediators of group affective evaluations, group goals, and collective efficacy. Group affective evaluations and collective efficacy completely mediated the relation between performance feedback and group effectiveness.

Environmental effects on worker behavior can occur at the group level, as well as the individual level described earlier. For example, the effects of contextual or group level measures on individual outcomes are mediated by the meanings of the group level measures to individuals (James, James, & Ashe, 1990). The centralization of a work unit may affect worker productivity through the mediating variable of perceived autonomy of the worker. The effects of group level measures may affect group-level perceptions of autonomy that may in turn affect worker behavior (Hofmann & Gavin, 1998). These types of multilevel effects in which a group level measure affects another group level measure that then affects an individual level measure will be discussed in chapter 9.

2.5 *Clinical Psychology and Psychiatry*

Several prominent clinical researchers have called for increased attention to mediating mechanisms of psychological treatment (Kazdin, 2000; Kazdin & Nock, 2003; Kazdin & Weisz, 2003; Kraemer, Wilson, Fairburn, & Agras, 2002; Weersing & Weisz, 2002) at least in part to test theory. As summarized by Kraemer et al. (2002, p. 877), "Rapid progress in identifying the most effective treatments and understanding on whom treatments work and do not work and why treatments work or do not work depends on efforts to identify moderators and mediators of treatment outcome. We recommend that randomized clinical trials routinely include and report such analysis." Kazdin (1989) has repeatedly called for more research on the mechanisms by which childhood treatment programs achieve effects. Kazdin (1989) outlined different models for childhood depression, including psychosocial models that postulate psychic and interpersonal causes of depression, psychoanalytic models that suggest intrapsychic influences, behavioral models that emphasize learning and environmental causes, cognitive models that emphasize perceptual and attributional styles that underlie depression, biochemical models that postulate chemical imbalances for the cause of depression, and genetic models that implicate genes as the cause of depression. In many cases, these theories have very clear predictions of the mediational mechanisms underlying depression. For example, it is hypothesized that effects of negative life events increase hopelessness that then leads to depression (Kazdin, 1989). Most recently, Weisz and Kazdin (2003, p. 445) concluded that, "The job of making treatments more efficient could be greatly simplified by an understanding of the specific change processes that make the treatments work. But a close review of child research reveals much more about what outcomes are produced than about what actually causes the outcomes."

The possible theoretical mechanisms by which effective psychotherapy works have been outlined by several researchers. Freedheim and Russ (1992) identified six mechanisms of change that occur in child psychotherapy: (a) labeling of feelings and the release of emotion (catharsis), make the feelings less overwhelming and more understandable, (b) corrective emotional experience, which consists of the acceptance of the child's emotions as valid and the discussion of the reasons for the emotions, (c) insight, the emotional resolution of conflict and trauma, (d) problem solving and coping strategies, which consist of learning methods to solve problems and the use of effective coping strategies, (e) object relations and internal representations, which consist of exposure to a stable, predictable, and caring therapist throughout the process of therapy, and (f) nonspecific factors such as expectations before therapy. Additional mediating mechanisms include the therapeutic alliance between therapist and client and a host of mediators related to compliance with prescription drug regimens.

As summarized by Weersing and Weisz (2002), few studies in clinical psychology estimate mediated effects even though most studies have the data available to examine mediation. Only a few researchers have conducted some form of mediation analysis to address mediating mechanisms in treatment research. Huey, Henggeler, Brondino, and Pickrel (2000) report that decreased affiliation with delinquent peers mediated the effects of their treatment program on delinquent behavior. Eddy and Chamberlain (2000) found that reductions in deviant peer associations and improved family management skills mediated the effects of their program on adolescent antisocial behavior. Hollon, Evans, and DeRubeis (1990) found evidence that attributional style mediated the effect of cognitive behavioral treatment. Hinshaw (2002) found evidence that changes in negative parental discipline mediated the effect of treatment programs among children with attention deficit hyperactivity disorder. In a study of treatment of substance abuse patients either with or without post-traumatic stress syndrome (PTSD), Ouimette, Finney, and Moos (1999) found evidence that PTSD was associated with poor coping strategies, which led to increased chance of remission. In a study of the effects of a Mississippi River flood on psychological distress and physical symptoms, Smith and Freedy (2000) found that loss of psychosocial resources mediated the effects of flood exposure on symptoms.

There are several unique aspects of mediation in clinical treatment research. In particular, there are several levels of intervention. Therapy may be delivered in groups or in an individual setting. The most recognized agent of change is the therapist who conducts several actions, including discussion designed to assist the client. The client also conducts several activities to change mediators based on his or her own actions and thoughts. In many respects, the mediators inside the client are likely to be the most powerful agents of change in therapy. In addition, clinical treatment may also include environmental changes designed to enhance treatment, such as a period of separation as part of marriage therapy. Often drug treatments are included and sometimes changed during the course of treatment. These different agents of change may work simultaneously or synergistically in a treatment program. As a result, clinical research may require more detailed development of theory relating treatment components to mediators compared with the application of the mediation model to other fields. Treatment is also often adaptive to the experience of the client so that the meaning of different actions may differ at different times for the client.

2.6 Communications Research

McGuire's (1999) theory of the effects of communication on behavior encompasses a large number of steps from noticing a communication to changing behavior as a result of the communication. Some of these steps include noticing the message, processing the message, remembering the message, and changing attitude in response to the information in the message. The model explains the small effects of most communications because of the large number of steps that must be passed in the chain of mediation for an effect to be observed. This mediation chain is a good example of a multiple path mediation model with many links between the independent variable and the dependent variable.

Mediation analysis has also been recommended for political and health communication research as summarized by Holbert and Stephenson (2003, p. 559), "The basis for much of today's mass communication study of political campaigns is built on a foundation of mediation" and McLeod and Reeves (1980, p. 18), "Mediating variables exist at every stage of the media effects process." An example in political communication is the extent to which exposure to information about political candidates leads to attitudes about the candidates that predicts voting or political participation. McLeod, Kosicki, and McLeod (2002) describe an orientation–stimulus–organism–response model for communication to reflect how an individual's orientation may act as a moderator of a stimulus–organism–response relation or their individual's orientation may lead to selective attention to different stimuli.

2.7 Sociology

The direct and indirect effects of independent variables on dependent variables is a focus of sociological research. Parental characteristics influence on offspring behavior (Duncan, 1966) has received sustained research attention for its importance in predicting future achievement based on background characteristics. Several of the example data sets in this book are classic sociological examples. In chapter 6, for example, mediation models for how father's education affects offspring education that then affects offspring income (Duncan, Featherman, & Duncan, 1972) are used to illustrate path analysis models. In a study of parent characteristics on drug abuse, Chassin, Pillow, Curran, Molina, and Barrera (1993) found that pathways for the effect of parental alcoholism on child alcohol use were mediated by stress and negative affect but not by temperamental sociability. Examples of other indirect effect hypotheses in sociology include the prediction that aid to families with dependent children leads to decreased school dropout rates, which lead to lower homicide rates (Hannon, 1997), that poverty reduces local social ties, which increases assault and burglary rates (Warner & Rountree, 1997), and that social status has an indirect effect on depression through changes in social stress (Turner, Wheaton, & Lloyd, 1995).

Several major advancements in statistical methodology have been made in the context of sociological research (Alwin & Hauser, 1975; Hyman, 1955; Sobel, 1982, 1986). One of the original articles on the decomposition of the effects of an independent variable into direct and indirect effects was discussed in sociology (Alwin & Hauser, 1975). The derivation of the standard error of indirect effects and detailed examination of indirect effects were published in sociology journals (Bollen, 1987; Sobel, 1982, 1986). Application of resampling methods in the estimation of indirect effects was described by Bollen and Stine (1990).

2.8 Agriculture

There are examples of mediation in agricultural studies. In these studies mediating variables such as amount of fertilizer and insecticide, which are hypothesized to be related to crop yield, are manipulated. This literature distinguishes among different types of covariates or concomitant variables (Rosenbaum, 1984). Some concomitant variables such as watering in different plots of land are generally not affected by the experimental manipulation and may be used as covariates to reduce unexplained variability in the dependent variable. Other concomitant variables serve as mediators in that they are affected by the experimental manipulation. Fertilizers, varieties, and insecticides provide examples of mediating variables (Cochran, 1957; Smith, 1957). For example, fertilization affects germination, which then affects yield. Delivery of fertilizer increases soil quality, which increases plant growth. Cochran and Cox (1957) described an experiment in which the effects of fumigation to reduce eelworms is used to increase oat yield. In this study, some fields were randomly assigned to receive fumigation (actually four types of fumigants), and others were not fumigated. Measures of the density of eelworms in each plot of land were measured before and after fumigation. Measures of oat yield were made at the end of the study. There was interest in the extent to which the control of eelworms leads to increases in oat yield. In another interesting agricultural example, the effects of feeding cows three preparations of alfalfa that differed in the concentration of carotene were examined. Cows were assigned to receive one of the different preparations, and the potency of vitamin A in the butter produced from each cow's milk was measured (Snedecor, 1946). The mediated effect was the extent to which the preparation of alfalfa affects carotene in the alfalfa, which then affects vitamin A in butter. Other agricultural examples are described in Shipley (2000).

2.9 Epidemiology

Although description rather than theory is often prioritized in epidemiology (Vandenbrouke, 1988), there are numerous examples of the importance of theory for the mechanism of transmission of disease. Examples are the mosquito theory for yellow fever, the germ theory for cholera, and related ideas (Gorgas, 1915). Susser (1973) described several examples of mediation models including the theory that maternal diet causes maternal weight that in turn causes birth weight. In epidemiology, mediating variables are called intermediate or intervening variables. An ideal aspect of mediation analysis in epidemiology is the face validity of the dependent variables, such as disease, death, and injury. Many of these dependent variables are binary, requiring logistic regression or some other method to accurately handle the analysis of relations in the data.

One of the best examples of mediation for design is the study of intermediate endpoints in epidemiological and medical studies. In many medical studies, the length of time for a disease to occur and low incidence rates of the disease make it very difficult to conduct research on predictors of disease. Instead, researchers advocate using a surrogate for disease as the dependent variable. This approach assumes that there is a causal relation between the surrogate and disease (Prentice, 1989). The surrogate is a mediator of the relation between a predictor and disease. For example, in the study of colon cancer, the lengthy development of the disease makes it very difficult to study the predictors of colon cancer. In this situation, the number of precancerous cells is investigated rather than colon cancer itself because the presence of these cells occurs earlier than colon cancer. The precancerous cells are known as a surrogate endpoint or intermediate endpoint in this literature. Prentice (1989, p. 432) defined a surrogate or intermediate endpoint as a "response variable for which a test of the null hypothesis of no relationship to the treatment groups under comparison is also a valid test of the corresponding null hypothesis based on the true endpoint." Once a valid surrogate is found, studies are designed to change the surrogate under the assumption that changing the surrogate will subsequently change the ultimate endpoint.

Examples of intermediate endpoints are shown in Table 2.1 based on Choi, Lagakos, Schooley, and Volberding (1993), Day and Duffy (1996), and Fleming and DeMets (1996, Table 2.1). Surrogate endpoints for cardiovascular disease include congestive heart failure, cholesterol levels, and blood pressure. A surrogate for breast cancer mortality is tumor size and level of malignancy at screening. A surrogate for osteoporosis is bone mineral density. These surrogate endpoints are generally easier to study than the ultimate disease outcome. They are easier to study

Table 2.1 Examples of Surrogates and Ultimate Endpoints

Disease	Surrogate
Death due to cardiovascular disease	Elevated lipid levels, congestive heart failure, arrhythmia, elevated blood pressure (Fleming & DeMets, 1996).
Death from breast cancer	Tumor size, malignancy, and invasion of lymph nodes by cancer cells (Day & Duffy, 1996)
Prostate cancer symptoms	Prostate biopsy (Fleming & DeMets, 1996)
HIV infection	CD4+ lymphocyte viral load (Choi et al., 1993)
Osteoporosis	Bone mineral density (Fleming & DeMets, 1996)
Ophthalmic conditions	Partial loss of vision (Buyse & Molenberghs, 1998)

because the mediating variables are affected earlier than the disease outcome and the incidence of cases is larger than those for the disease. In this way, surrogates are related to the idea of a micromediational chain described in chapter 1. The surrogate tends to be very close to the ultimate endpoint in the mediational chain, often making the theoretical relation between the surrogate and the ultimate endpoint very clear and the statistical relation large.

The extent to which a variable is a valid surrogate endpoint, of course, depends on the mediation assumption that the variable is intermediate in the causal sequence relating an independent variable to the ultimate disease outcome. The relation between the surrogate and the disease endpoint has been questioned on the basis of studies in which medication is used to reduce levels of surrogates (Fleming & DeMets, 1996), but no corresponding reduction in the outcome measures is observed. An example in which the surrogate was actually iatrogenic occurred in the Cardiac Arrhythmia Suppression randomized trial in which the surrogate for cardiac deaths was premature ventricular contractions (PVCs). PVCs are associated with sudden death, so it was reasonable to hypothesize that the use of drugs to prevent PVCs ought to reduce death rates. However, the opposite effect occurred. More persons treated with the drugs died from arrhythmia and shock after a heart attack in the group receiving the drugs to prevent PVCs (Echt et al., 1991).

In an important article on surrogate endpoints, Freedman, Graubard and Schatzkin (1992) concretized the criteria for surrogate endpoints described in Prentice (1989) as the proportion of the treatment effect explained by the surrogate endpoint as a measure of the surrogate endpoint effect for which a value of 100% indicates that the surrogate endpoint explains all of the relation between the treatment and the dependent variable. The proportion measure includes the size of the surrogate endpoint (i.e., mediated) effect as well at the amount of the treatment effect explained by the surrogate endpoint. The use of the proportion mediated has not been accepted without criticism, namely that accurate identification of surrogate endpoints requires measurement of the ultimate outcome (Begg & Leung, 2000), that values of the proportion mediated are often very small, and that additional causal mechanisms through other mediators may be neglected (Fleming & DeMets, 1996). Furthermore, other research has shown that the proportion mediated is an unstable measure unless sample size is large or effect size is large (Freedman, 2001; MacKinnon, Warsi, & Dwyer, 1995). The importance of this mediation assumption of surrogate endpoints for studies of disease was summarized by Begg and Leung (2000). Alternative measures of the surrogate endpoint effect are discussed in chapter 11.

Surrogate endpoints are often more closely related to the ultimate outcome variable than mediating variables described in other examples. In the long mediational chain relating variables to an ultimate outcome, surrogates are often biological measures closely related to the ultimate outcome. Other mediating variables are often more distal in the micromediational chain, and as a result are not as strongly related to the outcome variable. A surrogate that is more distal to the ultimate outcome will tend to have a weaker relation with the outcome because more steps in the mediational chain are necessary for it to affect the ultimate outcome variable. On the other hand, surrogates may occur much earlier than the ultimate endpoint, such as childhood obesity as a surrogate for adult heart disease.

2.10 Mediation in Program Development and Evaluation

Mediation analysis has been recommended in many fields of prevention and treatment including nursing, "Nurse scientists who are interested in exploring more than just the direct effects . . . should consider hypotheses about mediators that could provide additional information about why an observed phenomenon occurs" (Bennett, 2000, p. 419), children's programs, "Including even one mediator and one moderator in a program theory and testing it with the evaluation should not be overly expensive or impractical, but it will yield more fruit than the atheoretical and exploratory searches that have dominated outcome studies of children's programs to date" (Petrosino, 2000, p. 69), and nutrition, "Finally future nutrition intervention trials should include and analyze repeated measures of the hypothesized mediating factors that are the basis for their interventions. More detailed analyses of large studies, beyond reporting intervention effects alone, will support further advances in behaviorally based chronic disease prevention" (Kristal, Glanz, Tilley, & Li, 2000, p. 123).

Researchers from many fields have stressed the importance of assessing mediation in the evaluation of prevention and treatment studies for four major reasons (Baranowski, Anderson, & Carmack, 1998; Baranowski, Lin, Wetter, Resnicow, & Hearn, 1997; Baron & Kenny, 1986; Begg & Leung, 2000; Choi et al., 1993; Donaldson, 2001; Donaldson, Graham, & Hansen, 1994; Judd & Kenny, 1981a, 1981b; MacKinnon, 1994; Sandler, Wolchik, MacKinnon, Ayers, & Roosa, 1997; Shadish, 1996; Sussman, 2001; Weiss, 1997). First, mediation analysis provides a check on whether the prevention or treatment program has produced a change in the construct it was designed to change. If a program is designed to change norms, then program effects on norm measures should be found. Second, the results may suggest that certain program components need to be strengthened or measurements need to be improved. Failures to significantly change mediating variables occur either because the program was ineffective or the measures of the mediating construct were not adequate. Third, program effects on mediating variables in the absence of effects on dependent measures suggest that program effects on dependent variables may emerge later or that the targeted constructs were not critical in changing outcomes. Finally, and most importantly, evidence bearing on how the program achieved its effects can be obtained.

One common way to organize prevention activities is under the three headings of universal, selected, and indicated prevention. The mediation model applies in each of these prevention activities. Universal prevention refers to preventing disease prior to the biological origin of the disease, before the disease has had a chance to manifest itself. Examples of universal prevention include programs to prevent children from starting to smoke cigarettes and the promotion of healthy behaviors. Selected prevention is the prevention of the disease after the disease has been identified but before it has caused suffering and disability. Screening is an example of selected prevention such as mammography screening for breast cancer. Indicated prevention is the prevention of further deterioration after the disease has already caused suffering or disability. Treatment programs, in general, are examples of indicated prevention. Programs to prevent relapse from addiction, such as Alcoholic Anonymous, are examples of indicated prevention.

Prevention programs in a variety of substantive areas are designed to change mediating variables that are causally related to the outcome variable as shown in Table 2.2. If the assumption that the mediating variables are causally related to the outcome is correct, a prevention program that

Table 2.2   Examples of Mediators and Outcomes in Prevention Studies

Reference	Mediators	Outcomes
AIDS/HIV: Sexually Transmitted diseases (Coyle, Boruch, & Turner, 1991)	Safe sex practices Abstinence	Unprotected sexual relations Sexually transmitted diseases
Adolescent anabolic steroid use (Goldberg et al., 1996)	Nutrition alternatives Weight training alternatives	Anabolic steroid use
Mental illness (Heller, Price, Reinharz, Riger, & Wandersman, 1984)	Positive coping with stress social competency	Adjustment DSM–III diagnosis
Symptoms of children after divorce (Sandler et al., 1997)	Quality of parent–child relationship Child's active coping	Conduct problems Anxiety Depression
Drug abuse (Hansen, 1992)	Social norms Resistance skills	Cigarette use Alcohol use Marijuana use
Learning disabilities (Silver & Hagin, 1989)	General social competency skills specific to learning	School achievement Standardized test scores
Symptoms after disasters (Pynoos & Nader, 1989)	Affirm family support Facilitate through grief stages	Depression Anxiety Fear
Suicide (Shaffer, Philips, Garland, & Bacon, 1989)	Awareness of hotline services Referrals to general psychiatric care	Suicide ideation Deaths due to suicide
Delinquency (Dryfoos, 1990)	Educational achievement Parental support and guidance	Arrests
Cardiovascular disease (Multiple Risk Factor Intervention Trial Research Group, 1990)	Smoking Cholesterol Blood pressure	Death due to myocardial infarction
Nutrition (Kristal et al., 2000)	Beliefs, attitudes, motivations barriers, norms, social support	Percent fat intake Servings of fruit and vegetables
Physical exercise (Lewis, Marcus, Pate, & Dunn, 2002)	Self-efficacy Enjoyment Knowledge of behaviors	Weekly physical activity
Teenage pregnancy (Dryfoos, 1990)	Educational achievement Parent–child communication	Unintentional pregnancy Unprotected intercourse

substantially changes the mediating variables will, in turn, change the outcome. Mediating variables can be psychological such as norms, behavioral such as social skills, or biological such as serum cholesterol level. Many drug prevention programs, for example, are designed to increase communication skills, educate, and change norms to reduce drug use. AIDS prevention programs focus on increasing condom use, safe sex, and abstinence to reduce exposure to the human immunodeficiency virus (Miller & Downer, 1988). Selected prevention programs, such as campaigns to increase screening for cancer (Murray et al., 1986), educate, reduce barriers, and change health norms to increase screening rates. Indicated prevention in substance abuse treatment programs, such as Alcoholics Anonymous, increases communication, motivation, and support to prevent relapse (Prochaska, DiClemente, & Norcross, 1992). In each of these examples, a mediator is a variable that transmits the effect of an intervention variable on a dependent variable.

2.10.1 Drug Prevention

As an example of mediation in prevention programs, mediation in school-based drug prevention is described in more detail. Drug prevention has received major national attention, and considerable literature on the effects of school-based drug prevention programs exists. School programs based on social psychological principles have been shown to prevent or delay the onset of youth substance use (Botvin, Baker, Renick, Filazzola, & Botvin, 1984; Cuijpers, 2002; Flay, 1987; Pentz et al., 1989). Not all studies generated consistent results, however, with variation in the magnitude and duration of effects and in the social influences program evaluated (Flay, 1985; MacKinnon, Weber, & Pentz, 1989; Peterson, Kealey, Mann, Marek, & Sarason, 2000). The extent to which each component of these prevention programs is responsible for the program effects on drug use remains to be determined (Hansen, 1992; MacKinnon, Taborga, & Morgan-Lopez, 2002; Tobler, 1986).

Changing psychosocial mediating constructs is the basis of educational and behavioral approaches to universal drug prevention. Social influences programs, for example, are designed to teach social skills and engender a social environment less receptive to substance use. If these prevention programs work as planned, then favorable changes in mediating variables such as beliefs about drug use outcomes, normative beliefs, resistance skills, attitudes about drug use and related variables, and behavioral intentions are indicators of success. Understandably, the emphasis in drug prevention research has been on drug use outcomes, and much less attention has been paid to assessing program effects on the psychosocial variables hypothesized to mediate changes in outcomes. Less attention has been given to the relation between changes in mediating variables after program implementation and drug use outcomes. A better understanding of these mediating variables might help clarify inconsistent results among studies. In many cases, the data required to investigate these processes are available but the analyses have not been conducted.

The lack of attention to mediation has been noted by several prominent drug prevention researchers. McCaul and Glasgow (1985, p. 361) concluded that "little is known about the construct validity of successful programs, a problem that results from the neglect of process measurement and analysis." Flay (1987, p. 172) has argued that future prevention programming should move to "comparing programs derived from competing theoretical perspectives (with careful assessment of mediating variables presumed to be differentially affected by different treatments)." As recently summarized by Botvin (2000, p. 894), "While the research conducted thus far examining the impact of these preventive interventions on mediators as well as efforts to identify mediating mechanisms are important first steps, it is clear that additional research is needed." Social norms appear to be a critical component in successful drug prevention to date. Botvin, Eng, and Williams (1980) found the largest program effects in the grades with the largest reduction in need for group acceptance. McAlister, Perry, and Maccoby (1979) concluded anecdotally that a change in school norms regarding drug use may have caused the reduction in cigarette use. MacKinnon et al. (1991) found evidence that social norms were statistically significant mediators of drug prevention program effects. Social norms were also important mediators of a program effect on drug use among minority youth (Botvin et al., 1992). Similarly, Bachman, Johnston, O'Malley, and Humphrey (1988) found that a decline in marijuana use was due to changes in perceived approval of drug use. Hansen and Graham (1991) and Donaldson et al. (1994) found experimental evidence for the importance of social norms as a mediator of program effects on drug use. In a study of high school football players, norms and perceived severity of steroid use were important mediators of the program effect on intention to use steroids (MacKinnon, Goldberg, et al., 2001). Future studies have the potential of clarifying the mediating effects of social norms and other potential mediators of successful drug prevention programming.

2.10.2 *Theoretical Interpretation of the Links in a Mediation Model*

The mediation approach to prevention and treatment research is summarized in Fig. 2.1, based on theory for how a program changes the dependent

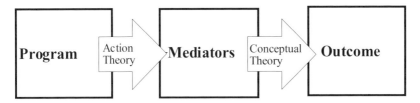

Figure 2.1. Prevention Program Model.

variable. Lipsey (1993), for example, argues that theory should be used to shed light on the black box (Ashby, 1956) representing how an intervention leads to changes in the dependent variable. Chen (1990) identifies two critical aspects of this type of intervening variable model. The first part is action theory, which refers to how the intervention changes the mediating variable. For example, a program component in drug prevention seeks to correct overestimation of drug use prevalence among adolescents; that is, most adolescents think more people smoke than actually do. The action theory is that a program component, such as correction of normative expectations, changes the social norm about smoking by reducing the perception of the number of smokers. The second theory is conceptual theory, which specifies how the mediating variables affect the dependent variable. For example, conceptual theory refers to the general result that perceptions of social norms affect behavior. Most research focuses on conceptual theory for the important predictors of an outcome and most theoretical models focus entirely on how variables are related to the outcome variable. For example, there are many studies of the correlates of tobacco use. Less attention is devoted to action theory, or how the intervention will change the mediating variables. Action theory is important because it forces researchers to consider how a program can change intervening variables. For example, even though personality variables may be the strongest predictors of drug use, they may be difficult to change, especially with the resources of many intervention programs. Similarly, media is often the intervention of choice because it is relatively easy to change, by placing counter-advertisements, but the conceptual theory relating media to the outcome may suggest small effects on actual behavior. Action and conceptual theory provide a useful way to conceptualize prevention and treatment activities.

Mediation analysis consists of tests of the action theory link, the conceptual theory link, and a simultaneous test of action and conceptual theory in the test of the process by which the program changes the mediating variable, which then changes the dependent variable. Hansen and McNeal (1996) add an interesting interpretation of the action and conceptual theory links. First, the association between the mediating variable and the dependent variable represents the maximum effect of the mediating variable on the dependent variable. The size of the program effect on the mediating variable will limit the size of the effect on the outcome variable. Similarly, the size of the mediating variable effect on the dependent variable limits the size of effects. This approach assumes that all mediators are consistent; that is, the program changes the mediators in a way that there is a beneficial effect on the dependent variable.

2.10.3 *Where Do Ideas for Mediators Come From?*

There are at least six overlapping ways in which possible mediators are identified for prevention and treatment projects. Often several different ways to identify mediators are combined in a single study. For the most part, mediators are selected on the basis of conceptual theory for what variables are related to the outcome variable of interest. It is important to consider action theory, the theory for how a manipulation would affect a mediator, while identifying potential mediators. It is also important to evaluate mediating mechanisms in program development so that information on beneficial and iatrogenic mediators can be obtained.

The first method, a seat-of-the-pants method, picks mediators on the basis of common sense or intuition about what seems to be the best target for a program. This may not be the best method, but in some cases may be the only method, such as the prevention activities when HIV/AIDS was first observed and knowledge of its cause was limited. Even if changing the mediator does not prove to affect the outcome, the failure of programs designed to change the mediators provides useful information about the mediating variables to be targeted in the next study.

A second method applies qualitative methods such as focus groups to discuss a problem outcome and ways to prevent it (Sussman, 2001). For example, a focus group might consist of a group of 10 adolescents convicted of driving under the influence of alcohol who are convened to discuss how and why they did it and ways other persons like them could be stopped from driving after drinking alcohol or using drugs. Focus groups typically include clear-cut goals and are directed by an effective leader who ensures that all persons are heard from. These meetings are coded and scored for variables such as sentiments, concerns, and subtopics and are classified into themes such as exploratory, clinical, and phenomenological. There is typically a written report of the results that includes extensive subjective information, and this report provides a basis for selecting mediating variables for a program.

A third way to identify mediators is through review of the research literature on a topic. Ideally there are reviews for the topic already published. If these reviews are not available, any available literature on the topic, such as popular articles and testimonials, is studied. If there are few studies on a topic, researchers typically look for program strategies for similar outcome measures. It is important to note that relevant literature may not be published or may not be easily accessible. Here the focus is on any information on empirical relations between mediating variables and the outcome variable of interest. It is surprising how few research articles present information useful for the design of prevention programs. Ideally, each research study would contain a section describing the implications of the study for the selection and importance of mediating variables.

A fourth way to identify mediators is based on theory. Many researchers have consistently argued for "theory-driven" evaluation (Chen, 1990; Lipsey, 1993; Sidani & Sechrest, 1999). For example, major theories in drug prevention include problem behavior theory, theory of reasoned action, and the health belief model (Hawkins, Catalano, & Miller, 1992; Jessor & Jessor, 1980). Theory provides a basis for mediators to target. For example, the health belief model would suggest that a program target barriers to performing a health behavior. A most important aspect of theory-based program development is that a theory successful in one situation is more likely to be successful in other situations (Bandura, 1977).

A fifth way to identify mediators is to conduct a study on the correlates of the outcome measure to shed light on the conceptual theory for the outcome. Here the purpose of the study is to identify variables that are potentially causally related to the outcome and are also potentially modifiable by a prevention strategy. A researcher may not need to know why a variable is related to the outcome variable, but the variable may still be an effective mediator. These studies then provide a quantitative measure of associations between mediators and outcome variables. Ideally, these studies include measures of effect size for the relation between the mediator and the outcome variable.

A sixth way to identify mediators is on the basis of prior mediational analyses of a prevention program. Ideally, successful mediators have been identified in prior research that will guide the selection of mediators. It may also be reasonable to design a study based on the most effective mediators in one study. The methodical evaluation of mediating mechanisms in a sequence of research studies is most likely to generate information on mediating mechanisms and more effective programs.

2.10.4 Steps in a Mediation Approach to Program Development

Table 2.3 outlines the steps in a mediation approach to program development. Step 1 illustrates the importance of preliminary research to help identify mediators and moderators of program effects. The six ways to identify mediators are reflected in steps 2 and 3, in which the action and

Table 2.3 Eight Steps in a Mediation Approach to Prevention and Treatment Program Development

1. Define the outcome measure. Investigate the epidemiology of the outcome. Identify high-risk groups. Develop theory for how the outcome occurs.
2. Identify the conceptual theory of how the outcome occurs. Identify correlates of the outcome variables by theory and empirical studies. Review prior literature for ideas on what is related to the outcome. Create a conceptual theory effect size table with the list of candidate mediators and the effect size for the relation between the mediator and outcome. Ideally, identify two or more theories about the mechanism by which the outcome occurs that have different predictions regarding mediating processes.
3. Link the mediators with the action needed to affect the mediator. Identify program components of studies that have attempted to change the outcome measure and related outcome measures. Is it reasonable to change the mediator given the resources available? Create an action theory table that lists the action that will change each mediator.
4. Study potential interaction effects of the program with subgroups. Are there groups for whom the action and conceptual theory make the most sense? Consider the possibility that the effect of the program will be greatest for those persons lowest or highest on the mediators at the baseline measurement.
5. Design the intervention to have the greatest chance of success by documenting and ensuring adequate implementation of the program and measurement of variables.
6. Conduct the study and evaluate action and conceptual theory of the program.
7. Repeat the study and improve the program by selecting effective components or adding new components.
8. Design a study in which subjects are randomly assigned to levels of mediating variables to more clearly understand the mechanism by which the program worked.

conceptual theory of project are specified. Step 4 addresses moderators of program effects, which is whether the program has differential effects by subgroups. An important moderator variable is the individual's mediator value before the study whereby a person lower on a mediator before an experiment may have more room for improvement when exposed to the program. Step 5 emphasizes the importance of satisfactory implementation of a program. Implementation may be considered as a variable in a mediation chain relating exposure to treatment to implementation of treatment to change in the mediator to change in the outcome. Statistical mediation analysis is used in step 6 to evaluate the action and conceptual theory of the program. Statistical mediation and moderation analysis results are used in step 7 to improve the program by deleting ineffective or counterproductive components and enhancing successful components. Decisions such as these are difficult because some mediators may not have been affected by the program because of poor measurement, or these mediators may actually contribute to a longer mediation chain such that change in these mediators may lead to change in other mediators. Ideally, step 8 consists of more detailed studies of mediators including random assignment of individuals to the level of the mediator or separate studies to evaluate individual program components or mediators.

2.11 Summary

This chapter described examples of the mediation model in a variety of disparate areas. The goal of the examples was not to be exhaustive but to give a view of types of mediation studies. The same general mediation model applies in all research areas such that an independent variable is related to a mediating variable that is related to a dependent variable. Although the mediator model applies in many fields, the examples in this chapter illustrate some specific issues in each field. In all research areas, the identification of mediating variables is best served by a program of research involving information from many sources.

Two overlapping uses of mediating variables were described, mediation for the explanation of observed relations and the design of manipulations based on mediating variables. In the mediation for explanation research, the relation of the independent variable to the dependent variable is considered to be known, and the task of the researcher is to explain the mediation process that translates exposure to the independent variable to change in the dependent variable. Mediation for design studies target mediating variables hypothesized to be causally related to the dependent variable. Surrogate endpoint, treatment, and prevention research are examples of mediation for design studies. In treatment and prevention studies, the relation of the mediator to outcome is assumed to be known, and the major task is designing actions to change the mediators. In the surrogate endpoint case, a relation between the mediator and dependent variable is considered to be known, but whether the relation is strong enough for the surrogate to be used instead of the ultimate outcome is investigated.

Some research, such as surrogate endpoint research, focuses on one mediator with the assumption that the single surrogate endpoint completely explains the mediation from the independent variable to the dependent variable. Other research areas such as prevention and treatment often target many mediators to change a dependent variable. The additional mediating variables may have complicated relations among each other and may have synergistic effects or counterproductive effects. Prevention and treatment studies may also have more than one dependent variable. The number of mediators and their potential relations often makes mediation of prevention and treatment programs more complex. The complexity is ideally addressed in a program of research involving replication studies, studies of individual mediators, qualitative research, longitudinal designs, and theory testing.

Mediators differ in many ways. Mediators may be behavioral, psychological, physiological, or biological. Mediators differ in ease of measurement. For example, measurement of the number of eelworms in a liter of soil may be simpler than measuring social norms among friends. Mediation analysis may be viewed as a measurement process in which the mediating process is more accurately measured as a field progresses. For example, brain processes first measured as self-report may be subsequently measured by brain scan activity. Mediators differ in ease of manipulation as well. For example, a pill may more easily and specifically alter blood chemicals than a cognitive behavior therapy program. More extensive actions are needed to alter personality than change attitudes. Similarly, surrogate endpoints are mediators selected to be used instead of the ultimate outcome. This differs from mediators in other contexts, which also lie along a causal chain but the purpose is not to identify mediators that can be used instead of the ultimate outcome.

A goal of this chapter was for you to find at least one content area that overlaps with your own interests. At this point you are probably ready to learn how to quantify mediated effects and test them for statistical significance. The rest of this book is concerned with quantifying mediation effects. Chapter 3 describes the single mediator model. Chapter 4 describes some details about the single mediator model, and chapter 5 describes the multiple mediator model. The rest of the book describes mediation analysis for more complicated designs.

2.12 Exercises

2.1. Why did Taylor and Fiske (1981) criticize the typical way to evaluate mediators in social psychological research?

2.2. Briefly describe action and conceptual theory. What are reasons for considering action theory in the design of a prevention program?

2.3. Describe the action and conceptual theory for the mediators of the Multiple Risk Factor Intervention Trial (MRFIT) cardiovascular disease prevention study.

2.4. Pick one of the substantive areas mentioned in this chapter and describe the mediational model in one of the cited studies.

2.5. Briefly describe and give one example of mediation for explanation and mediation for design.

2.6. Pick one content area and find one new study in that area. Describe the mediational hypothesis in that study.

2.7. How are surrogate endpoints different from mediators targeted in most prevention programs?

2.8. For one of the prevention programs in this chapter, describe how mediators could be selected.

2.9. In the context of a micromediational chain, where do mediators and surrogate endpoints lie?

2.10. Describe whether the following intermediate variables are more likely to be surrogates or mediators? Compare and contrast surrogate endpoints and mediating variables based on these examples.

    a. Seedlings is an intermediate variable for the effect of fertilizer on potato yield.

    b. Norms is an intermediate variable for the effect of socioeconomic status on assault.

    c. Carotene is an intermediate variable for the effect of alfalfa preparations fed to cows on vitamin A in butter made from cow milk.

    d. Fighting in sixth grade is an intermediate variable for the effect of an intervention on adult incarceration.

2.11. Describe the theory and the mediators targeted for a research project. Here are some possible examples: (a) school-based tobacco prevention programs, (b) Alcoholics Anonymous, (c) programs to prevent recidivism among juvenile offenders, (d) suicide prevention programs.

3

Single Mediator Model

> Instead of going to a drinking fountain, a thirsty man may simply "ask for a glass of water"; that is, may engage in behavior that produces a certain pattern of sounds, which in turn induces someone to bring him a glass of water. The sounds themselves are easy to describe in physical terms; but the glass of water reaches the speaker only as the result of a complex series of events including the behavior of the listener. . . . The consequences of such behavior are mediated by a train of events no less physical or inevitable than direct mechanical action
>
> **—Burrhus Frederic Skinner, 1961, p. 67**

3.1 Overview

The first two chapters provided verbal descriptions of mediating variables in diverse contexts including alfalfa growing, control of yellow fever, and educational achievement. These verbal descriptions of mediating variable models must be described more explicitly to quantify mediated effects and to judge whether a mediated effect substantially differs from zero. The purpose of this chapter is to translate the verbal description of mediation into regression equations and statistical procedures to conduct mediation analysis for the case of one mediator. In other words, chapter 3 describes a statistical model for the substantive aspects of mediation described in chapters 1 and 2. This chapter is important because subsequent chapters use the same notation and computational approach to mediation analysis. First, a visual representation of mediation is described along with symbols to represent different mediation relations. Next, the three regression equations that provide the information for mediation analysis are presented. Statistical tests for mediation are described as are procedures to compute confidence limits for the mediated effect. SPSS and SAS programs to estimate the single mediator model are shown, and mediation analysis is illustrated using data from a hypothetical study. Finally, assumptions for the mediator model to yield accurate results are presented along with sections of this book that deal with each assumption.

The material in this chapter may be more difficult than that in the first two chapters for some readers because it covers statistical aspects of mediation. Understanding the material in the chapter is worth the effort because it represents an approach to quantifying verbal descriptions of mediation.

3.2 The Mediation Model Diagram

Figure 3.1 shows a model relating an independent variable (X) to a dependent variable (Y) and represents the simplest model of the relation of one variable to another variable. Note that there is an arrow in figure 3.1 to represent that X predicts Y. Note also that the path from X to Y is given the symbol, c. An equation relating X to Y is shown below the figure and will be described in the next section. The coefficient, e_1, represents the part of Y that is not explained by its relation with X. Figure 3.1 is a total effect model because it represents the total relation between X and Y without consideration of other variables. Figure 3.1 is an example of a two-variable model where X causes Y.

Figure 3.2 represents the mediation model. In figure 3.2, the independent variable (X) is related to the mediator (M) which in turn, is related to the dependent variable (Y). Figure 3.2 represents a third-variable model where there is an underlying mediation relation of X to M to Y. Note that there is a relation of X to Y that is not through M and that is the direct effect of X on Y. As in figure 3.1, the arrows show the direction of the relation with X to M, M to Y, and X to Y. Note also that there are symbols above each arrow corresponding to the relation of X to M, a, the relation of M to Y, b, and the relation of X to Y, c'. Note that the relation of X to Y has a prime, c', to reflect adjustment for the mediator in figure 3.2 but does not have a prime in figure 3.1, c, because it is not adjusted for the mediator,

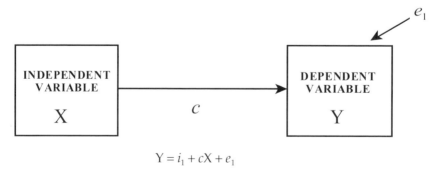

$$Y = i_1 + cX + e_1$$

Figure 3.1 Path diagram and equations for the regression model.

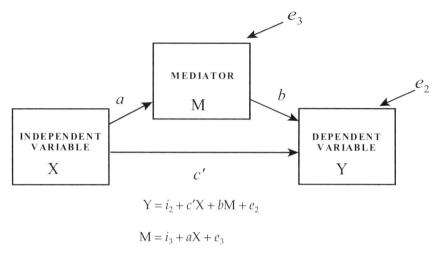

$$Y = i_2 + c'X + bM + e_2$$

$$M = i_3 + aX + e_3$$

Figure 3.2   Path diagram and equations for the mediation model.

M. The parameter e_2 represents the part of Y that is not explained by its relation with X and M. The parameter e_3 represents the part of M that is not explained by its relation with X. The two equations corresponding to figure 3.2 are also shown and described in the next section. Figure 3.2 represents the simplest mediation model, and it will be the primary model in much of this book. The mediation model in figure 3.2 looks simple and is simple in many respects, especially in its verbal description. However, the statistical specification of the model and application to real data has intriguing statistical and interpretational challenges.

3.3 Regression Equations Used to Assess Mediation

The three regression equations in figures 3.1 and 3.2 are used to investigate mediation,

$$Y = i_1 + cX + e_1 \tag{3.1}$$

$$Y = i_2 + c'X + bM + e_2 \tag{3.2}$$

$$M = i_3 + aX + e_3 \tag{3.3}$$

where Y is the dependent variable, X is the independent variable, M is the mediating variable or mediator, c represents the relation between the independent variable to the dependent variable in the first equation, c' is the parameter relating the independent variable to the dependent variable adjusted for the effects of the mediator, b is the parameter relating the mediator to the dependent variable adjusted for the effects of the independent variable, a is the parameter relating the independent variable to the mediating variable, e_1, e_2, and e_3 represent unexplained or error variability, and the intercepts are i_1, i_2, and i_3. The intercepts are not involved in the estimation of mediated effects and could be left out of the equations. However, they are included here because intercepts are important for other aspects of mediation such as plotting the mediated effect. Note that both c and c' are parameters relating the independent variable to the dependent variable, but c' is a partial effect, adjusted for the effects of the mediator. The parameters of this model can be estimated by multiple regression. Equation 3.1 defines the total effect model in figure 3.1, and Equations 3.2 and 3.3 define the mediation model in figure 3.2.

3.4 The Total Effect

The relation between the independent variable and the dependent variable represented by c in Equation 3.1 is often of primary interest in research studies. In experimental studies, for example, the c parameter represents the effect of the manipulation on the dependent variable. The interpretation of this relation is important in mediation studies as well. However, a mediated effect may exist whether or not there is a statistically significant effect of the independent variable on the dependent variable. Extra information can be extracted from a research study if a mediating variable is measured.

3.5 Mediated Effect

There are two approaches to quantifying mediated effects from the regression models based on different uses of the parameters a, b, c, and c'. The product of the a and b parameters, ab, is the mediated effect. Because X affects Y indirectly through M, the mediated effect is also known as the indirect effect. The effect of X on Y after adjustment for M, c', is known as the direct effect. The mediated effect is also equal to the difference between the c and c' parameters, $c - c'$. As a result, the total effect c can be decomposed into a direct effect, c', and an indirect effect, $ab = c - c'$. For the multiple regression equations described earlier, $c - c'$ is always equal to ab. The rationale behind the ab mediation quantity is that mediation depends on the extent to which the independent variable affects the mediator (parameter a) and the extent to which the mediator affects the dependent variable (parameter b). The ab quantity reflects how much a 1 unit change in X affects Y indirectly through M. Similarly, the change in the c parameter when adjusted for the mediator, c', reflects how much of the relation between the independent variable and the dependent variable is explained by the mediator.

The parameters in Equations 3.1, 3.2, and 3.3 can be estimated using ordinary least squares regression to obtain estimates of the mediated effect, $\hat{a}\hat{b}$ and $\hat{c} - \hat{c}'$. (Hats ˆ above coefficients represent estimates.) As described in later chapters, in some analyses such as logistic regression and multilevel analysis, the estimated $\hat{c} - \hat{c}'$ does not always exactly equal the estimated $\hat{a}\hat{b}$ because of different standardization across mediation regression equations. However, for the analysis of the equations described in this chapter, $\hat{c} - \hat{c}'$ always equals $\hat{a}\hat{b}$, unless the sample was different for the different regression equations. For example, if the sample size for Equation 3.3 differs from the sample size for Equations 3.1 and 3.2, then $\hat{c} - \hat{c}'$ will be based on a different set of subjects than $\hat{a}\hat{b}$, and consequently $\hat{c} - \hat{c}'$ may not equal $\hat{a}\hat{b}$. This would happen if some subjects were missing the mediator variable, for example, so that the sample size for Equations 3.2 and 3.3 is different from the sample size for Equation 3.1.

3.6 Confidence Intervals for the Mediated Effect

The estimate of the mediated effect and its standard error can be used to construct confidence intervals for the mediated effect. Confidence intervals are widely used because they incorporate the error in an estimate thereby providing a range of possible values for an effect rather than a single value of the effect. There is considerable movement toward the use of confidence intervals in research for several reasons (Harlow, Mulaik, & Steiger, 1997). These reasons include that it forces researchers to consider the value of the effect in addition to its statistical significance, the confidence interval has a valid probability interpretation, and a wide confidence interval implies inaccuracy in the value of the effect suggesting that the effect may not be easily replicated (Krantz, 1999).

As described earlier, the $\hat{c} - \hat{c}'$ or the $\hat{a}\hat{b}$ value provides an estimate of the mediated effect. There are several alternative formulas for the standard error of $\hat{a}\hat{b}$ and $\hat{c} - \hat{c}'$ that can be used to construct confidence limits for the estimates. The standard errors based on $\hat{a}\hat{b}$ are called product of coefficient standard errors, and standard errors based on $\hat{c} - \hat{c}'$ are called difference in coefficients standard errors. Each of these standard error formulas can be used to construct upper and lower confidence limits for the mediated effect based on the following equations,

$$\text{Lower confidence limit (LCL)} = \text{mediated effect} - z_{\text{Type 1 error}}\,(s_{\hat{a}\hat{b}}) \qquad (3.4)$$

$$\text{Upper confidence limit (UCL)} = \text{mediated effect} + z_{\text{Type 1 error}}\,(s_{\hat{a}\hat{b}}) \qquad (3.5)$$

where the mediated effect estimate is $\hat{a}\hat{b} = \hat{c} - \hat{c}'$, $z_{\text{Type 1 error}}$ is the value of the z (or t) statistic for the required confidence limits (e.g., 1.96 for 95% confidence limits for a large sample size) and $s_{\hat{a}\hat{b}}$ is an estimate of the standard error of the mediated effect based on one of the formulas for the standard error of the mediated effect described below. Critical values for the z rather than the t distribution are primarily used because the formulas for the standard errors are large sample approximations. Because $\hat{a}\hat{b}$ is algebraically equivalent to $\hat{c} - \hat{c}'$, these standard errors can be used to compute confidence limits for $\hat{c} - \hat{c}'$ as well as $\hat{a}\hat{b}$.

The most commonly used standard error of $\hat{a}\hat{b}$, $s_{\hat{a}\hat{b}}$, is the formula derived by Sobel (1982) based on first derivatives using the multivariate delta method (Folmer, 1981). The background for this formula is described in chapter 4. The resulting formula is shown below, where $s_{\hat{a}}^2$ and $s_{\hat{b}}^2$ correspond to the squared standard error of $\hat{a}$ and $\hat{b}$, respectively.

$$s_{\text{First}} = \sqrt{\hat{a}^2 s_{\hat{b}}^2 + \hat{b}^2 s_{\hat{a}}^2} \tag{3.6}$$

Equation 3.6 shows the formula that is used in many covariance structure computer programs, such as EQS (Bentler, 1997), Mplus (Muthén & Muthén, 2004) and LISREL (Jöreskog & Sörbom, 2001), to compute the standard error estimates for mediated effects. When regression coefficients and standard errors are small, as they often are, it is very easy for rounding errors to affect the accuracy of the hand calculation of the standard error using Equation 3.6. A computationally easier formula is based on the t values for the $\hat{a}$ and $\hat{b}$ effects, called $t_{\hat{a}}$ ($\hat{a}/s_{\hat{a}}$) and $t_{\hat{b}}$ ($\hat{b}/s_{\hat{b}}$), respectively:

$$s_{\text{First}} = \frac{\hat{a}\hat{b}\sqrt{t_{\hat{a}}^2 + t_{\hat{b}}^2}}{t_{\hat{a}} t_{\hat{b}}} \tag{3.7}$$

Standard Error of $\hat{c} - \hat{c}'$. The standard error of the difference between two regression coefficients (MacKinnon, Lockwood, Hoffman, West, & Sheets, 2002; McGuigan & Langholz, 1988), $\hat{c} - \hat{c}'$, is equal to:

$$s_{\hat{c}-\hat{c}'} = \sqrt{s_{\hat{c}}^2 + s_{\hat{c}'}^2 - 2rs_{\hat{c}}s_{\hat{c}'}} \tag{3.8}$$

where the covariance between $\hat{c}$ and $\hat{c}'$, $rs_{\hat{c}}s_{\hat{c}'}$, is the mean square error (MSE, the variance of the error term in Equation 3.2) divided by the sample size times the variance of the independent variable (MSE/(N $*$ s_X^2)). In most examples, the values from Equations 3.6 and 3.8 are very similar. Equation 3.6 (or 3.7) is usually preferred over Equation 3.8 as it is easier to compute and generalizes to more complicated models.

3.7 Asymmetric Confidence Limits for the Mediated Effect

The confidence limits for the mediated effect described above are symmetric, meaning that the upper and lower limits are an equal amount above and below the mediated effect. More accurate confidence limits for the mediated effect can be obtained with methods for asymmetric confidence limits that do not have equal distance above and below the estimate for the mediated effect. Asymmetric confidence limits are more accurate because the mediated effect does not always have a normal distribution. Using critical values from the distribution of the product of two variables to create confidence limits is more accurate because it appropriately adjusts confidence limits for the non-normality of the mediated effect. Another method to address the non-normality of the mediated effect is to use resampling methods. Both methods provide more accurate confidence limits for the mediated effect. The distribution of the product method is described in chapter 4, and chapter 12 describes resampling methods for mediation studies.

3.8 Significance Tests for the Mediated Effect

Researchers often want to test whether an observed mediated effect is significantly different from zero. One way to test the mediated effect for significance is to assess whether zero is included in the confidence interval. If zero is outside the confidence interval, then the mediated effect is statistically significant. The mediated effect can also be tested for statistical significance by dividing the estimate of the mediated effect by its standard error and comparing this value to tabled values of the normal distribution. If the absolute value of the ratio exceeds 1.96 then the mediated effect is significantly different from zero at the 0.05 level of significance. An alternative method is to test whether the $\hat{a}$ coefficient is statistically significant, and whether the $\hat{b}$ coefficient is statistically significant, but this method does not incorporate confidence limits. Chapter 4 describes more about statistical power and Type 1 error rates of these methods and several other alternative methods including methods based on the distribution of the product of two random variables that provide more accurate confidence limits and significance tests.

3.9 Assumptions of the Mediation Regression Equations

Each mediation regression equation requires the usual assumptions for regression analysis (Cohen, Cohen, West, & Aiken, 2003). Four of these assumptions are correct functional form, no omitted influences, accurate measurement, and well-behaved residuals. Each of these assumptions is described below. More information regarding assessing these assumptions and methods to remedy them are described in Cohen et al. (2003). Section 3.12 describes several additional assumptions and considerations related to the inference about mediation relations.

Correct Functional Form. Each mediation regression equation assumes linear relations among variables whereby a 1 unit change in the independent variable leads to a given change in the dependent variable. Using the X to M relation, for example, a 1 unit change in X leads to a change of $\hat{a}$ units in M. It is possible to model nonlinear relations among variables in these models with nonlinear transformations and specification of independent variables to reflect the nonlinear relation.

Another aspect of the correct functional form assumption is that relations among variables are additive, meaning that variables do not interact. An important interaction effect in the single mediator case is the interaction of X and M in the model where X and M predict Y. This interaction assesses whether the relation of M to Y is different at different levels of X and also whether the relation of X to Y differs across levels of M. This interaction can be tested by including the XM interaction in the prediction of Y as discussed in chapter 10. This type of interaction may also reflect important mediational processes (Judd & Kenny, 1981b; Kraemer, Wilson, Fairburn, & Agras, 2002). If X represents assignment to one of two experimental groups, then the XM interaction represents the different relation of M to Y for each experimental group, which may be very important in some situations.

No Omitted Influences. Stated concretely, it is assumed that the mediation regression equations reflect the correct underlying model. No important variables or other influences are omitted from the regression model. There are many ways that the model may fail to include all important influences as described later in section 3.12, which covers assumptions relating to inference from a mediation analysis.

Accurate Measurement. The third general assumption is that X, M, and Y are reliable and valid measures. There are several ways in which measurement may be compromised in a mediation analysis, and there are several methods to address this limitation. As described by Hoyle and Kenny (1999), measurement error can be especially problematic in the analysis of mediation because error in the mediator will lead to attenuated effects for the relation between M and Y. Using measures with adequate reliability and validity addresses this concern. Another alternative is to specify measurement models for constructs such that a latent construct is hypothesized to be measured by several fallible indicators. These types of measurement models are described in chapter 7.

Well-Behaved Residuals. Note that only two of the three mediation equations are estimated to test the mediated effect, that is, Equations 3.1 and 3.2 for $\hat{c} - \hat{c}'$ or Equations 3.2 and 3.3 for $\hat{a}\hat{b}$. The residuals in each equation are assumed to be uncorrelated with the predictor variables in each equation, are independent of each other, and the residuals are assumed to have constant variance at each value of the predictor variable. For the multiple equation case with Equations 3.2 and 3.3, it is also assumed that residual error terms are uncorrelated across equations. It is possible that errors could be correlated across equations if variables are omitted that are causes of both M and Y. There are situations in which it is possible to model these correlated errors (McDonald, 1997) using approaches such as instrumental variable estimation (Angrist, Imbens, & Rubin, 1996). Inferential assumptions related to residuals are discussed in Section 3.12.

3.10 Hypothetical Study of the Effects of Temperature on Water Consumption

In this section, a hypothetical data example is used to clarify the computation and interpretation of mediation analysis. The example is a stimulus–organism–response mediation study (Woodworth, 1928), in which the effect of a stimulus on a response is mediated by the organism. Here the stimulus was temperature, the response was water consumption, and the mediator was the subject's report of thirst. The hypothesis was that exposure to higher temperatures increases thirst, which then leads to water consumption. The mediated effect of temperature on water consumption through self-reported thirst provides an estimate of the extent to which persons were capable of gauging their own need for water. The purpose of the study was to investigate the effects of temperature on water consumption in self-contained environments such as those present in spacecraft, space suits, and submarines. Each of these environments can be set to different temperatures and water loss and ensuing fatigue are detrimental to optimal performance. As persons in this environment will need to monitor their own dehydration, self-reports of thirst are important indicators of water needs.

The data for the 50 subjects in this hypothetical study of the effects of room temperature on water consumption are shown in Table 3.1, where X is the temperature in degrees Fahrenheit, M is a self-report measure of thirst at the end of a 2-hour period, and Y is the number of deciliters of water consumed during the last 2 hours of the study. The 50 subjects were in a room for 4 hours doing a variety of tasks including sorting objects, tracking objects on a computer screen, and communicating via an intercom system. The tasks were selected to represent activities of persons alone

Table 3.1 Data for a Hypothetical Study
of Temperature on Water Consumption

S#	X	M	Y	S#	X	M	Y
1	70	4	3	26	70	3	4
2	71	4	3	27	70	2	3
3	69	1	3	28	69	3	4
4	70	1	3	29	69	4	3
5	71	3	3	30	70	3	3
6	70	4	2	31	71	2	1
7	69	3	3	32	70	1	3
8	70	5	5	33	70	2	5
9	70	4	4	34	70	2	1
10	72	5	4	35	71	4	3
11	71	2	2	36	68	2	1
12	71	3	4	37	72	4	3
13	70	5	5	38	69	3	2
14	71	4	5	39	70	3	3
15	71	4	5	40	68	3	2
16	70	2	2	41	68	3	3
17	70	4	4	42	70	4	3
18	69	3	5	43	71	4	4
19	72	3	4	44	69	2	2
20	71	3	3	45	69	3	3
21	71	2	4	46	71	3	4
22	72	3	5	47	71	4	4
23	67	1	2	48	71	3	2
24	71	4	4	49	72	4	5
25	71	3	2	50	70	2	2

in contained environments such as a submarine, spacecraft, or space suit. Before the experiment, each participant was acclimated to a standard temperature of 70°F. Temperature, the independent variable, was then manipulated such that each participant was exposed to a specific temperature in the room for the 4 hours of the experiment. At the end of 2 hours, the subjects reported how thirsty they were on a 1 to 5 scale from 1 (not at all thirsty) to 5 (very thirsty). During the last 2 hours of the experiment, water was made available in the room, and the number of the deciliters of water the subjects drank was recorded.

SPSS and SAS Programs. The variable names X, M, and Y were used to represent the variables temperature, thirst, and water consumed, respectively.

The following SAS statements were used to obtain the regression coefficient estimates used to compute the mediated effect and its standard error. Complete data were available for each of the 50 cases.

The SAS program and output are shown in Table 3.2. The values in the output are the numbers used in the calculation of the mediated effect and related quantities.

For SPSS, the statements in Table 3.3 were used to obtain the information necessary to compute the mediated effect, standard error, and confidence limits. Note that a new regression statement is required for each regression equation. The output from SPSS is also included in Table 3.3.

Table 3.2 SAS Program and Output for Equations 3.1, 3.2, and 3.3

```
proc reg;
model Y=X;
model Y=X M;
model M=X;
```

Output for Equation 3.1

Variable	DF	Parameter Estimate	Standard Error	T for H0: Parameter=0	Prob > |T|
INTERCEP	1	-22.050489	9.42792490	-2.339	0.0236
X	1	0.360366	0.13432191	2.683	0.0100

Output for Equation 3.2

Root MSE	0.98523	R-square	0.2772		
Dep Mean	3.24000	Adj R-sq	0.2465		
C.V.	30.40836				

Variable	DF	Parameter Estimate	Standard Error	T for H0: Parameter=0	Prob > |T|
INTERCEP	1	-12.712884	9.19690719	-1.382	0.1734
X	1	0.207648	0.13325967	1.558	0.1259
M	1	0.451039	0.14597405	3.090	0.0034

Output for Equation 3.3

Variable	DF	Parameter Estimate	Standard Error	T for H0: Parameter=0	Prob > |T|
INTERCEP	1	-20.702430	8.58884617	-2.410	0.0198
X	1	0.338593	0.12236736	2.767	0.0080

Table 3.3 SPSS Program and Output for Equations 3.1, 3.2, and 3.3

```
regression
    /variables X Y M
    /dependent=Y
    /enter=X.
regression
    /variables X Y M
    /dependent=Y
    /enter=X M.
regression
    /variables X Y M
    /dependent=M
    /enter X.
```

Output for Equation 3.1

	Unstandardized Coefficients		Standardized Coefficients		
	B	Std. Error	Beta	t	Sig
(Constant)	-22.050	9.428		-2.339	.024
X	.360	.134	.361	2.683	.010

a. Dependent Variable Y

Output for Equation 3.2

Model Summary

Model	R	R Square	Adjusted R Square	Std. Error of the Estimate
1	.5265	.2772	.2465	0.9852

	Unstandardized Coefficients		Standardized Coefficients		
	B	Std. Error	Beta	t	Sig
(Constant)	-12.713	9.197		-1.382	.173
X	.208	.133	.208	1.558	.126
M	.451	.146	.413	3.090	.003

a. Dependent Variable Y

Output for Equation 3.3

	Unstandardized Coefficients		Standardized Coefficients		
	B	Std. Error	Beta	t	Sig
(Constant)	-20.702	8.589		-2.410	.020
X	.339	.122	.371	2.767	.008

a. Dependent Variable M

As shown below, all SPSS estimates are identical (with rounding) to those in the SAS output. The SPSS output automatically includes the standardized beta coefficients, which represent the change in the dependent variable for a 1 standard deviation change in the independent variable. The standardized beta measure is one of the effect size measures for mediation described in the next chapter.

Mediation Analysis for the Temperature and Water Consumption Study. The unstandardized regression estimates and standard errors (in parentheses) from the SAS or SPSS output for the three models are:

$$\text{Equation 3.1:} \quad Y = i_1 + cX + \hat{e}_1$$
$$\hat{Y} = -22.0505 + 0.3604X$$
$$(0.1343)$$

$$\text{Equation 3.2:} \quad Y = i_2 + c'X + bM + e_2$$
$$\hat{Y} = -12.7129 + 0.2076X + 0.4510M$$
$$(0.1333)(0.1460)$$

$$\text{Equation 3.3:} \quad M = i_3 + aX + e_3$$
$$\hat{M} = -20.7024 + 0.3386X$$
$$(0.1224)$$

Temperature was significantly related to water consumption ($\hat{c} = 0.3604$, $s_{\hat{c}} = 0.1343$, $t_{\hat{c}} = 2.6783$), providing evidence that there is a statistically significant relation between the independent and the dependent variable. A 1°F increase in temperature was associated with roughly a third (0.36) of a deciliter of water consumed. There was a statistically significant effect of temperature on self-reported thirst ($\hat{a} = 0.3386$, $s_{\hat{a}} = 0.1224$, $t_{\hat{a}} = 2.767$). A 1°F increase in temperature was associated with change of 0.34 in the thirst rating scale. The relation of the self-reported thirst mediator on water consumption was statistically significant ($\hat{b} = 0.4510$, $s_{\hat{b}} = 0.1460$, $t_{\hat{b}} = 3.090$) when controlling for temperature. A 1 unit change in the thirst rating scale was associated with an increase of 0.45 deciliters consumed. The adjusted effect of temperature was not statistically significant ($\hat{c}' = 0.2076$, $s_{\hat{c}'} = 0.1333$, $t_{\hat{c}'} = 1.558$). There was a drop in the value of $\hat{c}'$ (0.2076) compared with $\hat{c}$ (0.3604).

The estimate of the mediated effect is equal to $\hat{a}\hat{b} = (0.33859)(0.45103) = \hat{c} - \hat{c}' = 0.36036 - 0.20765 = 0.1527$. The mediated effect of temperature through perceived thirst was equal to 0.15 deciliters of water consumed. Using Equation 3.6, the standard error of the mediated effect is equal to:

$$0.0741 = \sqrt{(0.3386)^2(0.1460)^2 + (0.4510)^2(0.1224)^2}$$

As seen in the preceding example, when the regression coefficients and standard errors are small, it is easy for rounding errors to affect the accuracy of the calculation of the standard error. Using Equation 3.7 gives the same answer, but it is less susceptible to computation errors because small numbers are not squared:

$$0.0741 = \frac{(0.3386)(0.4510)\sqrt{(2.767^2 + 3.090^2)}}{(2.767)(3.090)}$$

The 95% confidence limits for the mediated effect are equal to:

$$\text{LCL} = 0.1527 - 1.96\ (0.0741) = 0.0033$$

$$\text{UCL} = 0.1527 + 1.96\ (0.0741) = 0.2979$$

The standard error of $\hat{c} - \hat{c}'$ (where 1.293 is the variance of X) in Equation 3.8 shown below, is very close to the value for Equation 3.6. As in most situations, the estimates for the standard error formulas are very similar (MacKinnon, Warsi, & Dwyer, 1995):

$$0.0770 = \sqrt{0.1343^2 + 0.1333^2 - \frac{(2)(0.9852^2)}{(50)(1.293)}}$$

As described in chapter 4, asymmetric confidence limits based on the distribution of the product would use critical values of −1.6175 and 2.2540 rather than −1.96 and 1.96, respectively, and yield lower and upper confidence limits of 0.0329 and 0.3197. And as described in chapter 12, bootstrap confidence limits for these data were 0.0604 and 0.3322. In simulation studies, these confidence limits tend to be more accurate than the normal theory confidence limits, but in most cases the research conclusions are the same. Confidence limits based on critical values from the normal distribution tend to be very similar to the asymmetric confidence limits if either or both of the ratios $\hat{a}/s_{\hat{a}}$ or $\hat{b}/s_{\hat{b}}$ are equal to or greater than 6.

Note that whenever complete data are used in a mediation analysis, the two quantities $\hat{a}\hat{b}$ and $\hat{c} - \hat{c}'$ are equal. However, if different subjects are included for the analysis of different equations, then $\hat{a}\hat{b}$ may not equal $\hat{c} - \hat{c}'$. In the SAS program for the water consumption example, all regression statements were included under one PROC REG statement. This procedure differs from regression analysis in SPSS in which equations are all run separately. As a result, a researcher is more likely to have unequal numbers of subjects in the different regression models when SPSS is used, and consequently the researcher will not find that $\hat{a}\hat{b} = \hat{c} - \hat{c}'$ because of the slight difference in sample sizes for each regression. The researcher is advised to remove cases that do not have measures of all three variables before estimating the regression models in SPSS if it is desired that $\hat{a}\hat{b} = \hat{c} - \hat{c}'$.

An important test for the single mediator model is whether there is an interaction between the independent variable and the mediator. This interaction can be tested by including the independent variable (X) by mediator (M) interaction as an additional predictor in Equation 3.2. If the interaction is statistically significant, then there is evidence that the relation of the mediator to the dependent variable differs across the levels of the independent variable. The interaction effect was not statistically significant for the water consumption example as described in chapter 10.

3.11 Plots of the Mediated Effect

Several plots may be useful for illustrating mediation effects and investigating model assumptions. Plots for the regression analysis of the water consumption example data are shown in Figs. 3.3, 3.4, and 3.5. The dots in the figures represent observations, with larger dots representing more observations. Figure 3.3 shows a plot of the relation of X to Y corresponding to Equation 3.1. In this figure, the slope of the line is 0.3604, reflecting

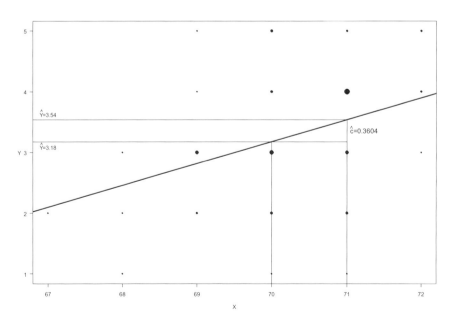

Figure 3.3 Relation of X and Y.

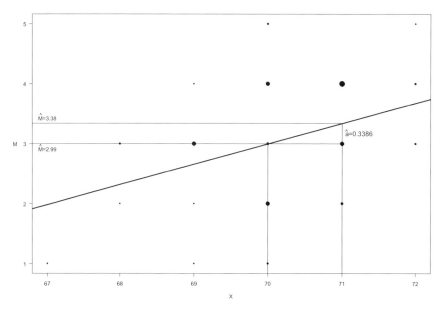

Figure 3.4   Relation of X and M.

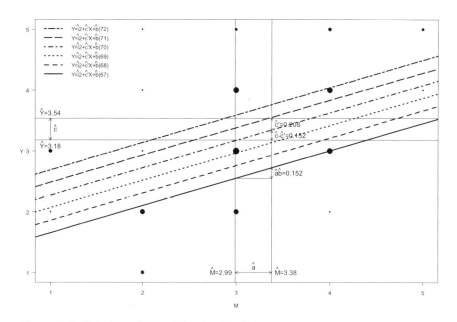

Figure 3.5   Relation of M and Y at levels of X.

the $\hat{c}$ coefficient, the change in Y for a 1 unit change in X. The horizontal lines in the plot demonstrate that the mean for 70°F was 3.18 and for 71°F equaled 3.54, corresponding to the $\hat{c}$ difference of 0.3604. Figure 3.4 shows the plot of X and M, corresponding to Equation 3.3. In Fig. 3.4, the relation of X to M, indicates that a 1 unit change in X corresponds to a 0.3386 change in M. The horizontal line in Fig. 3.4 for X equal to 70, the predicted M is 2.99, and for X equal to 71, the predicted M is 3.38.

Figures 3.3 and 3.4 are relatively straightforward in that they represent the simple relation between two variables. Figure 3.5 is more complicated and summarizes the mediation model graphically for X, M, and Y. Information from Figs. 3.3 and 3.4 is also shown in Fig. 3.5. The $\hat{c}$ coefficient is shown in the plot by the difference between the horizontal lines. The difference between the horizontal lines represents the predicted values of Y for a 1 unit change in X. In Fig. 3.3, the predicted Y score was 3.18 for an X equal to 70 and 3.54 for X equal to 71, reflecting the change in 0.3604 units for a 1 unit change in X. The predicted scores for X of 71 and 72 were chosen to illustrate effects in the model. Other adjacent values of X could have been used and each adjacent value of X would differ by 0.3604. In Fig. 3.5, the $\hat{a}$ coefficient is represented by the difference in the vertical lines in the plot for the predicted M value for X equal to 2.99 for 70°F, and the predicted M value for X equal to 3.38 for 71°F. The difference between the predicted M for X equal to 70 and 71 equals the $\hat{a}$ coefficient of 0.3386.

Figure 3.5 is more complicated than Figs. 3.3 and 3.4, because it shows the relation of M to Y at each level of X, the $\hat{c}$ and $\hat{a}$ effects, as well as the mediated effect, $\hat{a}\hat{b} = \hat{c} - \hat{c}'$. Because there are six temperatures of X for the water consumption example, there are six lines on the plot, and all of these lines have a slope equal to the $\hat{b}$ coefficient, 0.4510. That is, each line represents the linear relation of M to Y for one of the six different temperatures in the study. Each line has a different intercept corresponding to the value of water consumed, Y, when self-reported thirst, M, equals 0. The distance between adjacent parallel lines is equal to the $\hat{c}'$ effect, 0.1416. That is, the difference in the water consumed for a 1 unit change in temperature is 0.1416, holding self-reported thirst constant. As described earlier, the value of $\hat{c}$ can be seen as the distance between horizontal lines and the value of $\hat{a}$ can be seen as the distance between the vertical lines. As shown in the graph, the distance between $\hat{c}$ and $\hat{c}'$ is the mediated effect in these plots. The value of the mediated effect, $\hat{a}\hat{b}$, is the change in Y for a change of $\hat{a}$ units in M, as shown in the plot.

In the preceding plot, lines for all six values of X were presented. If X was continuous with many values, some decision must be made about what levels of X to plot. One option would be to plot lines for values of X that are 1 unit apart. Another alternative would be to plot lines for the most common values of X. In Fig. 3.5, the most common values were 70 and 71, so plotting only these two lines would provide a simpler plot. It is useful to plot lines 1 unit apart on X because the difference between the lines relating M and Y represents the $\hat{c}'$ coefficient. The $\hat{c}$, $\hat{a}$, $\hat{b}$, $\hat{a}\hat{b}$, and $\hat{c} - \hat{c}'$ estimates are obtained in the same manner as for the more comprehensive plot discussed earlier. Another alternative would be to plot the values of X 1 standard deviation above and 1 standard deviation below the average. The same procedure would be used to assess mediation, but the values, $\hat{c}$, $\hat{a}$, $\hat{b}$, $\hat{a}\hat{b}$, and $\hat{c} - \hat{c}'$, would be more difficult to specify because the difference between the lines is no longer in terms of 1 unit but is in terms of 1 standard deviation of X.

If X is a binary variable coding exposure to an independent variable, then the resulting plots are considerably simpler than the above case where X has many values. The plots for the effect of X on M and X on Y now have only two points, one for each level of X. The plot relating M to Y now includes two lines representing the $\hat{b}$ coefficient for the two levels of X. The difference between the two lines is again the $\hat{c}'$ coefficient. The $\hat{c}$ and $\hat{a}$ coefficients can be seen in the same way as for the continuous X variable, as the difference between the group means in Y on the ordinate and the difference between the group means in X for the abscissa, respectively. Again, the value of $\hat{c} - \hat{c}'$ is shown in the plot, and the change in Y for a change of $\hat{a}$ units reflects the $\hat{a}\hat{b}$ measure of mediation.

Another interesting aspect of the plot in Fig. 3.5 is the parallel lines for each value of the X variable, temperature. Because the interaction of X and M is not estimated in the model, the different lines relating M to Y are parallel. If the interaction between X and M was in the model and was nonzero, then the lines would not be parallel (Merrill, 1994).

3.12 Inferential Assumptions of the Single Mediator Model

There are several other overlapping assumptions and considerations for the single mediator model in addition to the ones mentioned earlier. Like any statistical analysis, it is important to interpret mediation analysis in the context of the validity of the assumptions of the mediation model. In any mediation study, these assumptions must be addressed to provide a reasoned argument for or against evidence of mediation.

Temporal Precedence. The single mediator model assumes an ordering of variables such that X comes before M, which comes before Y. In this regard, assessment of mediation with cross-sectional data is problematic as generally no information regarding temporal precedence is available, but must be based on theory or some other means. There are situations in which the meaning of variables measured in a cross-sectional study do imply some temporal precedence that may shed light on mediation such as when X is measured before M (Smith, 1982). Comprehensive models of time dependence in longitudinal data have been used in the past, and more methods are under development. Mediation models for longitudinal data are described in chapter 8.

Micro Versus Macro Mediational Chain. An assumption of the single mediator model related to temporal precedence is that the variables represent logical parts of a mediational chain. A mediational chain may consist of a large number of links or steps; the researcher must decide which of these steps to measure. Similar decisions must be made about the ultimate dependent variable studied. This distinction between the macromediational chain and the micromediational chain was discussed in the earliest applications of path analysis models. It is likely that research progresses by measuring more of the steps in a micromediational chain. It is also possible that a research study may not have measured the correct steps in the chain so that a real mediation effect will be missed. A research study may also investigate only a small part of a much longer mediational chain.

Measurement Timing. Related to micromediational chain and temporal precedence is the assumption that the timing of measurement of the mediator and the dependent variable appropriately matches the true timing of the relation between change in the independent variable, change in the mediator, and change in the outcome. Many experimental manipulations are expected to lead to immediate changes in mediators that subsequently lead to changes in the outcome. In some cases, the change in the mediator occurs long before the change in the ultimate outcome such as change in dietary calcium among young women, which may have its effects much later on the development of osteoporosis. Other more complicated aspects of change including a triggering of a mediating mechanism whereby a single event triggers an entire mediation mechanism or a cumulative effect mediation mechanism in which each change in a mediator increases effects over time (Howe, Reiss, & Yuh, 2002; Tang & DeRubeis, 1999). For example, most change in clinical psychotherapy appears to occur after early sessions (Tang & DeRubies, 1999).

Normally Distributed X, M, and Y. It is generally assumed that X, M, and Y have a normal distribution (Darlington, 1990). If X is binary, then the statistical methods outlined in the chapter remain accurate, but the size of effects may be reduced from when X is a continuous variable, unless X is truly binary. If Y is binary, then estimates of the mediated effect can be inaccurate as described in chapter 11, which describes mediation analysis for a binary dependent variable. In general, resampling methods that do not make as many assumptions regarding the distribution of X, M, and Y are appropriate when mediation variables do not have a normal distribution, as described in chapter 12. The appropriate mediation analysis may differ for different distributions of the variables in the mediation model.

Normally Distributed Product of Coefficients. The application of the standard errors in chapter 3 assumes that the product of $\hat{a}$ and $\hat{b}$, $\hat{a}\hat{b}$, has a normal distribution. In fact, the distribution of the product of two random variables does not have a normal distribution in several situations. Two alternative ways to address this problem are the creation of confidence limits based on the distribution of the product of two random variables and resampling methods as described in chapter 12. More information about a method based on the distribution of the product is described in chapter 4.

Omitted Influences. The single mediator model assumes that no other variables affect the relations in the model. For the single mediator model, this means that there are no other variables related to the three variables in the mediation model. Omitted variables may consist of unmeasured, but important, variables or interactions among variables that are not included in the statistical analysis.

With real data, it is unlikely that the three variables in the single mediator model are the only relevant variables. As described in chapter 5, the single mediator model can be easily extended to multiple mediators, thereby incorporating additional mediation effects. A more general model with multiple mediators, multiple independent variables, and multiple dependent variables is described in chapter 6. It is still possible that these more comprehensive models with many mediators may not contain all relevant variables because there may be an unmeasured variable that may explain a pattern of effects. Approaches to this problem based on programs of research, careful interpretation of relations among variables, and replications are described in chapters 13 and 14. For example, a program of research based on experimental and nonexperimental studies can reduce the plausibility of omitted variable explanations of observed mediated effects.

The model also assumes the same relations for all participants in a research study; that is, there are not subgroups of participants with different mediational processes. However, it is possible that important moderators may not have been included in the analysis. Mediation may differ across groups. For example, the mediated effect may differ for males and females. As described in chapter 10, one way to assess the assumption of no moderation is to test potential moderator effects. In some cases, the moderator effects are predicted on the basis of theory and are included in the analysis, so they serve as not merely assumptions to be tested but also as a primary focus of the research study. For example, a treatment program may be more successful for persons already low on a mediator at baseline so that program effects are expected to be larger for participants with the lowest scores on a mediator. And if a mediated effect differs across subgroups, it suggests that other mediating variables may explain these moderator effects.

Causal Inference. Another assumption related to omitted effects is that the relation between X and M, $\hat{a}$, between M and Y adjusted for X, $\hat{b}$, between X and Y, $\hat{c}$, and between X and Y adjusted for M, $\hat{c}'$, reflect true causal relations of the correct functional form (Holland, 1988a; Rubin, 2004). If X represents random assignment to conditions, the $\hat{a}$ relation and the $\hat{c}$ relation represent causal effects under certain assumptions described in chapter 13. However, there are situations in which these coefficients may not reflect a true causal relation such as if X does not represent random assignment to conditions or the random assignment has been compromised in some way. In this X nonrandomized case, the $\hat{a}$ coefficient may reflect other effects besides the effect of level of X on M. Even if X represents random assignment, the $\hat{b}$ and $\hat{c}'$ coefficients are still potentially problematic because M is not randomly assigned but is determined or self-selected by study participants, as discussed in chapter 13. In many situations, the results of a mediation analysis are descriptive rather than implying causal relations.

Theoretical Versus Empirical Mediator. Even though there is evidence for a variable as a mediator, such as a statistically significant mediated effect, it is possible that the mediator identified does not reflect the true mechanism by which an effect occurs. One simple explanation of such an effect is a Type I error, whereby the effect was significant by chance alone. Another option is that the mediator identified is actually a proxy for the true mediator (Kraemer et al., 2002). For example, in a study of the effects of cognitive therapy on depression, cognitive attributions about health may function as a mediator in an analysis when it is really a proxy for the more general mediator of general negative cognitive attributions.

It is not likely that a true mechanism can be demonstrated in one statistical analysis. The point is that mediation analysis provides information regarding possible mediating mechanisms. These analyses inform the next experiment that provides more information until a series of studies provides convincing evidence of a mediating mechanism.

3.13 Other Tests for Mediation

The methodology for testing mediation described in this chapter reflects ideas from several different prior mediation tests and the results of simulation studies comparing tests. Several other tests are described in this section because you may encounter these statistical tests in the research literature. These tests may be the mediation test of choice in some situations. This section provides optional background for mediation analysis.

Three general types of tests are described in this section. Tests of mediation based on the $\hat{a}\hat{b}$ estimator of the mediated effect are called product of coefficients tests and tests based on the $\hat{c} - \hat{c}'$ estimator are called difference in coefficients tests (MacKinnon, 2001). A third group of tests are based on testing hypotheses consistent with mediation. These step tests are described in the next section. As described in chapter 13, the definition of a causal relation is controversial and will often require more criteria than are described in these tests.

Baron and Kenny (1986) Steps to Establish Mediation. The most widely used method to assess mediation was described by David Kenny and colleagues (Baron & Kenny, 1986; Judd & Kenny, 1981b; Kenny, Kashy, & Bolger, 1998). The Baron and Kenny (1986) article is one of the most cited articles in the social sciences, largely because of its guidance regarding testing for mediation. This method consists of a series of statistical tests of relations among variables corresponding to significance tests of the $\hat{a}$, $\hat{b}$, $\hat{c}$, and $\hat{c}'$ regression coefficients described earlier. The series of tests of causal steps described by Kenny and colleagues is essentially the same across all of the articles:

1. The independent variable (X) must affect the dependent variable (Y), as indicated by coefficient $\hat{c}$ in Equation 3.1.

    The purpose of this first test is to establish that there is an effect to mediate. If the effect is not statistically significant, then the analysis stops in the causal steps approach. This test is controversial because it is possible that the relation between the independent variable and the dependent variable may be nonsignificant, yet there can still be substantial mediation. This will occur in cases of what is called inconsistent mediation (suppression models). Inconsistent mediation occurs when the mediated effect and the direct effect have opposite signs. In these models the relation of X to Y actually increases in magnitude when it is adjusted for the mediator. As mentioned by Rosenberg (1968, p. 84), "one can be equally misled in assuming that an absence of relation between two variables is real, whereas it may be due . . . to the intrusion of a third variable."

2. The independent variable (X) must affect the mediator (M), evaluated by coefficient $\hat{a}$ in Equation 3.3.

    This test requires that the independent variable is significantly related to the mediator. In the case of an X variable coding an experimental manipulation, this requires that there is an experimental effect on the mediating variable. As described in chapter 2, in an experimental study this provides a test of the action theory of the manipulation, that is, whether the theory of how the independent variable changes the mediator is accurate.

3. The mediator (M) must affect the dependent variable (Y) when the independent variable (X) is controlled, coefficient $\hat{b}$ in Equation 3.2.

This test requires a significant relation between the mediator and the dependent variable, providing a test of the conceptual theory of how the mediator is related to the dependent variable as described in chapter 2. It makes sense that the mediator must be significantly related to the dependent variable for there to be mediation. If the mediator is unrelated to the dependent variable, the effect of the independent variable on the mediator cannot be carried through to the dependent variable. Clogg, Petkova, and Shihadeh (1992) concluded that the test of significance of $\hat{b}$ is a test for mediation at least in terms of testing whether adding the mediator changes the relation between the independent variable and the dependent variable. Generally, the test of $\hat{b}$ is not sufficient to demonstrate a mediation effect because a researcher will typically require the relation between the independent variable and the mediator, the $\hat{a}$ regression coefficient, to be statistically significant.

4.   The direct effect, coefficient $\hat{c}'$, must be nonsignificant, in Equation 3.2.

Across the articles on the causal step mediation approaches, there is some difference regarding the fourth step, relating to the extent to which an effect is completely mediated or partially mediated. The Judd and Kenny (1981b) method requires total mediation or that the independent variable does not have a significant effect on the dependent variable when the mediator (M) is controlled. In this case, the $\hat{c}'$ or direct effect must not be significantly different from zero. There is motivation for this requirement based on detailed causal analysis of the mediation model described in chapter 13. The Judd and Kenny (1981b) description also assumes that X represents an experimental manipulation. The Baron and Kenny (1986) method and later descriptions of this approach allow for partial mediation, or that the effect of the independent variable on the dependent variable is larger when the mediator is not partialled than when it is partialled, that is, that $\hat{c}'$ is less than $\hat{c}$. The partial mediation case allows $\hat{c}'$ to be significant and makes sense given that complete mediation is probably unrealistic in many research areas such as social science research because of the many causes of behavior (Baron & Kenny, 1986). As a result, the requirement that $\hat{c}'$ be less than $\hat{c}$, that is, $\hat{a}\hat{b} > 0$, rather than $\hat{c}' = 0$, is included in most recent applications of these causal step methods. There are often situations, however, in which it can be demonstrated that $\hat{c}'$ is not significantly different from zero, lending support for complete mediation.

In a recent simulation study, MacKinnon, Lockwood, et al. (2002) found results suggesting that the most important conditions for mediation are that the $\hat{a}$ coefficient is statistically significant (step 2) and that the $\hat{b}$ coefficient is statistically significant (step 3) based on Type 1 error rates and statistical power. Such a procedure was mentioned by Cohen and Cohen (1983, p. 366) in the slightly different context of a mediation effect with a chain of two or more mediators. As a result, for many mediation analyses, only steps 2 and 3 are required to establish mediation. The statistical test for mediation described earlier in this chapter focuses on information from steps 2 and 3. The additional conditions relating to steps 1 and 4 are not critical, but there are situations in which these conditions are very important. If a researcher is interested only in direct and mediated effects of the same sign, then the first step, that there is a significant effect of X on Y, is important. The interpretation of the mediated effect is also clearer if there is evidence for total mediation, step 4.

The causal step approach is the most widely used method to test for mediation because of the clear conceptual link between the causal relations and the aforementioned statistical tests. It is worth emphasizing that steps for establishing mediation were outlined earlier in Judd and Kenny (1981a) but with three notable differences. First, the X variable represented an experimental design so that the $\hat{a}$ and $\hat{c}$ relations represent effects of an experimental manipulation. Second, the $\hat{c}'$ coefficient was required to be nonsignificant, indicating a complete mediation model. Third, testing the interaction between the mediator and the independent variable was discussed.

MacArthur Mediation Framework. A recent example of a mediation framework containing steps for establishing mediation is the MacArthur model as described by Kraemer and colleagues (Kraemer et al., 2002; Kraemer, Kiernan, Essex, & Kupfer, 2004). The MacArthur framework is similar to the causal steps tests of mediation. The main difference is that the Mac-Arthur framework does not attempt to specify underlying mediating mechanisms beforehand but uses observed relations among variables to explore possible mediation and moderation relations. Temporal precedence and association are the two primary criteria necessary (but not sufficient) to indicate a causal relation between two variables. The goal of the MacArthur approach is to generate hypotheses about a possible causal role to be tested in future studies. First, the MacArthur model explicitly states that nonlinear relations among variables qualify as mediation as long as there is a relation between X and M. If there is not a relation between X and M, but the interaction is statistically significant, then the variable is considered as a moderator. Second, the existence of the interaction indicating that the relation between M and Y differs across levels of M is explicitly included in the model and is taken as evidence of mediation. Third, a defining characteristic of a moderator is that it is measured before any experimental manipulation is delivered. The time when the moderator is measured is not explicitly defined (although it is generally contemporaneous; Baron, & Kenny, 1986, p. 1174) but is implied in the Baron and Kenny mediation steps methods and is usually based on theory. In the MacArthur framework, any variable measured at the baseline of the study is a potential moderator, and a mediator must change after the independent variable. But any measure obtained after the study starts is not a moderator in this framework. Third, there must be evidence that there was change in the mediator before the change in the dependent variable for a variable to function as a mediator. This requirement explicitly addresses the temporal relation assumption. Any variable that changes over time is a potential mediator in this framework.

The Baron and Kenny (1986) steps test is criticized in the MacArthur approach, but these criticisms are addressed, primarily as assumptions of the Baron and Kenny model. For example, additive relations among variables are not explicitly excluded and the possibility of a differential relation between M and Y across levels of X was described in some detail by Judd and Kenny (1981a) as part of a steps method. It is unlikely that the steps approach would not consider additive or nonlinear relations among variables as mediation and do consider temporal precedence a characteristic of a mediating variable.

The definition of moderator and mediator in terms of when they are measured can lead to some ambiguity in the MacArthur framework. In the MacArthur framework, a theoretical moderator variable is considered a mediator if it is not measured before treatment. Similarly, the strict requirement for measurement of a mediator before the outcome prohibits using cross-sectional data to study mediating processes. This would seem to prohibit the work of detectives, psychotherapists, and physicians who seek to untangle the process of events after they have occurred. Despite these limitations, in most cases the MacArthur framework is a way to organize exploratory analyses of many potential variables in the evaluation of randomized clinical trials (MTA Cooperative Group, 1999). Most importantly, it has raised awareness of the importance of investigating mediation and moderation in the analysis of randomized trials.

Another aspect of the MacArthur approach is the identification of five types of risk factors: proxy, overlapping, independent, moderator, and mediator. A proxy risk factor is one that serves as proxy for the true causal risk factor. For example, attributional style for events at the workplace is a proxy for general attributional style across many domains. In the MacArthur framework, proxy risk factors are replaced by the true causal factor if there is a better measure of the causal risk factor. In other approaches, proxy measures would be used as additional measures of a construct to improve its reliability and validity. Overlapping risk factors refer to two risk factors that are correlated. The other type of risk factors, independent risk factors, are uncorrelated and represent unique relations with the outcome measure. In practice, some criterion value of the correlation must be defined for factors to be judged independent. Table 3.4 shows the steps in the MacArthur approach as described by Kraemer (2003), in which a criterion value for the Spearman correlation is used as a threshold to determine the relation of a risk factor with an outcome. These criteria are based on an unpublished presentation and may be refined in later versions of this approach.

Confirmatory Test of Complete Mediation. James, Mulaik, and Brett (2006) describe a confirmatory approach to mediation analysis based on the complete versus partial mediation models. The authors argue that the complete mediation model should generally be the first model tested because it is a more parsimonious representation of mediation, and a χ^2 test of model fit is available. Essentially, the complete mediation model consists of testing whether or not the $\hat{c}'$ coefficient is statistically significant. The complete mediation model is also important because it reduces the possibility that some important mediation variables have been omitted from the analysis (given adequate statistical power, valid measurement, and other assumptions). A two-step process is proposed. First, the researcher hypothesizes a complete or partial mediation model. If theory or prior research is insufficient, the complete mediation model should be tested first because it is a more parsimonious model. A noteworthy aspect of this first step is that the c' path is specified to be zero for theoretical reasons before analysis rather than after statistical analysis of the $\hat{c}'$ coefficient. In the second step, for a complete mediation model, the path relating X to M, $\hat{a}$, and the path relating M to Y (note that this is not adjusted for the mediator) $\hat{b}_{unadjusted}$, should be statistically significant. For the complete mediation model, a statistical test of model fit is obtained comparing the covariances

---

Table 3.4 Steps in the MacArthur Framework for the Single Mediator Model

1. Test the Spearman rank order correlation between X and Y. Decide whether to discard the variable if the correlation does not attain a specified value. (Note that the authors of this approach mention that this requirement can be dismissed if necessary.)

2. Test the Spearman rank order correlation between X and M. Decide whether to discard the variable if the correlation does not attain a specified value.

3. Test whether the regression coefficient relating M to Y is statistically significant when both X and M are in the same regression model. This is equivalent to testing whether the $\hat{b}$ path is statistically significant. Partial mediation is present if the relation between X and Y is statistically significant in the model with both X and M as predictors.

among X, M, and Y predicted by the complete mediation model with the observed covariances among X, M, and Y. If a partial mediation model is hypothesized, then the $\hat{a}$, $\hat{b}$, and $\hat{c}'$ coefficients in Equations 3.2 and 3.3 are estimated and the coefficients $\hat{a}$ and $\hat{b}$ must be statistically significant for mediation to exist. If the $\hat{c}'$ coefficient is statistically significant, then there is evidence of partial, not complete mediation. An important aspect of this test for mediation is its focus on specifying complete or partial mediation before the study is conducted. Practically, the test of complete mediation can be obtained with the methods described earlier in this chapter with the significance test of the $\hat{c}'$ coefficient.

Product of Coefficients Tests for Mediation. The standard error of the mediated effect is given in Equation 3.6. However, there are other standard error estimators for the mediated effect based on the product of coefficients, $\hat{a}\hat{b}$. One of these is the standard error of the product of $\hat{a}$ and $\hat{b}$ which is equal to:

$$s_{\text{Second}} = \sqrt{\hat{a}^2 s_{\hat{b}}^2 + \hat{b}^2 s_{\hat{a}}^2 + s_{\hat{a}}^2 s_{\hat{b}}^2} \tag{3.9}$$

based on the first- and second-order derivatives (Baron & Kenny, 1986; MacKinnon & Dwyer, 1993). The formula in Equation 3.6 is based on first derivatives. In fact, the use of second derivatives in the Taylor series for the variance of the product involves a mixed derivative equal to 1, which leads to the additional term, $s_{\hat{a}}^2 s_{\hat{b}}^2$, in Equation 3.9 that is not in Equation 3.6. This formula for the variance of the product of two random variables is also given in several mathematical statistics textbooks (Mood, Graybill, & Boes, 1974; Rice, 1988). An alternative formula for the second-order solution is shown in Equation 3.10. Although the standard error from Equation 3.9 is based on a more elaborate derivation, the two standard errors are usually very close and are sometimes not as accurate as the formula in Equation 3.6 (Allison, 1995b):

$$s_{\text{Second}} = \frac{\hat{a}\hat{b}\sqrt{t_{\hat{a}}^2 + t_{\hat{b}}^2 + 1}}{t_{\hat{a}}t_{\hat{b}}} \tag{3.10}$$

Goodman (1960) and Sampson and Breunig (1971) derived the unbiased variance of the product of two normal variables, which subtracts the product of variances $s_{\hat{a}}^2 s_{\hat{b}}^2$ shown in Equation 3.11, and Equation 3.12 shows an alternative computational formula.

$$s_{\text{Unbiased}} = \sqrt{\hat{a}^2 s_{\hat{b}}^2 + \hat{b}^2 s_{\hat{a}}^2 - s_{\hat{a}}^2 s_{\hat{b}}^2} \tag{3.11}$$

$$s_{\text{Unbiased}} = \frac{\hat{a}\hat{b}\sqrt{t_{\hat{a}}^2 + t_{\hat{b}}^2 - 1}}{t_{\hat{a}}t_{\hat{b}}} \qquad (3.12)$$

The Sampson and Breunig (1971) unbiased standard error takes into account the sample size associated with the $\hat{a}$ and $\hat{b}$ coefficients. One drawback of the unbiased estimator of the standard error is that it is sometimes undefined at sample sizes <200 in simulation studies because the variance is negative (MacKinnon, Lockwood, et al., 2002; MacKinnon, Lockwood, & Williams, 2004). In this case, the mediated effect is likely to be nonsignificant, because small values of $\hat{a}$ and $\hat{b}$ make the two elements in Equation 3.11 very small compared to the $s_{\hat{a}}^2 s_{\hat{b}}^2$ term.

It has been suggested that the standard error formula in Equation 3.6 can be used to test the statistical significance of the product of $\hat{a}$ and $\hat{b}$ standardized coefficients (Russell, Kahn, Spoth, & Altmaier, 1998). However, the standard error formula in Equation 3.6 was derived for unstandardized regression coefficients, not standardized coefficients. Using the above formulas to test the significance of the product of standardized $\hat{a}$ and $\hat{b}$ regression coefficients (based on unstandardized standard errors) can lead to misleading results. Bobko and Rieck (1980) present a formula for the standard error of the product of regression coefficients from path analysis, in which variables are standardized before analysis. The method uses the formula for the product of the standardized regression coefficients for $\hat{a}$ and $\hat{b}$, calculated using the three correlation coefficients involved (i.e., the correlation between the independent variable and the dependent variable, r_{XY}, the correlation between the independent variable and the mediator, r_{MX}, and the correlation between the mediator and the dependent variable, r_{MY}). The large sample covariance matrix among these three correlations (Olkin & Siotani, 1976) is required for the standard error computation, making the formula quite cumbersome because the covariance formulas are complicated.

The other product of coefficient standard errors for $\hat{a}\hat{b}$ yields standard errors that are very close to those obtained from Equation 3.6. Simulation studies of the different standard errors suggest that the standard error formula in Equation 3.6 performs better than other formulas for the standard error. The product of coefficients for standardized variables suggested by Bobko and Rieck (1980) is also not better than the standard error formula in Equation 3.6.

Difference in Coefficients Tests for Mediation. A difference in coefficients test for mediation estimates the difference between the correlation between the independent variable and the dependent variable, r_{XY}, with the partial correlation between the independent and dependent variable corrected for the effect of the mediator, $r_{XY.M}$ (Olkin & Finn, 1995). The difference between the correlations is the mediated effect, and its standard error is found using the multivariate delta method. This method uses the covariance matrix among the three correlations, r_{XY}, r_{MX}, and r_{MY} in the standard error, making it cumbersome to compute. The requirement for a correlation to range from –1 to 1 can lead to failure to find true mediated effects in some cases (see Kenny http://users.rcn.com/dakenny/mediate.htm). As a result the difference between the raw and partial correlation is not recommended as a test of mediation.

3.14 Summary

This chapter presents a basic statistical framework that can be used to evaluate mediational models. Two estimators, $\hat{c} - \hat{c}'$ and $\hat{a}\hat{b}$, which are equivalent for most analyses, can be used to calculate the mediated effect. Several different formulas for the standard error of the mediated effect were presented, which led to negligibly different estimates for the water consumption example in this chapter. Additional approaches to testing mediation were also described, which may be appropriate in certain research situations. The remainder of this book elaborates this general framework, at least in part, to address violations of assumptions described in this chapter. It is important to remember that the statistical model is an abstraction of a verbal description. A verbal description of mediation is limited because it does not explicitly describe relations among variables in a way that they can be tested. The statistical model is also limited as it reduces verbal concepts to numerical relations and assumptions. Both approaches are incomplete. It is the researcher's task to interpret the results of the mediation analysis in the context of substantive and conceptual aspects of the mediation model studied.

Subsequent chapters expand upon the analysis presented here. In the next chapter, effect size measures and some statistical background for the single mediator model are described. Later chapters expand the model to categorical outcomes, multiple mediators, measurement models for mediators, multiple independent variables, and multiple dependent variables.

3.15 Exercises

3.1. Compute the standard error from Equation 3.6 and the ratio of the mediated effect estimate to its standard error for the following values:
   a. $\hat{a} = 0.2$, $s_{\hat{a}} = 0.1$, $\hat{b} = 0.4$, and $s_{\hat{b}} = 0.01$.
   b. $\hat{a} = 0.22$, $s_{\hat{a}} = 0.1$, $\hat{b} = 0.22$, and $s_{\hat{b}} = 0.1$.
   c. $\hat{a} = 0.2$, $s_{\hat{a}} = 0.2$, $\hat{b} = 0.4$, and $s_{\hat{b}} = 0.01$.
   d. $\hat{a} = 0.2$, $s_{\hat{a}} = 0.01$, $\hat{b} = 0.4$, and $s_{\hat{b}} = 0.4$.

e. How does the significance levels of the individual coefficients relate to the significance test of the mediated effect? Is it more important to have one of the paths highly significant or both paths about the same size?

3.2. Data from an evaluation of a program designed to increase healthy nutrition among high school football players are used to illustrate the estimation of mediated effects (Goldberg et al., 1996). In this example, the data are from 1,227 subjects measured immediately after about half received a program designed to improve nutrition behaviors. The dependent variable is a summary measure composed of six measures of healthy nutrition. The mediator is a three-item measure of the extent to which subjects felt that their peers were a source of information about nutrition. The program was designed to change peer norms regarding nutrition behavior, which was then hypothesized to improve nutrition behaviors. The regression estimates and standard errors (in parentheses) for the three models are presented below.

Equation 3.1: $Y = i_1 + cX + e_1$
$$\hat{Y} = 4.016 + 0.3552X$$
$$(0.0631)$$

Equation 3.2: $Y = i_2 + c'X + bM + e_2$
$$\hat{Y} = 3.258 + 0.1856X + 0.1711M$$
$$(.0642) \ (.0195)$$

Equation 3.3: $M = i_3 + aX + e_3$
$$\hat{M} = 4.423 + 0.9912X$$
$$(0.0896)$$

a. Compute the mediation effect using two methods.
b. Compute the standard error using Equations 3.6, 3.7, 3.8, 3.9, 3.10, 3.11, and 3.12. The mean square error for model 2 was 1.1289, and the variance of the independent variable was 0.2459. How much do the standard errors differ? Which formula is easiest to compute?
c. What is the 95% confidence interval for the mediated effect?
d. Evaluate each step in the causal steps approach to establishing mediation.
e. What is your conclusion about whether peers as an information source is a significant mediator of the program effect on nutrition behaviors?

3.3. Compare and contrast the causal step method to directly testing whether the ratio of the mediated effect to its standard error is larger than a certain z value.

3.4.   Evaluate each assumption for the water consumption example.

3.5.   Find a research article mentioned in the first three chapters of this book and summarize how mediation was tested.

3.6.   For the water consumption example, dichotomize X so that 67, 68, or 69, have X equal to 0 and X equals 1 for 70, 71, or 72. Conduct a mediation analysis for the binary X variable and make the same plots as in figures 3.3, 3.4, and 3.5. Indicate mediation coefficients, $\hat{a}$, $\hat{b}$, $\hat{c}$, $\hat{c}'$, $\hat{a}\hat{b}$, and $\hat{c} - \hat{c}'$ in the plot.

4

Single Mediator
Model Details

> Emmie: Mom, I'm not going back to school this year.
> Mom: Why not?
> Emmie: Because last year the teacher said three plus
>   seven made ten. Then he said five plus five
>   made ten. And then he said eight plus two
>   made ten.
> Mom: So?
> Emmie: So, I'm not going back till he makes up his
>   mind!
>
> **—Lisa Eisenberg & Katy Hall, 1994, p. 10**

4.1 Overview

The first two chapters defined mediating variables and described substantive applications of mediating variables. Chapter 3 introduced the single mediator model regression equations and outlined assumptions of the model. Chapter 4 provides technical details and advanced information about the single mediator model, including measures of effect size, expected variances and covariances among X, M, and Y, derivation of standard errors, and a Monte Carlo study investigating the statistical properties of mediated effect estimators.

4.2 Meaning of Effects in the Single Mediator Model

The estimate of the mediated effect ($\hat{a}\hat{b}$ or $\hat{c} - \hat{c}'$) is one meaningful statistic from mediation analysis. Remember that the value for the mediated effect in the single mediator model is the effect of the independent variable on the dependent variable that is indirect, through the mediating variable. The value of the mediated effect is more interpretable if the unit of measurement of the dependent variable involved is clear; for example, for the water consumption example in chapter 3, the unit was deciliters of water. Confidence limits provide more information about a mediated effect because a range of possible values for the mediated effect are considered rather than one single value (Krantz, 1999; Kline, 2004).

Significance tests aid in the evaluation of whether an observed effect is larger than expected by chance alone. A large critical value (estimate divided by the standard error of the estimate) for a significance test suggests that the observed effect is not consistent with chance and is likely to be a real effect. The conclusion from a significance test depends on sample size, however, where very small effects can be highly statistically significant if sample size is large enough and very large effects may be nonsignificant for a small sample size. As described by many researchers (Cohen, 1988; Rosnow & Rosenthal, 1989), significance tests do not provide good measures of the size or the meaningfulness of an effect.

Measures of effect size provide an indication of the size and meaningfulness of an effect that does not depend on sample size. The effect size can be the same across studies with different conclusions regarding tests of significance. The importance of effect size measures in psychology and other fields has been emphasized by several researchers (Cohen, 1988; Rosnow & Rosenthal, 1989; Wilkinson et al., 1999). Although alternative effect size measures have been proposed for mediated effects (Taborga, MacKinnon, & Krull, 1999), the ideal effect size measure for mediation and the statistical properties of the potential effect size estimators are not yet resolved. The measures described here provide a survey of current measures to be evaluated in future studies.

4.3 Effect Size Measures of Individual Paths in the Mediated Effect: Partial Correlation

Effect size measures can be specified for each path in the two-path mediated effect, the $\hat{a}$ path from the independent variable to the mediator and the $\hat{b}$ path from the mediator to the dependent variable. One of the most widely used measures of effect size is the correlation coefficient. For the regression model with one predictor, the correlation between the independent and dependent variables is the correlation effect size measure. For example, the correlation between the independent variable and the mediating variable is the correlation effect size measure for the relation between the independent variable and the mediator. Cohen (1988) provided guidelines for small, medium, and large effects in social sciences corresponding to correlations of 0.1, 0.3, and 0.5, respectively. For the model that includes both the mediator and the independent variable predicting the dependent variable, there are two regression coefficients and as a result, two partial correlations. The partial correlation effect size measure is the correlation between one predictor and the dependent variable with the relation of the other predictor and the dependent variable removed. Of primary interest for the mediated effect is the correlation between the mediating variable and the dependent variable adjusted for the correlation between the independent variable and the dependent variable, thus providing a partial correlation for the $\hat{b}$ coefficient. Equations 4.1 and 4.2 show the formulas for the partial correlations for $\hat{c}'$, $r_{YX.M}$ (correlation between X and Y partialled for M) and $\hat{b}$, $r_{YM.X}$ (correlation between Y and M, partialled for X), respectively. For the water consumption example, the raw correlations among X, M, and Y were $r_{XY} = 0.361$, $r_{MY} = 0.490$, and $r_{XM} = 0.371$. The correlation for the $\hat{a}$ coefficient was 0.371, and the partial correlation for the $\hat{b}$ coefficient was 0.411, corresponding to effects between medium and large in the social sciences. The correlation for the total effect $\hat{c}$ was 0.361 and the partial correlation for $\hat{c}'$ was 0.208. Because guidelines for the effect size of correlations in the social sciences are available, simulation studies have often used the correlation effect size measures (MacKinnon, Lockwood, Hoffman, West, & Sheets, 2002) in the generation of data. In this way, the statistical power to detect small, medium, and large effects in the social sciences can be studied in statistical simulations, as will be described in section 4.18:

$$r_{YX.M} = \frac{r_{XY} - r_{MY}r_{XM}}{\sqrt{(1 - r_{MY}^2)(1 - r_{XM}^2)}} \qquad (4.1)$$

$$r_{YM.X} = \frac{r_{MY} - r_{XY}r_{XM}}{\sqrt{(1 - r_{XY}^2)(1 - r_{XM}^2)}} \qquad (4.2)$$

4.4 Effect Size Measures of Individual Paths in the Mediated Effect: Standardized Regression Coefficients

Another type of effect size measure for individual coefficients is the standardized regression coefficient. The standardized regression coefficient is a rescaled regression coefficient that represents the change in the dependent variable for a 1 standard deviation change in the independent variable. A standardized $\hat{a}$ coefficient represents the change in the mediating variable for a 1 standard deviation change in the independent variable. For the $\hat{b}$ coefficient, the standardized regression coefficient represents the change in the dependent variable for a 1 standard deviation change in the mediating variable adjusted for the X variable in the model. The standardized regression coefficients are commonly presented in covariance structure model results. For a mediation example, Hansen and McNeal (1997) reported a standardized coefficient from exposure to a Drug Abuse and Resistance Education (DARE) program to commitment to avoid drugs of .160 and a standardized coefficient for the relation between commitment to avoid drugs and tobacco use of −0.134. Equations 4.3 and 4.4 show the formulas for the $\hat{c}'$ and $\hat{b}$ regression coefficients in terms of correlations and standard deviations of X, M, and Y. Note that the right side of each equation includes the ratio of the standard deviation of the variables. For standardized coefficients, these variances are equal to 1 (i.e., $s_Y = s_X = 1$). Also note the equations to the left of (s_Y/s_X) in Equation 4.3 and (s_Y/s_M) in Equation 4.4 are equal to the regression coefficients $\hat{c}_s'$ and $\hat{b}_s$, for standardized variables, respectively. For the water consumption example, the standardized regression coefficient for $\hat{a}_s$ was 0.371 and the standardized regression coefficient for $\hat{b}_s$ was 0.413. The standardized regression coefficients were 0.361 for $\hat{c}_s$ and 0.208 for $\hat{c}_s'$:

$$\hat{c}_s' = \frac{r_{XY} - r_{XM}r_{YM}}{1 - r_{XM}^2}\left(\frac{s_Y}{s_X}\right) \tag{4.3}$$

$$\hat{b}_s = \frac{r_{MY} - r_{XM}r_{XY}}{1 - r_{XM}^2}\left(\frac{s_Y}{s_M}\right) \tag{4.4}$$

4.5 Effect Size Measures for the Entire Mediated Effect

Other measures of effect size for mediation models focus on a single measure of the mediated effect, $\hat{a}\hat{b}$, as a way to gauge the size of the effect (Taborga, 2000). There are three major types of effect size measures for the overall mediated effect: (a) proportion and ratio measures, (b) R-squared measures, and (c) standardized effect measures. These effect size measures differ in meaning and statistical properties.

4.6 Ratio and Proportion Mediated Effect Measures

One of the most common mediation effect size measures is the proportion of the total effect that is mediated, $\hat{a}\hat{b}/\hat{c}$, which is algebraically equivalent to $1 - \hat{c}'/\hat{c}$ and $\hat{a}\hat{b}/(\hat{c}' + \hat{a}\hat{b})$ in the ordinary least squares regression model. Alwin and Hauser (1975) suggested this measure as a way to gauge the size of mediated effects. A researcher could state that a mediated effect explains about 30% of the total effect of an independent variable on a dependent variable. For the water consumption example, the proportion mediated was 42% (0.1527/0.3604 = 0.42). MacKinnon et al. (1991) found that norms among friends explained about 37% of a school-based prevention effect on tobacco use. Wolchik et al. (1993) found that 43% of the effect of a children of divorce program on child mental health was mediated by changes in the mother–child relationship.

In some models, the mediated effect and the direct effect have opposite signs, complicating the interpretation of the mediated effect because the proportion value can be greater than 1 or even negative. In this case, the total effect may be very close to zero, and the proportion mediated can then be very large. These models are inconsistent mediation models because there are both positive and negative effects on the dependent variable (MacKinnon, Krull, & Lockwood, 2000). One effect size option in these scenarios, suggested by Alwin and Hauser (1975), is to take the absolute values of the quantities before computing the proportion mediated, leading to a different interpretation of the proportion mediated as the proportion of the absolute total effect that is mediated. For the water consumption example, if the $\hat{c}'$ coefficient was actually -0.2076, then the proportion mediated would equal $0.1527/(-0.2076 + 0.1527)$, which equals -2.78. Taking absolute values would yield a proportion mediated equal to 0.42.

A related measure is the ratio of the mediated effect to the direct effect, $\hat{a}\hat{b}/\hat{c}'$, which equals 0.736 ($0.1527/0.2076$) for the water consumption example. Sobel (1982) suggested that this measure may be useful to compare direct and indirect effects. With this measure, a researcher could state that the mediated effect is twice as large as the direct effect or that the mediated effect is one-third as large as the direct effect. For example, Leigh (1983) reported that the mediated effect of schooling to healthy habits to health was 18 times larger than the direct effect of schooling on health. Ratio measures may also be useful for comparing mediated effects. In a study of guinea pigs, Wright (1934) investigated whether size of litter affects birth weight through a shorter gestational period or by competition for growth among developing fetuses. He found evidence that the mediated effect through growth was three times larger than the mediated effect through length of the gestation period.

Buyse and Molenberghs (1998) suggest a ratio measure $\hat{c}/\hat{a}$ (which is equal to $(\hat{c}' + \hat{a}\hat{b})/\hat{a}$ in ordinary least squares regression) that is useful for identifying surrogate (mediator) endpoints. The ratio of the effect of X and Y, $\hat{c}$, to the effect of X on M, $\hat{a}$, is expected to be 1, as a valid surrogate should have the same relation with an independent variable as the ultimate outcome variable. An additional requirement for this framework is that the correlation between the mediator and the ultimate outcome should be close to 1. These two measures, $\hat{c}/\hat{a}$ and r_{MY}, could be used to judge the effect size of a mediated effect. For the water consumption data, $\hat{c}/\hat{a}$ equals 0.613 ($0.2076/0.3386$) and r_{MY} equals 0.361. So in terms of a surrogate effect, the effect of X on M is about 60% of the size of the effect of X on Y, and X and M have about 10% shared variance. No guidelines are yet available to judge whether these relations are large or small.

4.7 R-Squared Measures

There are several possible *R*-squared measures for the mediated effect. These measures partition the observed amount of variance in the dependent variable into parts; the part that is explained by the direct effect, the part that is not explained, and the part that is explained by the mediated effect. Equation 4.5 represents an *R*-squared measure designed to localize the amount of variance in Y that is explained by M specific to the mediated effect. The *R*-squared measure is obtained by identifying the variance in Y explained by both M and X but not by X alone or M alone. Equation 4.6 represents a measure that corresponds to the squared correlation between X and M times the squared partial correlation between M and Y partialled for the effect of X. Equation 4.7 represents a proportion measure such that the product of *R*-squared values in Equation 4.6 is divided by the total amount of variance in Y explained by both M and X. Note that the notation is the same as that used earlier with the difference that capital R is used for the effect size measures and $R^2_{Y,MX}$ is the amount of variance explained in Y by X and M. All three of these measures require more development, but it appears that they have minimal bias even at relatively small sample sizes for the model studied by Taborga (2000) and Taborga et al. (1999). For the water consumption example, values of (0.2401 − (0.2772 − 0.1303)) = 0.0932, (0.1376)(0.1689) = 0.0232, and ((0.1376)(0.1689))/(0.2772) = 0.0838 were obtained for Equations 4.5, 4.6, and 4.7, respectively. Applying Equation 4.5 to the water consumption example suggests that about 9% of the variance in Y is explained by X and M together:

$$R^2_{Y.\text{Mediated}} = r^2_{YM} - (R^2_{Y,MX} - r^2_{YX}) \tag{4.5}$$

$$R^2_{Y.\text{Mediated}} = (r^2_{MX})(r^2_{YM.X}) \tag{4.6}$$

$$R^2_{\text{Proportion}} = ((r^2_{MX})(r^2_{YM.X}))/(R^2_{Y,MX}) \tag{4.7}$$

4.8 Standardized Effect

Some alternative measures of effect size in mediation models include the product of standardized coefficients and *d* effect size measures suggested by Cohen (1988) and others for analysis of variance, that reflect the effect in standardized units. One possible *d* effect size measure is the ratio of the mediated effect to the standard deviation of the Y variable, as shown in Equation 4.8. The measure indicates the size of $\hat{a}\hat{b}$ in terms of standard deviation units in Y. For the water consumption example, the mediated effect is associated with a change of 0.1343 (0.1527/1.137) standard deviation units in Y:

$$\text{Standardized}_{\hat{a}\hat{b}} = \hat{a}\hat{b}/s_Y \tag{4.8}$$

4.9 Summary of Effect Size Measures

Simulation studies of the effect size measures indicate that correlation and standardized coefficient measures have low bias even at small sample sizes. The proportion mediated and the ratio measures require much larger sample sizes. In general, a sample size of 500 is needed for the proportion measure to stabilize, but lower values are required if the direct effect is larger (MacKinnon, Warsi, & Dwyer, 1995). Smaller sample sizes are also adequate if all estimates are statistically significant. The results for the ratio measure are less encouraging with sample sizes of at least 1,000 required for stable findings for the set of sample sizes studied. The R-squared measures generally had low bias for a sample size of at least 50. These effect size measures have been primarily studied with a single mediator model that has consistent effects. It is unclear how accurate they will be in more complicated models, especially inconsistent mediation models.

There are also some conceptual difficulties with the interpretation of some effect size measures. The ratio and proportion can be large when the total effect is very small. That is, both the mediated effect and the total effect can be very small, yet the proportion or ratio may be large. One way to reduce this possibility is to test effects for statistical significance before computing these values. The R-squared measures can be very small, suggesting that only a tiny percentage of variance in the dependent variable is explained by the mediated effect. Even small effects can be important (Abelson, 1985; Rosnow & Rosenthal, 1989), and small effects may be more common for mediated effects because they are products of coefficients, which will be smaller than the individual coefficients (if the coefficients are less than 1).

The standardized effect size measure for the mediated effect is new but is promising in simulation studies. Other potential measures of effect size include the percentage of persons with patterns of responses consistent with mediation. It may also be useful to test contrasts between effects in a mediation model such as testing whether the mediated effect is significantly different than the direct effect (see Equation 4.32 for the variance of this difference). Meta-analysis effect sizes based on the significance levels of mediation coefficients may also be useful as mediation effect size measures. Another important tool for the interpretation of these effect size measures is the creation of confidence limits for the effects as described in chapter 3. Methods to determine the standard error of the mediated effect and related quantities are described later in this chapter. Methods to calculate more accurate confidence limits than those described in chapter 3 are also described later in this chapter.

4.10 *Derived Variances and Covariance for the Single Mediator Model*

Given assumptions, it is possible to derive the population or true variances and covariances among X, M, and Y for the single mediator model. These variances and covariances are useful for the investigation of several statistical aspects of mediation analysis, as will be done later in this chapter. The derivation is accomplished using covariance algebra based on Equations 3.2 and 3.3 and the assumption of uncorrelated error terms across equations, normally distributed variables, and a linear system of relations among variables (McDonald, 1997). With the true covariance matrix, it is then possible to determine the true values of many quantities in mediation analysis on the basis of the values of the parameters, a, b, and c', and values of e_2 and e_3 error terms in Equations 3.2 and 3.3. This expected covariance matrix can also be used to determine the true values of several mediation analysis quantities, such as the variance of the mediated effect and true effect sizes described earlier in this chapter. These true values can then be used in statistical simulation studies to evaluate the accuracy of estimators of mediation quantities in a sample as a function of sample size, population parameter values, and violations of mediation model assumptions.

To illustrate the derivation of covariances among X, M, and Y, three covariances are derived in detail as follows. For example, the covariance of X and Y, Cov[X,Y], is defined as $E[(X - E(X))(Y - E(Y))]$ and the variance, Cov[X,X], is defined as $E[(X - E(X))^2]$, where E represents the expectation of the quantity or the value of the quantity that is most likely to occur. There are several rules of covariance algebra that will be applied in the derivations assuming that c is a constant: $Cov[c,X] = 0$, $Cov[cX,M] = c\ Cov[X,M]$, and $Cov[X + M,Y] = Cov[X,Y] + Cov[M,Y]$. For example, the covariance between X and M (Cov[X,M]) is expanded to include the equations for X and M as shown below. The covariance between X and aX is equal to $a\sigma_X^2$. The covariance between X and e_3 is zero based on the assumption of uncorrelated error terms yielding the expected covariance between X and M in Equation 4.9:

$$Cov[X,M] = Cov(X, aX + e_3)$$

$$Cov[X,M] = Cov(X, aX) + Cov(X, e_3)$$

$$Cov[X,M] = a\sigma_X^2 + 0 \tag{4.9}$$

The covariance between X and Y, Cov[X,Y] is derived by first writing the equations for X and Y, forming the product of these equations, and then reducing terms such as Cov[X,bM] to b Cov(X,M), which is equal to b times the covariance of X and M from Equation 4.9 ($a\sigma_X^2$), which is equal to $b\ a\sigma_X^2$. The terms Cov(X,c'X) and Cov(X,e_2) are reduced in a similar manner:

$$Cov[X,Y] = Cov(X,bM + c'X + e_2)$$

$$Cov[X,Y] = Cov(X,bM) + Cov(X,c'X) + Cov(X,e_2)$$

$$Cov[X,Y] = b\ Cov(X,M) + c'\ Cov(X,X) + 0$$

$$Cov[X,Y] = b\ a\sigma_X^2 + c'\sigma_X^2 \tag{4.10}$$

Using the same methods gives the covariance between M and Y (Cov[M,Y]):

$Cov[M,Y] = Cov(aX + e_3,\ bM + c'X + e_2)$

$Cov[M,Y] = Cov(aX,bM) + Cov(aX,c'X) + Cov(aX,e_2) + Cov(e_3,bM) + Cov(e_3,c'X) + Cov(e_3,e_2)$

$Cov[M,Y] = abCov(X,M) + ac'\ Cov(X,X) + 0 + b\ Cov(e_3,M) + 0 + 0$

$Cov[M,Y] = aba\sigma_X^2 + ac'\sigma_X^2 + 0 + b\ Cov(e_3,\ aX + e_3) + 0 + 0$

$Cov[M,Y] = a^2b\sigma_X^2 + ac'\sigma_X^2 + b\sigma_{e_3}^2 \tag{4.11}$

The covariances (called variances if it is covariance of a variable with itself) of X, M, and Y are shown in Equations 4.12, 4.13, and 4.14, respectively:

$$Cov[X,X] = Var[X] = \sigma_X^2 \tag{4.12}$$

$$Cov[M,M] = Var[M] = a^2\,\sigma_X^2 + \sigma_{e_3}^2 \tag{4.13}$$

$$Cov[Y,Y] = Var[Y] = b^2\,(a^2\sigma_X^2 + \sigma_{e_3}^2) + 2bc'a\sigma_X^2 + c'^2\sigma_X^2 + \sigma_{e_2}^2 \tag{4.14}$$

The values of these covariances can be represented as the covariance matrix shown in Equation 4.15.

$$\begin{array}{c}
 \quad \underline{X} \qquad\qquad\qquad \underline{M} \\[4pt]
\begin{array}{c} X \\ M \\ Y \end{array}
\left[\begin{array}{cc}
\sigma_X^2 & \\
a\sigma_X^2 & a^2\sigma_X^2 + \sigma_{e_3}^2 \\
ba\sigma_X^2 + c'\sigma_x^2 & a^2b\sigma_X^2 + ac'\sigma_X^2 + b\sigma_{e_3}^2
\end{array}\right]
\end{array}$$

$$\underline{Y}$$

$$Y[b^2(a^2\sigma_X^2 + \sigma_{e_3}^2) + 2bc'a\sigma_X^2 + c'^2\sigma_X^2 + \sigma_{e_2}^2] \qquad (4.15)$$

As an example of how these covariances are used, consider the first step in the Baron and Kenny (1986) causal steps test of mediation, which requires that there is a statistically significant relation between X and Y for mediation to be present; that is, $r_{XY} = \text{Cov}[X,Y]/(\text{Var}[X]^{\frac{1}{2}}\,\text{Var}[Y]^{\frac{1}{2}})$. The expected values of Cov[X,Y], Var[X], and Var[Y] shown earlier are used to compute the population value of this correlation. Assuming that 2% of the variance in M explained by X for a and 13% of the variance in Y explained by M adjusted for X for b (based on Cohen's guidelines) yields a true value of this correlation of 0.0474, it would require at least 3,488 participants to have 0.8 power to detect this correlation and pass the first step of this approach. This demonstrates why the causal steps test has low power to detect effects. The expected correlations among X, M, and Y can be obtained in the same manner by dividing the covariance between the two variables by the standard deviation of each variable. These values can then be used to compute the expected effect size measures to get population correlations and partial correlations for example.

4.11 Single Mediator Model Coefficients and Standard Errors

The variances and covariances derived in section 4.10 can be used to calculate population parameters and the true variance of estimates. The population a coefficient is given in Equation 4.16. Sample estimates of Cov[X,M] and Var[X] are used to estimate $\hat{a}$.

$$a = \frac{\text{Cov}[X,M]}{\text{Var}[X]} \qquad (4.16)$$

The theoretical or true variance of the estimator of $\hat{a}$, $\sigma_{\hat{a}T}^2$ (sample values are used for the variance of the estimate, $s_{\hat{a}}^2$) is shown in Equation 4.17.

$$\sigma_{\hat{a}T}^2 = \frac{\sigma_{e_3}^2}{(N-1)\text{Var}[X]} \qquad (4.17)$$

where $\sigma^2_{e_3}$ is the population variance of the errors in the equation where X predicts M. An estimator of the population residual variance, σ^2_{e}, is shown in Equation 4.18, where p is the number of X variables, which is equal to 1 for the one predictor case here. For the single predictor case, $\Sigma^2_{e_i}$ is the sum of the squared difference between the predicted and observed M, that is, the sum of the squared residual score for each subject, divided by $N - 2$. The same formulas are used to determine the population value c and the variance of the estimator of $\hat{c}$:

$$\hat{\sigma}^2_e = \frac{\Sigma^2_{e_i}}{N - p - 1} \tag{4.18}$$

In Equation 3.2, where both X and M are used to predict Y, the population c' and b coefficients are shown in Equations 4.19 and 4.20, respectively. Sample values of the variances and covariances are used to calculate $\hat{c}'$ and $\hat{b}$.

$$c' = \frac{Var[M]Cov[XY] - Cov[XM]Cov[MY]}{Var[X]Var[M] - Cov[XM]^2} \tag{4.19}$$

$$b = \frac{Var[X]Cov[MY] - Cov[XM]Cov[XY]}{Var[X]Var[M] - Cov[XM]^2} \tag{4.20}$$

The true variances (sample values are used to estimate $s^2_{\hat{c}}$ and $s^2_{\hat{b}}$) of estimators of $\hat{c}'$ and $\hat{b}$ are equal to 4.21 and 4.22, respectively;

$$\sigma^2_{\hat{c}'T} = \frac{\sigma^2_{e2}}{N - 1} \frac{\dfrac{1}{Var[X]}}{1 - r^2_{XM}} \tag{4.21}$$

$$\sigma^2_{\hat{b}T} = \frac{\sigma^2_{e2}}{N - 1} \frac{\dfrac{1}{Var[M]}}{1 - r^2_{XM}} \tag{4.22}$$

where N is the number of observations and $\sigma_{e2}{}^2$ is estimated by the sum of the squared difference between the observed and predicted Y score for each subject divided by $N - 3$, analogous to Equation 4.18 but for two predictors, X and M.

4.12 True Variance of $\hat{a}\hat{b}$

The population value of ab is the product of Equations 4.16 and 4.20 and the sample value $\hat{a}\hat{b}$ is obtained using sample values of variances and covariances. The true variance of the estimator of $\hat{a}\hat{b}$ can be obtained by substituting the population values of $\sigma_{e_2}^2$, $\sigma_{e_3}^2$, Var[X], and Var[M] into 4.17 and 4.22 and using the values in Equations for the standard error of $\hat{a}\hat{b}$ described in chapter 3. As an example, the theoretical or true variance of the estimator $\hat{a}\hat{b}$ based on Equation 3.9 is shown in Equation 4.23, with population values a and b and true variance of the estimators, $\sigma_{\hat{a}T}^2$ and $\sigma_{\hat{b}T}^2$ instead of sample estimates.

$$\sigma_{\hat{a}\hat{b}T}^2 = a^2\sigma_{\hat{b}T}^2 + b^2\sigma_{\hat{b}T}^2 + \sigma_{\hat{a}T}^2\sigma_{\hat{b}T}^2 \qquad (4.23)$$

The population values a, b, c', σ_x^2, $\sigma_{e_2}^2$, and $\sigma_{e_3}^2$ can be used to generate sample data to investigate statistical mediation analysis. Because population or true quantities are known, the extent to which mediation tests give the right answer can be evaluated in a Monte Carlo study as described in section 4.18. For example, the square root of Equation 4.23 provides a true or theoretical standard error to compare with the standard error of $\hat{a}\hat{b}$ from sample estimates. Using $N - p - 1$ instead of $N - 1$ in Equations 4.17, 4.21, and 4.22 yields more accurate true values.

4.13 Covariance Among Parameter Estimates

Each of the coefficients in the single mediator model, $\hat{a}$, $\hat{b}$, $\hat{c}$, and $\hat{c}'$, has a variance that is the squared value of the standard error, as shown in the last section. There are also covariances among these coefficients. The covariances among the coefficients in the three mediation regression equations are used to calculate the standard error of several useful quantities for mediation analysis. The covariance matrix has four rows and four columns corresponding to the four coefficients in the mediation regression equations, $\hat{a}$, $\hat{b}$, $\hat{c}$, and $\hat{c}'$. For the covariance between $\hat{b}$ and $\hat{c}'$, the covariance is computed as part of the analysis of Equation 3.2. The covariance between $\hat{b}$ and $\hat{c}'$ in Equation 3.2 is equal to the negative of the correlation between X and M times the standard error of $\hat{b}$ and the standard error of $\hat{c}'$ (Hanushek & Jackson, 1977). The covariances among other estimates in the mediation equations, $\hat{a}$, $\hat{b}$, $\hat{c}$, and $\hat{c}'$, are complicated because some coefficients are from separate regression equations, including the case where the coefficient is for the same X variable in different equations, such as $\hat{c}$ and $\hat{c}'$ and $\hat{a}$ and $\hat{c}$. The covariance of coefficients across different linear regression equations has been examined in several articles (Allison, 1995a; Clogg, Petkova, & Cheng, 1995; Tofighi, MacKinnon, & Yoon, 2006).

Two covariances between coefficients are especially important for mediation, the covariance between $\hat{a}$ and $\hat{b}$, and the covariance between $\hat{c}$ and $\hat{c}'$. The coefficients $\hat{a}$ and $\hat{b}$ are independent in the single mediator model (MacKinnon et al., 1995; Sobel, 1982) so the covariance between a and b is zero (see exercise problem 4.10 for an approach to deriving this covariance). The covariance between $\hat{c}$ and $\hat{c}'$ is complicated but has been examined by several researchers (Clogg et al., 1992; Freedman & Schatzkin, 1992; McGuigan & Langholz, 1988). McGuigan and Langholz (1988) and Clogg et al. (1995) derived the covariance between $\hat{c}$ and $\hat{c}'$ shown in Equation 4.24, where $\hat{\sigma}_{e_2}^2$ is the residual mean square from Equation 3.2.

$$s_{\hat{c}\hat{c}'} = \frac{\hat{\sigma}_{e_2}^2}{(N(\text{Var}(X)))} \quad (4.24)$$

The covariance between $\hat{a}$ and $\hat{c}'$ is zero for the single mediator model (MacKinnon et al., 1995; see exercise 4.10). The covariance between $\hat{a}$ and $\hat{c}$ ($\hat{b}\,\text{Var}(\hat{a})$) is discussed in Buyse and Molenberghs (1998).

An important use of the covariance matrix among the regression coefficients is the derivation of the standard errors of functions of mediation regression coefficients such as the proportion mediated. For the linear regression models described in chapter 3 and this chapter, the covariance of coefficients across equations must be computed by hand outside the software program. For covariance structure analysis programs discussed in chapter 6, the covariances among all coefficients in a model are calculated as part of the statistical analysis and are available in the computer printout. The next section describes a general method to derive the variance of any function, given the covariance matrix among coefficients in the function and partial derivatives of the function.

4.14 Variance of Functions of Parameters

Many important quantities in mediation analysis require finding the variance of functions of regression coefficients. The delta method is a general method to find the variance of a function of random variables such as regression coefficients (see Bishop, Fienberg, & Holland, 1975, chapter 14, and Rao, 1973, for more details). The delta method is most clearly described for the variance of a function of a variable X as shown in Equation 4.25. For the single delta method, the variance of a function of one random variable is equal to the square of its first derivative times the variance of the original variable. For example, the variance of 5X is equal to the variance of X times the square of the first derivative of 5X with respect to X, $(\partial f/\partial X)^2 = (5)^2$, yielding the result that the variance of 5X is equal to 25 times the variance of X.

$$\text{Var(function)} = (\partial f/\partial X)^2\,(\text{Var}(X)) \quad (4.25)$$

The multivariate delta method is used to find the variance of functions of more than one random variable by pre- and post-multiplying the covariance matrix among the parameter estimates, V, by a vector of first partial derivatives, D, as shown in Equation 4.26. The covariance matrix V includes the covariances among regression parameter estimates such as the covariance between $\hat{c}$ and $\hat{c}'$. For the variance of the product of the $\hat{a}$ and $\hat{b}$, $\hat{a}\hat{b}$, the partial derivative with respect to $\hat{a}$ is $\partial f/\partial \hat{a} = \hat{b}$, and the partial derivative with respect to $\hat{b}$ is $\partial f/\partial \hat{b} = \hat{a}$, to form the 1×2 vector of partial derivatives, $\mathbf{D}' = [\hat{b} \ \hat{a}]$. The covariance matrix among $\hat{a}$ and $\hat{b}$ has off-diagonal values of 0 because $\hat{a}$ and $\hat{b}$ are uncorrelated. The diagonal of the covariance matrix has the squared values of the standard errors of $\hat{a}$ and $\hat{b}$. Applying formula 4.26 yields the multivariate delta solution for the variance of $\hat{a}\hat{b}$ in Equation 4.27 as derived by Sobel (1982):

$$\text{Var(function)} = \mathbf{D}' \, \mathbf{V} \, \mathbf{D} \qquad (4.26)$$

$$s_{\hat{a}\hat{b}}^2 = \hat{a}^2 s_{\hat{b}}^2 + \hat{b}^2 s_{\hat{a}}^2 \qquad (4.27)$$

If there is a nonzero covariance between $\hat{a}$ and $\hat{b}$ corresponding to nonzero off-diagonal elements in the $\mathbf{V}$ matrix, then $2\hat{a}\hat{b} \, \text{Cov}(\hat{a},\hat{b})$ must be added to the covariance formula in Equation 4.27. In some models, such as latent variable mediation models, the covariance between $\hat{a}$ and $\hat{b}$ is nonzero, so this extra term, $2\hat{a}\hat{b} \, \text{Cov}(\hat{a},\hat{b})$, must be included in the formula.

Applying the multivariate delta method for the difference in regression coefficients $\hat{c} - \hat{c}'$, with partial derivatives of $\partial f/\partial \hat{c} = 1$ and $\partial f/\partial \hat{c}' = -1$ and the covariance between $\hat{c}$ and $\hat{c}'$, gives the variance formula in Equation 3.8. The quantity $s_{\hat{c}\hat{c}'}$ is the covariance between $\hat{c}$ and $\hat{c}'$ in Equation 4.28:

$$s_{\hat{c}-\hat{c}'}^2 = s_{\hat{c}}^2 + s_{\hat{c}'}^2 - 2s_{\hat{c}\hat{c}'} \qquad (4.28)$$

The multivariate delta method can also be used to find the variance of other functions that are useful for mediation analysis. As these functions become more complicated, the derivation of partial derivatives can be more complicated because of the need to apply several rules for differentiation such as the product and quotient rules. Detailed information on finding these partial derivatives can be obtained in any calculus textbook such as Stewart (1999, chapter 14). Without showing the details of finding the partial derivatives, the variance of the ratio effect size measure, $\hat{a}\hat{b}/\hat{c}'$, has partial derivatives equal to $\partial f/\partial \hat{a} = \hat{b}/\hat{c}'$, $\partial f/\partial \hat{b} = \hat{a}/\hat{c}'$, and $\partial f/\partial \hat{c}' = -\hat{a}\hat{b}/\hat{c}'^2$. The 3 by 3 covariance matrix now includes the covariances among $\hat{a}$, $\hat{b}$, and $\hat{c}'$ with the squared standard errors of each coefficient along the diagonal of the matrix and a nonzero covariance between $\hat{b}$ and $\hat{c}'$. Applying Equation 4.26 yields the variance of $\hat{a}\hat{b}/\hat{c}'$, equal to Equation 4.29. The standard error is the square root of the variance:

$$s_{\hat{a}\hat{b}/\hat{c}'}^2 = (\hat{b}/\hat{c}')^2 s_{\hat{a}}^2 + (\hat{a}/\hat{c}')^2 s_{\hat{b}}^2 + 2 \, (\hat{a}/\hat{c}')(-\hat{a}\hat{b}/\hat{c}'^2)s_{\hat{c}'\hat{b}} + (-\hat{a}\hat{b}/\hat{c}'^2)^2 s_{\hat{c}'}^2 \qquad (4.29)$$

The variance of $\hat{a}\hat{b}/(\hat{a}\hat{b} + \hat{c}')$, has a variance equal to Equation 4.30:

$$
\begin{aligned}
s^2_{\hat{a}\hat{b}/(\hat{c}'+\hat{a}\hat{b})} = {} & ((\hat{b}\hat{c}')/(\hat{c}' + \hat{a}\hat{b})^2)^2 s^2_{\hat{a}} + ((\hat{a}\hat{c}')/(\hat{c}' + \hat{a}\hat{b})^2)^2 s^2_{\hat{b}} \\
& + 2((-\hat{a}\hat{b})/(\hat{c}' + \hat{a}\hat{b})^2)((\hat{a}\hat{c}')/(\hat{c}' + \hat{a}\hat{b})^2) s_{\hat{c}'\hat{b}} \\
& + ((-\hat{a}\hat{b})/(\hat{c}' + \hat{a}\hat{b})^2)^2 s^2_{\hat{c}'}
\end{aligned}
\tag{4.30}
$$

The variance of $(\hat{c}' + \hat{a}\hat{b})/\hat{a}$, has a variance equal to Equation 4.31:

$$
s^2_{(\hat{c}'+\hat{a}\hat{b})/(\hat{a})} = (-\hat{c}'/\hat{a}^2)^2 s^2_{\hat{a}} + (1)^2 s^2_{\hat{b}} + 2(1)(1/\hat{a}) s_{\hat{c}'\hat{b}} + (1/\hat{a})^2 s^2_{\hat{c}'}
\tag{4.31}
$$

The variance of contrasts among effects in a mediation model may also be derived. The contrasts are comparable because they are in the same metric as the dependent variable (MacKinnon, 2000). For example, the variance of the difference between the mediated effect and the direct effect, $\hat{a}\hat{b} - \hat{c}'$, has a variance equal to Equation 4.32.

$$
s^2_{(\hat{a}\hat{b}-\hat{c}')} = \hat{b}^2 s^2_{\hat{a}} + \hat{a}^2 s^2_{\hat{b}} + s^2_{\hat{c}'} - 2\hat{a}\hat{c}s_{\hat{c}'\,\hat{b}}
\tag{4.32}
$$

To illustrate the calculation of these standard errors, the formula for the difference between the mediated effect and the direct effect for the water consumption example is shown in the following. The difference $\hat{a}\hat{b} - \hat{c}' = 0.1527 - 0.2076 = -0.0549$ and the standard error of the difference is equal to 0.1494 substituting sample estimates into Equation 4.32.

$$
s^2_{(\hat{a}\hat{b}-\hat{c}')} = 0.4510^2\,0.1224^2 + 0.3386^2\,.1460^2 + 0.1333^2 - 2(0.3386)(0.2076)(0.0066)
$$

The multivariate delta method in this section was described for the case of functions of regression coefficients but is also applicable to functions of correlation coefficients such as the difference between the raw correlation between X and Y and the correlation between X and Y partialled for the mediator (see MacKinnon, Lockwood, et al., 2002, for a simulation study of this measure). Similarly, the variance of the R-squared measures described earlier in this chapter can be derived using the multivariate delta method. The partial derivatives are obtained in the same manner for functions of correlation coefficients as for functions of regression coefficients using Equation 4.26. The application of the multivariate delta method for functions of correlations requires the specification of the covariance matrix among correlation coefficients. The variance of correlation coefficients and the covariances among correlations were derived by Olkin and Siotani (1976). The covariance matrix among correlations in the single mediator model are given in Appendix A of MacKinnon, Lockwood, et al. (2002). The standard error of any function of correlations can be obtained using this method, although the accuracy of these methods appears to depend on sample size (MacKinnon et al., 2002).

Standard errors based on the multivariate delta are generally based on large sample theory and are best checked in a statistical simulation. The standard error for the mediated effect is generally accurate at sample sizes as low as 25. As discussed earlier, the standard errors for the proportion mediated and ratio of the mediated to direct effect are much less stable and require at least 500 or 1000 sample size, respectively.

4.15 Confidence Limits Based on the Distribution of the Product

The application of the standard error of $\hat{a}\hat{b}$ in chapter 3 assumes that the product of $\hat{a}$ and $\hat{b}$, $\hat{a}\hat{b}$, has a normal distribution. In fact, the distribution of the product of two random variables does not have a normal distribution in all situations, and information regarding the distribution of the product of two random variables has been shown to provide more accurate confidence limits and statistical tests (MacKinnon, Lockwood, & Williams, 2004). The method based on the distribution of the product is described here as it will be used elsewhere in this book. A second method for improving confidence limits and statistical tests based on resampling methods is described in chapter 12.

Although the variance and standard error estimates of the mediated effect may be unbiased at small sample sizes, there is evidence that confidence limits based on these estimates do not always perform well. Three simulation studies (MacKinnon et al., 1995; MacKinnon et al., 2004; Stone & Sobel, 1990) show an imbalance in the number of times a true mediation value falls to the left or right of the confidence limits. For positive values of the mediated effect, where population values of *a* and *b* are both positive or both negative, sample confidence limits are more often to the left than to the right of the true value. The imbalance is also demonstrated in asymmetric confidence intervals from bootstrap analysis of the mediated effect (Bollen & Stine, 1990; Lockwood & MacKinnon, 1998). The implication of the imbalance is that there is less power to detect a true mediated effect. Stone and Sobel (1990, p. 349) analytically demonstrate that part of the imbalance may be due to use of only the first-order derivatives in the solution for the multivariate delta method standard error of the indirect effect. However, MacKinnon et al. (1995) found that the second-order Taylor series solution in Equation 3.9 also had similar imbalances in confidence intervals. MacKinnon et al. (2004) showed that confidence limits based on the distribution of the product were the best single sample method in terms of Type I error rates, statistical power, and accuracy of confidence limits.

4.16 The Distribution of a Product

The assumption that the indirect (mediated) effect divided by its standard error has a normal distribution is incorrect in some situations. In these situations, using the standard normal distribution described earlier for $z = \hat{a}\hat{b}/s_{\hat{a}\hat{b}}$ will be incorrect. An alternative method for testing indirect effects can be developed on the basis of the distribution of the product of two normally distributed random variables (Aroian, 1947; Craig, 1936; Springer, 1979). As the indirect effect is the product of regression estimates that are normally distributed (Hanushek & Jackson, 1977), the distribution of the product can be applied to the use of the product $\hat{a}\hat{b}$ as a test of the indirect effect based on the product, $z_a z_b$, where $z_a = \hat{a}/s_{\hat{a}}$ and $z_b = \hat{b}/s_{\hat{b}}$.

The product of two normal variables is not normally distributed (Lomnicki, 1967; Springer & Thompson, 1966). In the null case, in which both a and b (or z_a and z_b) have zero means, the distribution is symmetric with kurtosis of 6 (Craig, 1936), and the predicted kurtosis is 6 for any sample size including very large sample sizes. When the product of the population means, ab or $z_a z_b$, is nonzero, the distributions are skewed and have excess kurtosis, although Aroian, Taneja, and Cornwell (1978) showed that the product approaches the normal distribution as either z_a, z_b or both get large in absolute value. The four moments of the product of two correlated normal variables were given by Craig (1936) and Aroian et al. (1978). Following are the moments of $z_a z_b$ when the variables are uncorrelated as for the single mediator model case described in chapter 3. The non-normality of the distribution of the product can be easily shown with these formulas. For example, if the zs are zero, then the kurtosis will equal 6.

$$\text{Moment}_1 = \text{Mean} = z_a z_b \tag{4.33}$$

$$\text{Moment}_2 = \text{Variance} = z_a^2 + z_b^2 + 1 \tag{4.34}$$

$$\text{Moment}_3 = \text{Skewness} = \frac{6(z_a z_b)}{(z_a^2 + z_b^2 + 1)^{3/2}} \tag{4.35}$$

$$\text{Moment}_4 = \text{Kurtosis} = \frac{12(z_a + z_b) + 6}{(z_a^2 + z_b^2 + 1)^2} \tag{4.36}$$

The distribution of the product of two independent standard normal variables does not approximate familiar distributions commonly used in statistics, although Aroian (1947) showed that the gamma distribution can provide an approximation in some situations. Instead, the analytical solution for the product distribution is a Bessel function of the second kind with a purely imaginary argument (Aroian, 1947; Craig, 1936). Although computation of these values is complex, Springer and Thompson (1966) provided a table of the values of this function when $z_a = z_b = 0$. Meeker, Cornwell, and Aroian (1981, see pp. 129–144 for uncorrelated variables) presented tables of the distribution of the product of two standard normal variables based on an alternative formula more conducive to numerical integration. Tables of fractiles of the standardized distribution function for $(\hat{a}\hat{b} - ab)/\sigma_{ab}$ for different values of a, b, σ_a, and σ_b are given in Meeker et al. (1981). The tables assume that the population values of σ_{ab}, a, and b are known, but the authors suggest that sample values can be used in place of the population values as an approximation, e.g., $t_a = \hat{a}/s_{\hat{a}}$ and $t_b = \hat{b}/s_{\hat{b}}$.

An alternative method to find critical values for the distribution of the product is to use a FORTRAN program, fnprod.f90 (http://users.bigpond.net.au/amiller/), written by Alan Miller based on Meeker and Escobar (1994) to iteratively find the critical value. This program was edited to automate the iterative selection of critical values to form the PRODCLIN program (MacKinnon, Fritz, Williams, & Lockwood, 2007, http://www.public.asu.edu/~davidpm/ripl/index.htm). The input to the PRODCLIN program is the value of $\hat{a}$, $s_{\hat{a}}$ (sea in the program), $\hat{b}$, $s_{\hat{b}}$ (seb in the program), the correlation between $\hat{a}$ and $\hat{b}$, and the Type I error rate for the desired confidence interval as described in the next section.

4.17 Asymmetric Confidence Limits for the Mediated Effect

As described in chapter 3, confidence limits for the normal distribution are obtained using Equations 3.4 and 3.5, where $z_{\text{Type I error}}$ is the critical value from the z distribution. For 95% confidence limits, the z is equal to 1.96. Because the distribution of the product is not always symmetric and is often skewed, these confidence limits can be inaccurate. A more accurate method takes the shape of the distribution of the product into account when the confidence limits are calculated.

The computation of confidence limits using the distribution of the product requires different critical values for the upper and lower confidence limits when the distribution of the product is not symmetric. When the distribution of the product is symmetric, the upper and lower critical values are the same value but are not the same as those for the normal distribution. The critical values, ProdUpper and ProdLower in Equations

4.37 and 4.38, respectively, are both added to the point estimate because the lower critical value is negative:

Lower confidence limit (LCL) = mediated effect
$$+ \text{ProdLower}_{\text{Type 1 Error}} (s_{\hat{a}\hat{b}}) \qquad (4.37)$$

Upper confidence limit (UCL) = mediated effect
$$+ \text{ProdUpper}_{\text{Type 1 Error}} (s_{\hat{a}\hat{b}}) \qquad (4.38)$$

The values for the upper and lower critical values are obtained from the PRODCLIN program by inputting $\hat{a}$, $s_{\hat{a}}$, $\hat{b}$, $s_{\hat{b}}$, the correlation between $\hat{a}$ and $\hat{b}$, and Type I error rates for the desired confidence limits. So for the water consumption example, the following values served as input to the program: 0.3386 0.1224 0.4510 0.1460 0 0.05. As shown in the following, the resulting critical values were −1.6175 and 2.2540 for upper and lower critical values, respectively. Note the substantial discrepancy in critical values based on the normal distribution that are −1.96 and 1.96. These confidence limits based on the distribution of the product were found to be more accurate than normal theory confidence limits in a large statistical simulation (MacKinnon et al., 2004):

$$\text{LCL} = \text{mediated effect} - 1.6175 \, (0.0741) = 0.0329$$

$$\text{UCL} = \text{mediated effect} + 2.2540 \, (0.0741) = 0.3197$$

4.18 Monte Carlo Study of Mediation Regression Equations

The mediation regression methods described in chapters 3 and 4 are typically applied to one data set. But the data from a study are a sample from the population. Each sample of data contains error, making the results of any single study potentially an inaccurate representation of the population. How can a researcher know whether the formulas for different statistical quantities such as the ones described in this book yield values that are close to population values? Similarly, which method yields the most statistical power to detect mediation effects?

Monte Carlo studies assess the accuracy of statistical methods. In a Monte Carlo study, the researcher determines the true population model, and data sets are generated on the basis of this true model. The data sets are generated based on Equations 3.2 and 3.3 for specific values of the population coefficients and error terms. Because the population model is known, the accuracy of statistical methods can be assessed by determining whether the method leads to the correct conclusions for each simulated data set. For example, a Monte Carlo study can be used to compare the estimates of the regression coefficient to the population value of the regression coefficient. The value of the population regression coefficient and other mediation quantities are obtained on the basis of the population covariance matrix described in section 4.15. The standard errors can be evaluated in the same manner by comparing the true value of the standard error to the calculated standard error. Monte Carlo studies typically follow three steps: (a) a dataset of a certain sample size is generated under a known population model, (b) statistical methods are used to estimate parameters and standard errors for that sample and the results are saved, and (c) a new dataset is generated and the same statistics are calculated as in step 2. A large number of datasets are then generated and model coefficient estimated in this manner. The number of times the dataset is generated is called the number of replications. The average estimated regression coefficients across the replications should be very close to the population regression coefficient used to generate the data.

A Monte Carlo study of the mediation regression Equations 3.1 through 3.3 is summarized in Tables 4.1 and 4.2. Table 4.1 shows the average regression coefficients across 200 replications for sample sizes of 50, 100, 200, and 500 for a true regression model with $a = 0.4$, $b = 0.7$, $c' = 0.2$, $\sigma_x^2 = 1$ and residual error variances, $\sigma_{e_2}^2$ and $\sigma_{e_3}^2 = 1$. The average regression coefficients across the 200 replications are quite close to the true values.

Table 4.2 shows the true standard errors for $\hat{a}$, $\hat{b}$, $\hat{c}'$, and $\hat{a}\hat{b}$. Another measure of the true standard error, the empirical standard error, is the standard deviation of each statistic across the 200 replications. These two measures of the true standard error are compared with the average estimate of each of the standard errors, across the 200 replications. As a result, three standard error values are shown for $\hat{a}$, $\hat{b}$, $\hat{c}'$, and $\hat{a}\hat{b}$, (a) true value based on the analytical formula, e.g., $\sigma_{\hat{a}T}$ (b) true value based on the standard deviation of each statistic across the 200 replications, e.g., $\sigma_{\hat{a}}$ and (c) the average of the estimated standard error across the 200 replications, e.g., $\bar{s}_{\hat{a}}$. In all cases, the average of the estimated standard error is very close to the true standard error and the standard deviation across the 200 replications. For example,

Table 4.1   Average Coefficient by Sample Size

	True	50	100	200	500
a	0.4	0.4067	0.3938	0.4008	0.4024
b	0.7	0.7071	0.7097	0.7026	0.7000
c'	0.2	0.1872	0.1856	0.2065	0.2022
ab	0.28	0.2887	0.2803	0.2817	0.2817

Table 4.2 Standard Error by Sample Size

	50	100	200	500
Theoretical standard errors **(standard deviation of the estimator)**				
$\sigma_{\hat{a}T}$	0.1443	0.1010	0.0711	0.0448
$\sigma_{\hat{b}T}$	0.1459	0.1015	0.0712	0.0449
$\sigma_{\hat{c}T}$	0.1459	0.1015	0.0712	0.0449
$\sigma_{\hat{a}\hat{b}T}$	0.1188	0.0822	0.0575	0.0362
Standard deviation of estimates				
$\sigma_{\hat{a}}$	0.1390	0.0986	0.0762	0.0456
$\sigma_{\hat{b}}$	0.1449	0.1079	0.0744	0.0456
$\sigma_{\hat{c}}$	0.1470	0.1049	0.0755	0.0464
$\sigma_{\hat{a}\hat{b}}$	0.1188	0.0829	0.0616	0.0370
Average estimate of the standard errors				
$\bar{s}_{\hat{a}}$	0.1440	0.1011	0.0708	0.0449
$\bar{s}_{\hat{b}}$	0.1446	0.1015	0.0718	0.0447
$\bar{s}_{\hat{a}\hat{b}}$	0.1552	0.1090	0.0770	0.0482
$\bar{s}_{\hat{c}-\hat{c}'}$	0.1217	0.0834	0.0580	0.0363

Table 4.3 Approximate Sample Size Required for 0.8 Power to Detect a Mediated Effect as a Function of a and b Effect Size for a Completely Mediated Model

	Small	Medium	Large
Causal steps			
Baron & Kenny	20,886	397	92
Joint test	535	75	35
Product			
Sobel $s_{\hat{a}\hat{b}}$	667	90	42
Asymmetric confidence limits	509	70	33
Difference			
$s_{\hat{c}-\hat{c}'}$	675	94	42

Note: Small refers to both a and b small effects, medium refers to both a and b medium effects, and large refers to both a and b large effects. Sample sizes are for a complete mediation model, i.e., $c' = 0$.

the average of all the estimates of the standard error of ab equals 0.0580 for a sample size of 200, which is very close to the true standard error of 0.0575 and the standard deviation across the 200 replications, 0.0616. This Monte Carlo method has been used to study the statistical properties of mediation tests (Allison, 1995b; Bobko & Rieck, 1980; MacKinnon, Lockwood, et al., 2002; MacKinnon et al., 1995; Stone & Sobel, 1990). A SAS program to conduct this Monte Carlo study is included in the CD for this book.

The simulation methodology can also be used to compare different tests for the mediated effect in terms of statistical power to detect effects and Type I error rates. It is possible to use the simulation program to empirically find the sample size required to have 0.8 power to detect a mediated effect of a certain size. Sample size is varied and iterations are conducted to determine the sample size empirically (Fritz & MacKinnon, 2007). With the use of this method, Table 4.3 shows the approximate sample sizes necessary to find effects of different effect sizes, where effect size is determined by the correlation for the a coefficient and the partial correlation coefficient for the b coefficient. Note that for small effects of a and b, 20,886 subjects are required for the Baron and Kenny causal steps approach. Note that this sample size is based on a zero direct effect, $c' = 0$, so the total effect is equal to ab in the population. The excessive sample size is obtained because the total effect, c, for a small value of a and a small value of b is the product of these two coefficients. In step 1 of the Baron and Kenny method, the total effect, c, is tested, but this is a very small value because it is the product of small values for a and b. If c' is nonzero, smaller sample sizes are needed for the Baron and Kenny causal steps approach. The asymmetric CL approach described in section 4.17 required the smallest sample size for any effect size.

4.19 Summary

This chapter presented several technical aspects of the single mediator regression model including effect size, the background for the derivation of standard errors, and the use of a Monte Carlo study to evaluate the accuracy of mediation methods. In the next chapter, the mediation regression equations for multiple mediators are described. More complicated mediation models are described in later chapters. Effect size measures, use of statistical simulations, and derivation of true quantities are important for these more advanced models.

4.20 Exercises

4.1. Describe the effect size measures for the single mediation model. Which effect size measure do you prefer?

4.2. How does taking absolute values of quantities before computing the proportion mediated change the meaning of the proportion mediated?

4.3. The following data were generated using the Monte Carlo methods as described in section 4.18. Compute regression coefficients, standard errors, and effect size measures. What is unique about these data? Is this a consistent or inconsistent mediation model? The data were generated to demonstrate issues described in Hamilton (1987). Look at the title of the Hamilton paper for a hint about one unique aspect of these data.

X	M	Y
4.83	5.75	5.23
4.97	5.14	5.05
4.94	5.19	5.01
5.11	4.74	5.07
5.05	4.95	5.11
4.98	5.22	5.17
4.86	5.43	5.00
4.94	5.28	5.12
4.97	5.17	5.06
4.92	5.27	5.06
5.00	4.72	4.73
4.84	5.22	4.76
5.07	4.76	4.99
5.11	4.61	4.92
5.14	4.65	5.09

4.4. Using the formula for the true covariance between X and Y, compute the t-value for $a = 0.5$ and $b = 0.1$, error variances $= 1$. Use this value to demonstrate why large sample sizes are required for the Baron and Kenny causal steps method when c' is zero.

4.5. Compute and interpret the proportion mediated and ratio of mediated to direct effect or exercise 4.3.

4.6. (Technical Question) Complete the steps for the covariance algebra for the single mediator model variances for X, M, and Y.

4.7. (Technical Question) Derive the following quantities using the multivariate delta method:
   a. variance of the proportion mediated, $\hat{a}\hat{b}/(\hat{c}' + \hat{a}\hat{b})$.
   b. variance of the product of three independent random variables, $\hat{a}\hat{b}\hat{d}$.

4.8. (Technical Question) What are the values of $\hat{a}$ and $\hat{b}$ for standard-
      ized values? Bobko and Rieck (1980) derived the standard error of
      the product of standardized $\hat{a}$ and $\hat{b}$ using the multivariate delta
      method. Derive the variance using the multivariate delta method.

4.9. (Technical Question) What are the values of $\hat{c}$ and $\hat{c}'$ for standardized
      variables? Derive the standard error of the difference between $\hat{c}$ and
      $\hat{c}'$ for standardized variables.

4.10. (Advanced Technical Question) On pp. 107–109 in Bollen (1989), the
      matrix equation for the covariance among maximum likelihood esti-
      mates is given as $\Sigma_\theta = [(2/(N-1))\ \{E[(\partial^2 F_{ML})/(\partial\theta\ \partial\theta')]\}]$, where $\partial^2 F_{ML}$ is
      the second derivatives of the fit function from maximum likelihood,
      $F_{ML} = \log|\Sigma_\theta| + \text{trace}(S\Sigma^{-1}(\theta)) - \log|S| - (p+q)$ where I is an iden-
      tity matrix, S is the covariance matrix (the true covariance matrix in
      Equation 4.15 will be substituted here), p is the number of dependent
      variables ($p = 2$ for the single mediator model), and q is the num-
      ber of independent variables ($q = 1$ for the single mediator model).
      The resulting matrix contains the asymptotic variances of $\hat{a}$, $\hat{b}$, and $\hat{c}'$
      along the diagonal and the covariances among $\hat{a}$, $\hat{b}$, and $\hat{c}'$ in the off-
      diagonal elements of the matrix. Derive this asymptotic covariance
      among the estimates for the single mediator model using the true
      covariance matrix in Equation 4.15.

4.11. (Advanced Technical Question) McGuigan and Langholz (1988)
      derived the covariance $\text{Cov}(\hat{c},\hat{c}')$ where the estimate of $\hat{c} = (X_1^T X_1)^{-1}$
      $X_1^T y$, the estimate of $\hat{c}' = 1/s\ (X_2^T X_2)\ X_1^T y - (X_2^T X_1)\ X_2^T y$, $t = (X_1^T X_1)^{-1}$, and
      $s = (X_1^T X_1)(X_2^T X_2) - (X_2^T X_1)(X_1^T X_2)$. Using $\text{Cov}(a, b-c) = \text{Cov}(a,b) - \text{Cov}(a,c)$
      and $\text{Cov}(X_1^T y, X_1^T y) = \text{Var}(X_1^T y) = X_1^T\ \text{Var}(y) = X_1^T X_1 \sigma^2 y$ from Rao (1973, p.
      107) and then expanding the product of the estimators of and $\hat{c}$ and $\hat{c}'$,
      they obtained Equation 4.24 (actually $\text{MSE}/(\Sigma X^2)$) for the covariance
      of $\hat{c}$ and $\hat{c}'$. Supply the missing steps in the derivation. This result
      is important because it shows how covariances among coefficients
      across equations can be obtained.

5

Multiple Mediator Model

> There are multiple pathways to persuasion, each involv-
> ing a different subset of mediating processes. . . .
>
> **—William McGuire, 1999, p. 116**

5.1 Overview

This chapter extends the analysis of the single mediator model to a model with two or more mediators. Examples of multiple mediator models are described and the equations for the two mediator model are given along with formulas for standard errors of effects in the model. A hypothetical study of teacher expectations on student achievement is then used to illustrate the analysis using both the SAS and SPSS computer languages.

5.2 The Multiple Mediator Model

Often more than one mediational process is hypothesized in the relation between an independent variable and a dependent variable. One example of a multiple mediator model is the four-mediator model of how teacher's expectancies for a student affect student performance (Rosenthal, 1987). Harris and Rosenthal (1985) conducted a meta-analysis of 135 studies of the mediators of the relation between teacher expectancy and student achievement. Four major groups of mediators were identified: (a) warmer social climate for high-expectancy students, (b) more differentiated feedback to high-expectancy students, (c) tendency to teach more material and more difficult material to high-expectancy students and (d) tendency to give high-expectancy students more opportunities to respond. There was evidence for each mediational pathway, but smaller effects were obtained for the feedback mediator because of a relatively weaker relation between feedback and student achievement. The four-mediator model summarized a wide range of research on the topic and demonstrated multiple mediational processes in the relation between an independent and dependent variable.

Studies of health outcomes are also often based on more than one mediator. The Multiple Risk Factor Intervention Trial (MRFIT) was designed to change three mediators, smoking, cholesterol, and blood pressure, to prevent heart disease (Multiple Risk Factor Intervention Trial Research Group, 1990). Hansen (1992) outlined the 12 mediators most commonly targeted by drug prevention curricula: information, decision making, pledges, values clarification, goal setting, stress management, self-esteem, resistance skills training, life skills training, norm setting, assistance, and alternatives. Not all programs target all of these mediators and few research studies measure all of them. Nevertheless, the multiple mediator model is the theoretical basis of many prevention programs. As a result, the multiple mediator model described in this chapter is often the correct model for the evaluation of such programs. The detailed examination of the contributions of multiple mediators to changes in a dependent variable may clarify the critical mediators as well as help resolve discrepancies among studies.

Mediation analysis is most compelling when alternative theories predict different mediational pathways for program effects on drug use. Hansen and Graham (1991), for example, found evidence for the norm setting mediator but not the resistance skills mediator after experimental manipulation of these mediators. Similarly, social influence approaches have been more successful than affective based programs (Flay, 1985), and these different approaches hypothesize different mediational pathways for reduction of drug use.

The complexity of relations between most variables also suggests that the multiple mediator model may be a more reasonable approach than the single mediator models described in chapter 3. Fortunately, the analysis of the multiple mediator model is a straightforward extension of the single mediator model.

5.3 Diagram of the Two Mediator Model

The two-mediator model is shown in figure 5.1, in which an independent variable (X) is related to two mediators (M_1 and M_2) that are both related to the dependent variable (Y). Note that there are other potential multiple mediator models such as X to M_1 to M_2 to Y, which is discussed in chapter 6. The multiple mediator model described first includes two mediators that come between the independent variable and the dependent variable.

5.4 Regression Equations Used to Assess Mediation in the Two-Mediator Model

Four regression equations are used to investigate mediation in the two mediator model,

$$Y = i_1 + cX + e_1 \tag{5.1}$$

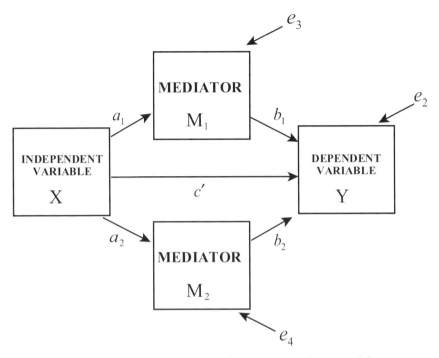

Figure 5.1. Path diagram and equations for the two mediator model.

$$Y = i_2 + c'X + b_1M_1 + b_2M_2 + e_2 \tag{5.2}$$

$$M_1 = i_3 + a_1X + e_3 \tag{5.3}$$

$$M_2 = i_4 + a_2X + e_4 \tag{5.4}$$

where Y is the dependent variable, X is the independent variable, M_1 is the first mediator, M_2 is the second mediator, c is the parameter relating the independent variable and the dependent variable in the first equation, c' is the parameter relating the independent variable to the dependent variable adjusted for the two mediators, b_1 is the parameter relating the first mediator to the dependent variable adjusted for the independent variable and the second mediator, b_2 is the parameter relating the second mediator to the dependent variable adjusted for the independent variable and the first mediator, a_1 is the parameter relating the independent variable to the first mediating variable, a_2 is the parameter relating the independent variable to the second mediating variable, e_1, e_2, e_3, and e_4 represent error variability, and the intercepts are i_1, i_2, i_3, and i_4. Note that both c and c' are parameters relating the independent variable to the dependent variable, but c' is adjusted for the effects of the mediators. The covariance between M1 and M2 is also included as part of Equation 5.2. Equations 5.2 through 5.4 are the equations that define the mediation model in figure 5.1.

5.5 Total Effect

As for the single mediator model, the overall relation of X to Y is important in multiple mediator models as well. The parameter c again represents the change in Y for a 1 unit change in X. If X represents an experimental manipulation, then the c parameter represents the effect of the manipulation. As for the single mediator model, adding measures of mediating variables provides a way to extract more information from a research study than just the overall relation of the X to Y.

5.6 Mediated Effects

The product of the a_1 and b_1 parameters, a_1b_1, and the product of the a_2 and b_2 parameters, a_2b_2, are the two mediated effects in the model. The effect of X on Y after adjustment for the two mediators, c', is the direct effect just as it was for the single mediator model; thus, $a_1b_1 + a_2b_2 = c - c'$. The total mediated effect, a_1b_1 plus a_2b_2 equals the difference between the c and c' coefficients, where c is the total effect of X on Y, thus $c = c' + a_1b_1 + a_2b_2$. As a result, the total effect c can be decomposed into a direct effect, c', and two mediated effects, a_1b_1 and a_2b_2. The parameters in Equations 5.1, 5.2, 5.3, and 5.4 can be estimated using ordinary least squares regression to obtain estimates $\hat{c}$, $\hat{c}'$, $\hat{b}$, $\hat{a}$, $\hat{a}_1\hat{b}_1$, $\hat{a}_2\hat{b}_2$, and $\hat{c} - \hat{c}'$. As described in chapter 3, there are times when researchers will find that $\hat{c} - \hat{c}'$ does not equal $\hat{a}_1\hat{b}_1$ plus $\hat{a}_2\hat{b}_2$, usually because of different sample sizes across equations.

  With more than one mediated effect, an approach to specifying each mediated effect is necessary. Bollen (1987) calls each mediated effect such as $\hat{a}_1\hat{b}_1$ and $\hat{a}_2\hat{b}_2$ for the two-mediator model specific indirect effects to clarify the distinction between the total mediated effect, which is the sum of $\hat{a}_1\hat{b}_1$ and $\hat{a}_2\hat{b}_2$ and the individual mediated effects. As the number of mediators increases, the number of specific mediated effects increases so that there are four mediated effects for a four-mediator model for example. In this book, a specific mediated effect will refer to a mediated effect transmitted through the product of regression coefficients corresponding to a single mediated effect.

5.7 Confidence Limits for the Mediated Effect

The estimate of the mediated effect and its standard error can be used to construct confidence limits as described in Equations 3.4 and 3.5 for symmetric intervals and Equations 4.37 and 4.38 for asymmetric intervals. The total mediated effect, $\hat{c} - \hat{c}' = \hat{a}_1\hat{b}_1 + \hat{a}_2\hat{b}_2$ and each specific mediated effect, $\hat{a}_1\hat{b}_1$ and $\hat{a}_2\hat{b}_2$, are the estimates of the mediated effects in the two-mediator model. The alternative formulas for the standard error of the mediated effect described in chapter 3 can be used for confidence limits of specific mediated effects, $\hat{a}_1\hat{b}_1$ and $\hat{a}_2\hat{b}_2$, and the standard error for the total mediated effect, $\hat{c} - \hat{c}' = \hat{a}_1\hat{b}_1 + \hat{a}_2\hat{b}_2$, as described later.

5.8 Standard Error of the Mediated Effects

The formula for the standard error of each specific mediated effect in the multiple mediator model is the same formula as that for the standard error of the single mediated effect described in Equation 3.6. For example, the standard error of $\hat{a}_1\hat{b}_1$ is equal to

$$s_{\hat{a}_1\hat{b}_1} = \sqrt{\hat{a}_1^2 s_{b1}^2 + \hat{b}_1^2 s_{\hat{a}1}^2} \qquad (5.5)$$

and Equation 5.6 provides a formula less susceptible to computation errors, where t is the t-value for the $\hat{a}$ and $\hat{b}$ coefficients in the respective mediated effect:

$$s_{\hat{a}_1\hat{b}_1} = \frac{\hat{a}_1\hat{b}_1\sqrt{t_{\hat{a}_1}^2 + t_{\hat{b}_1}^2}}{t_{\hat{a}_1} t_{\hat{b}_1}} \qquad (5.6)$$

Any of the other formulas for the standard error of the mediated effect described in chapter 3 can be applied in the multiple mediator case with corresponding notation change to indicate the correct mediated effect.

The multivariate delta solution for the standard error of the total mediated effect, $\hat{a}_1\hat{b}_1 + \hat{a}_2\hat{b}_2$, is equal to

$$s_{\hat{a}_1\hat{b}_1+\hat{a}_2\hat{b}_2} = \sqrt{s_{\hat{a}_1}^2\hat{b}_1^2 + s_{\hat{b}_1}^2\hat{a}_1^2 + s_{\hat{a}_2}^2\hat{b}_2^2 + s_{\hat{b}_2}^2\hat{a}_2^2 + 2\hat{a}_1\hat{a}_2 s_{\hat{b}_1\hat{b}_2}} \qquad (5.7)$$

which can be simplified to

$$s_{\hat{a}_1\hat{b}_1+\hat{a}_2\hat{b}_2} = \sqrt{s_{\hat{a}_1\hat{b}_1}^2 + s_{\hat{a}_2\hat{b}_2}^2 + 2\hat{a}_1\hat{a}_2 s_{\hat{b}_1\hat{b}_2}} \qquad (5.8)$$

where $s_{\hat{b}_1\hat{b}_2}$ the covariance between the $\hat{b}_1$ and $\hat{b}_2$ regression estimates. In some situations, there will be a nonzero covariance between $\hat{a}_1$ and $\hat{a}_2$, so $2\hat{b}_1\hat{b}_2 s_{\hat{a}_1\hat{a}_2}$ should be added to Equations 5.7 and 5.8.

The standard error of the total mediated effect, $\hat{c} - \hat{c}'$, for the multiple mediator case is equal to the following formula:

$$s_{\hat{c}-\hat{c}'} = \sqrt{s_{\hat{c}}^2 + s_{\hat{c}'}^2 - 2rs_{\hat{c}}s_{\hat{c}'}} \tag{5.9}$$

where the covariance between $\hat{c}$ and $\hat{c}'$, $rs_{\hat{c}}s_{\hat{c}'}$, is the mean square error in Equation 5.2 divided by the product of the variance of the independent variable and sample size as in Equation 3.8.

For models with more than two mediators, formulas for the standard error of the specific mediated effects are the same as Equation 5.5 and 5.6. The formula for the total mediated effect includes the standard errors of each specific mediated effect and the product of each pair of $\hat{a}$ coefficients and the corresponding covariance between the two $\hat{b}$ coefficients.

5.9 Significance Tests for the Mediated Effect

As described in chapter 3, the mediated effect can be tested for statistical significance by dividing the estimate of the mediated effect by its standard error. The value of the mediated effect divided by its standard error is then compared to tabled values of the normal distribution. If the absolute value of the ratio exceeds 1.96, for example, then the mediated effect is significantly different from zero at the .05 level of significance. Any of the aforementioned standard errors can be used for this test. As for the single mediator case, more accurate statistical tests can be obtained with the distribution of the product.

The equality of pairs of mediated effects can be tested using the formula for the standard error of the difference between the mediated effects shown in Equation 5.10. This test is justified because both mediated effects are in the metric of the dependent variable. The difference between the two mediated effects is divided by the standard error and the resulting ratio is compared to tabled z values. Note that this formula is very similar to the standard error of the total mediated effect (Equation 5.7) except that the last element of the equation is subtracted. In some situations, there will be a nonzero covariance between $\hat{a}_1$ and $\hat{a}_2$, so $2\hat{b}_1\hat{b}_2 s_{\hat{a}_1\hat{a}_2}$ should be subtracted as well, as described in chapter 6:

$$s_{\hat{a}_1\hat{b}_1-\hat{a}_2\hat{b}_2} = \sqrt{s_{\hat{a}_1}^2\hat{b}_1^2 + s_{\hat{b}_1}^2\hat{a}_1^2 + s_{\hat{a}_2}^2\hat{b}_2^2 + s_{\hat{b}_2}^2\hat{a}_2^2 - 2\hat{a}_1\hat{a}_2 s_{\hat{b}_1\hat{b}_2}} \tag{5.10}$$

$$s_{\hat{a}_1\hat{b}_1-\hat{a}_2\hat{b}_2} = \sqrt{s_{\hat{a}_1\hat{b}_1}^2 + s_{\hat{a}_2\hat{b}_2}^2 - 2\hat{a}_1\hat{a}_2 s_{\hat{b}_1\hat{b}_2}} \tag{5.11}$$

5.10 Baron and Kenny (1986) Steps to Establish Mediation

The causal steps method to assess mediation described in chapter 3 for one mediator also applies in multiple mediator models with a few limitations. The causal step method in models with more than one mediator consists of a series of statistical tests of relations among variables corresponding to significance tests of the $\hat{a}_1$, $\hat{a}_2$, $\hat{b}_1$, $\hat{b}_2$, $\hat{c}$, and $\hat{c}'$ regression coefficients described earlier. These steps are described here because the shortcomings of the steps demonstrate several unique aspects of the multiple mediator model.

1. The independent variable (X) must affect the dependent variable (Y), coefficient $\hat{c}$ in Equation 5.1.

As in the single mediator case, the purpose of this first test is to establish that there is an effect to mediate. If the effect is not statistically significant, then the analysis for consistent mediation stops. As for the single mediator model, it is possible that the relation between the independent variable and the dependent variable may be nonsignificant, yet there can still be substantial mediation. This will occur in cases of what is called inconsistent mediation (suppression models), and these types of models can be very complicated with multiple mediator models as some mediated effects may have different signs from each other and from the direct effect.

2. The independent variable (X) must affect the first mediator (M_1), coefficient $\hat{a}_1$ in Equation 5.3, and the independent variable (X) must affect the second mediator (M_2), coefficient $\hat{a}_2$ in Equation 5.4.

This test requires that the independent variable be significantly related to the mediators. In the case of an X variable coding an experimental manipulation, this requires that there is an experimental effect on each mediating variable. As described in chapter 2, in an experimental study this provides a test of the action theory of the manipulation, of whether the theory of how the independent variable changes the mediators is accurate. It is possible that the $\hat{a}$ coefficient may not be significant for one or more mediated effects, implying that the corresponding mediating variable is not a mediator of the relation between X and Y.

3. The mediator must affect the dependent variable (Y) when the independent variable (X) is controlled: coefficient $\hat{b}_1$ for the first mediator and $\hat{b}_2$ for the second mediator in Equation 5.2.

This test requires a significant relation between the mediators and the dependent variable, providing a test of the conceptual theory of how the mediator is related to the dependent variable as described in chapter 2. It makes sense that the mediator must be significantly related to the dependent variable for there to be mediation. If the mediator is unrelated to the dependent variable, the effect of the independent variable on the mediator cannot be transmitted to the dependent variable. Clogg, Petkova, and Shihadeh (1992) concluded that the test of significance of either $\hat{b}_1$ or $\hat{b}_2$ is a test for mediation because that is equivalent to testing whether adding either mediator changes the relation between the independent variable and the dependent variable. Unfortunately, this Clogg et al. test will be significant whenever any of the mediators in a multiple mediator model has a significant relationship to the dependent variable so it is not possible to distinguish mediated effects through each mediator (Allison, 1995a).

4. The direct effect must be nonsignificant: coefficient $\hat{c}'$ in Equation 5.2.

As for the single mediator model, when the direct effect is nonsignificant and either $\hat{a}_1\hat{b}_1$ or $\hat{a}_2\hat{b}_2$ or both are significant, there is evidence for complete mediation. If the direct effect remains statistically significant, there may still be a significant partial mediation of the effect.

There are several limitations of this causal hypotheses test for mediation effects with more than one mediator. First, no estimate of either mediated effect ($\hat{a}_1\hat{b}_1$ or $\hat{a}_2\hat{b}_2$) is available, although the causal hypotheses method can be combined with other approaches that do provide estimates of the mediated effect as described earlier. In general, multiple mediators are difficult to incorporate in the causal steps mediation analysis. Only the total mediated effect can be obtained from $\hat{c} - \hat{c}'$. There is not a procedure in the causal hypotheses method to obtain adjusted estimates of the specific mediated effects. A second limitation of the causal step method is that estimates of the standard errors of the mediated effects are not available, but the standard error formulas in chapter 3 are accurate in the multiple mediator case. It is possible to obtain estimates of the individual mediated effects and standard errors for multiple mediators using Equations 5.5 and 5.7.

A third limitation of the causal hypotheses method is the requirement that there must be a significant total effect, $\hat{c}$, for mediation analysis to proceed. Actually, significant mediation effects may be present when the total effect, $\hat{c}$, is equal to zero, but this requires that some of the mediated effects, $\hat{a}_1\hat{b}_1$, $\hat{a}_2\hat{b}_2$, and the direct effect, $\hat{c}'$, have opposite signs. Models with positive and negative mediated effects are called inconsistent models (Blalock, 1969; Davis, 1985). Inconsistent effects are likely with multiple mediators. As the number of mediators increases, the number of possible combinations of consistent and inconsistent mediation effects increases. As a result, the requirement of a significant total effect, $\hat{c}$, may be incorrect for some models.

It is helpful to consider examples for which the total effect is nonsignificant, yet mediation is present. The effects of age, X, on performance, Y, is one common substantive multiple mediator example of this effect whereby aging reduces physical capabilities, M_1, and performance but age also increases cognitive and other skills, M_2, which improve performance. For example, there is generally a nonsignificant relation of age on typing proficiency because of two opposing mediational processes (Salthouse, 1984). Age increases reaction time which in turn reduces typing proficiency, but age also increases cognitive skills such as chunking words which improves typing proficiency. In this case, the overall relation between X and Y is nonsignificant because of opposing mediational processes. Sheets and Braver (1999) described an experimental study of sexual harassment in which the organizational status of a person increased his or her perceived power, which increased perceived harassment, but organizational status increased social dominance, which reduced perceived harassment. As shown in figure 5.2, the overall relation between organizational status and perceived harassment may be close to zero, but the

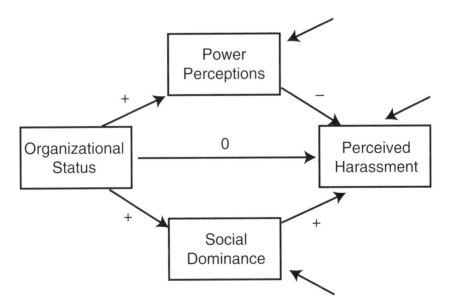

Figure 5.2. Opposing Mediational Process for Organizational Status and Harassment.

addition of two mediators to the analysis, power perceptions and social dominance, reveals important opposing mediational processes.

A total effect may be statistically significant yet one or more mediated effects may be inconsistent. In an evaluation of a steroid prevention program, the program increased knowledge of the reasons to use steroids that led to increased intentions to use steroids (MacKinnon, Krull, & Lockwood, 2000). Fortunately, there were changes in other mediators that led to a significant total effect of reducing intentions to use steroids. Without a multiple mediator model, it would not have been possible to expose this counterproductive mediation relation.

5.11 Hypothetical Study of Teacher Expectancies on Student Achievement

This example is based on Harris and Rosenthal's (1985) four-mediator model for how teacher expectancies affect student achievement. Two mediators were examined in this study, social climate, a measure of verbal and nonverbal warmth, and input, the tendency to teach more material and more difficult material to high-expectancy students. It was hypothesized that teacher expectancy leads the teacher to create a more positive social climate and input more material to high-expectancy students. A total of 40 students and 40 teachers provided the data. One student was picked from 1 of 40 classes taught by 40 separate teachers. Each student was randomly assigned an ability score and the teacher was told that this ability score reflected the student's true ability. The dependent variable was the score on a test of basic skills after one semester in the classroom. The social climate and teacher input to the student were measured four times during the semester and the four scores were averaged to obtain each score for the mediator. It is hypothesized that the general social warmth provided to the student is what leads him or her to achieve more. On the other hand, teacher expectancy may lead the teacher to teach more material and more difficult material that may lead to increased student achievement.

The data for the 40 subjects in this hypothetical study of teacher expectancies and student achievement are shown in Table 5.1, where X is the teacher expectancy based on an intelligence test given to the student the previous year, M_1 is the average observer rating of social warmth, M_2 is the average observer rating of input to the student, and Y is the score on the test at the end of the semester.

SPSS and SAS Programs. The variable names X, M1, M2, and Y were used to code the variables teacher expectancy, social climate, input, and test score at the end of the semester, respectively. The SAS statements in Table 5.2 were used to obtain the regression coefficient estimates used

Table 5.1 Data for Hypothetical Study of Teacher Expectations and Student Achievement

S#	X	M1	M2	Y	S#	X	M1	M2	Y
1	51	41	54	59	21	53	69	44	84
2	40	34	51	60	22	53	67	40	82
3	55	42	53	60	23	40	49	45	74
4	35	22	56	61	24	34	40	37	62
5	47	34	45	47	25	32	40	49	54
6	58	52	79	84	26	56	60	51	81
7	56	57	55	69	27	55	46	65	89
8	53	49	55	85	28	51	58	54	83
9	38	42	46	75	29	50	53	56	75
10	73	80	48	87	30	45	61	52	72
11	57	42	65	85	31	63	42	40	63
12	54	62	55	73	32	46	39	51	69
13	68	54	55	77	33	60	62	53	66
14	46	41	62	50	34	48	41	56	72
15	48	44	43	58	35	46	40	46	68
16	56	54	54	69	36	50	51	52	73
17	67	73	61	99	37	49	51	55	69
18	47	61	38	64	38	35	39	46	46
19	60	59	42	65	39	50	44	46	70
20	54	51	55	68	40	47	40	68	76

to compute the mediated effects and standard errors. Because the model statements are all under one PROC REG statement, only cases with data for all three variables will be included in the analysis. Note that the covb option is included in the SAS commands for Equation 5.2 in order to get the covariance between the $\hat{b}_1$ and $\hat{b}_2$ regression estimates necessary for the computation of the standard error of the total mediated effect and the test of the difference between mediated effects.

The output from SAS is also shown in Table 5.2. The coefficients and standard errors are the numbers used in the calculation of the mediated effect, standard error, and confidence limits as shown in the following.

For SPSS, statements for the two mediator model are shown in Table 5.3. The SPSS output is also shown in Table 5.3, and all estimates are identical (with rounding) to those found in the SAS output. The SPSS output automatically includes the standardized beta coefficients that represent the change in the dependent variable for a 1 standard deviation change in the independent variable. The standardized beta measure is one of

Table 5.2   SAS Program and Output for Equations 5.1, 5.2, 5.3, and 5.4

```
proc reg;
model Y=X;
model Y=X M1 M2/covb;
model M1=X;
model M2=X;
```

SAS Output for Equation 5.1
Dependent Variable: Y

Parameter Estimates

Variable	DF	Parameter Estimate	Std Error	T for H0: Parameter=0	Prob > |T|
INTERCEP	1	34.726935	8.92472341	3.891	0.0004
X	1	0.707760	0.17342970	4.081	0.0002

SAS Output for Equation 5.2
Dependent Variable: Y

Analysis of Variance

Source	DF	Sum of Squares	Mean Square	F Value	Prob>F
Model	3	2906.95288	968.98429	13.773	0.0001
Error	36	2532.82212	70.35617		
C Total	39	5439.77500			

Root MSE:	8.38786	R-squared:	0.5344
Dep Mean:	70.57500	Adj R-squared:	0.4956
C.V.:	11.88503		

Parameter Estimates

Variable	DF	Parameter Estimate	Std Error	T for H0: Parameter=0	Prob > |T|
INTERCEP	1	9.123327	10.47839358	0.871	0.3897
X	1	0.112152	0.20731147	0.541	0.5919
M1	1	0.569029	0.15681205	3.629	0.0009
M2	1	0.529720	0.16963747	3.123	0.0035

Covariance of Estimates

Variable	Intercept	x	M1	M2
Intercept	109.79673207	-0.387895193	-0.495870555	-1.227545009
X	-0.387895193	0.0429780463	-0.022410629	-0.013017423
M1	-0.495870555	-0.022410629	0.02459002	0.0078936364
M2	-1.227545009	-0.013017423	0.0078936364	0.0287768709

Table 5.2 (Continued)

```
SAS Output for Equation 5.3
Dependent Variable: M1
```

```
                         Parameter Estimates
                                         T for H0:
                     Parameter
Variable   DF         Estimate    Std Error    Parameter=0    Prob >  |T|

INTERCEP    1         7.097020    8.12852544   0.873          0.3881
X           1         0.840138    0.15795758   5.319          0.0001
```

```
SAS Output for Equation 5.4
Dependent Variable: M2
```

```
                         Parameter Estimates
                                         T for H0:
                     Parameter
Variable   DF         Estimate    Std Error    Parameter=0    Prob >  |T|

INTERCEP    1         40.710601   7.51396948   5.418          0.0001
X           1         0.221903    0.14601522   1.520          0.1369
```

the effect size measures described in chapter 4. A new regression statement is required for each regression equation. As a result, a researcher is more likely to have unequal numbers of subjects in the different regression models when SPSS is used, and consequently the researcher may not find that $\hat{c} - \hat{c}' = \hat{a}_1\hat{b}_1 + \hat{a}_2\hat{b}_2$ only because of the slight difference in sample sizes for each regression. The researcher is advised to remove cases (or use missing data analysis) that do not have measures of all four variables before estimating the regression models in SPSS if it is desired that $\hat{c} - \hat{c}' = \hat{a}_1\hat{b}_1 + \hat{a}_2\hat{b}_2$.

Mediation Analysis for the Expectancies and Achievement Study. The regression estimates and standard errors (in parentheses) from the SAS or SPSS output for the four models are given in the following equations and are displayed in figure 5.3:

Equation 5.1: $Y = i_1 + cX + e_1$
$$\hat{Y} = 34.7269 + 0.7078\ X$$
$$(0.1734)$$

Equation 5.2: $Y = i_2 + c'X + b_1M_1 + b_2M_2 + e_2$
$$\hat{Y} = 9.1233 + 0.1122X + 0.5690\ M_1 + 0.5297\ M_2$$
$$(0.2073)\quad (0.1568)\qquad (0.1696)$$

Table 5.3   SPSS Program and Output for Equations 5.1, 5.2, 5.3, and 5.4

```
regression
/variables= X Y M1 M2
    /dependent=Y
    /enter=X.
regression
    /variables= X Y M1 M2
    /dependent=Y
    /enter=X M1 M2
    /statistics=defaults bcov.
regression
    /variables= X Y M1
    /dependent=M1
    /enter= X.
regression
    /variables X Y M2
    /dependent=M2
    /enter X.
```

Output for Equation 5.1

	Unstandardized Coefficients		Standardized Coefficients		
	B	Std. Error	Beta	t	Sig
(Constant)	34.727	8.925		3.891	.000
X	.708	.173	.552	4.081	.000

a. Dependent variable Y

Output for Equation 5.2

Model Summary

Model	R	R Square	Adjusted R Square	Std. Error of the Estimate
1	.731	.534	.496	8.3879

	Unstandardized Cocfficients		Standardized Coefficients		
	B	Std. Error	Beta	t	Sig
(Constant)	9.123	10.478		0.871	.390
X	.112	.207	.087	0.541	.592
M1	.569	.157	.571	3.629	.001
M2	.530	.170	.383	3.123	.002

a. Dependent variable Y

Table 5.3 (Continued)

```
Output for Equation 5.3
```

	Unstandardized Coefficients		Standardized Coefficients		
	B	Std. Error	Beta	t	Sig
(Constant)	7.097	8.129		0.873	.388
X	.840	.158	.653	5.319	.000

a. Dependent variable M1

```
Output for Equation 5.4
```

	Unstandardized Coefficients		Standardized Coefficients		
	B	Std. Error	Beta	t	Sig
(Constant)	40.711	7.514		5.418	.000
X	.222	.146	.239	1.520	.137

a. Dependent variable M2

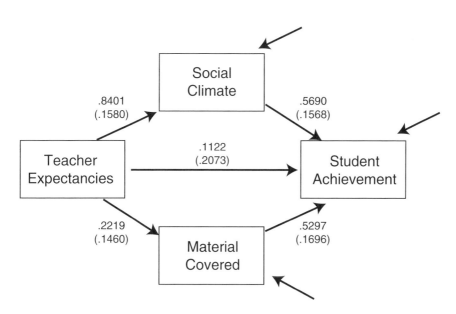

Figure 5.3.   Expectancy to Achievement Mediation Model.

Equation 5.3: $M_1 = i_3 + a_1 X + e_3$
$\hat{M}_1 = 7.0970 + 0.8401X$
                         (0.1580)

Equation 5.4: $M2 = i_4 + a_2 X + e_4$
$\hat{M}2 = 40.7106 + 0.2219X$
                         (0.1460)

Teacher expectancy was significantly related to student achievement ($\hat{c} = 0.7078$, $s_{\hat{c}} = 0.1734$, $t_{\hat{c}} = 4.081$), providing evidence that there is a significant relation between the independent and the dependent variable. A 1 unit increase in the teacher expectancy scale was associated with about two-thirds of a point on the achievement test. This result is surprising because the ability scores were randomly assigned to students so that ability should be unrelated to student achievement unless teacher expectancy alters performance. Perhaps this total effect can be explained by mediated effects through climate and input. There was a statistically significant effect of expectancy on social climate ($\hat{a}_1 = 0.8401$, $s_{\hat{a}1} = 0.1580$, $t_{\hat{a}1} = 5.319$) but not for the input mediating variable ($\hat{a}_2 = 0.2219$, $s_{\hat{a}2} = 0.1460$, $t_{\hat{a}2} = 1.520$). Teacher expectancy was associated with a 0.8401 increase in the score on the social climate mediator and 0.2219 change in the input mediator. The effect of the social climate mediator ($\hat{b}_1 = 0.5690$, $s_{\hat{b}1} = 0.1568$, $t_{\hat{b}1} = 3.629$) and the feedback mediator ($\hat{b}_2 = 0.5297$, $s_{\hat{b}2} = 0.1696$, $t_{\hat{b}2} = 3.123$) on student achievement was statistically significant when controlling for teacher expectancy. A 1 unit change in the social climate mediator was associated with a 0.5690 increase in the score on the test and a 1 unit increase in the feedback mediator was associated with a 0.5297 increase on the test. The adjusted effect of expectancy on student achievement was not statistically significant, ($\hat{c}' = 0.1122$, $s_{\hat{c}'} = 0.2073$, $t_{\hat{c}'} = 0.541$) consistent with a random association of ability score and test performance at the end of the semester. Apparently the overall significant relation between expectancy and achievement was due to the effects of expectancy on the mediators. There was a drop in the value of $\hat{c}'$ ($\hat{c}' = 0.1122$) compared with $\hat{c}$ ($\hat{c} = 0.7078$) of 0.5956.

The estimate of the two mediated effects are equal to $\hat{a}_1\hat{b}_1 = (0.8401)(0.5690)$ = 0.4781 for mediation through social climate and $\hat{a}_2\hat{b}_2 = (0.2219)(0.5297)$ = 0.1175 for mediation through input. The total mediated effect of $\hat{a}_1\hat{b}_1$ (0.4781) plus $\hat{a}_2\hat{b}_2$ (0.1175) equals 0.5956, which is equal to $\hat{c} - \hat{c}' = 0.7078 - .1122 = 0.5956$. The total mediated effect of expectancy on student achievement is 0.5956 so that a 1 unit change in teacher expectancy is associated with a 0.5956 effect on student achievement through the two mediating variables. Using Equation 5.5, the standard error of the specific mediated effect $\hat{a}_1\hat{b}_1$ is equal to

$$0.1595 = \sqrt{(0.8401)^2(0.1568)^2 + (0.5690)^2(0.1580)^2}$$

As seen in the preceding example, when the regression coefficients and standard errors are small, it is very easy for rounding errors to affect the accuracy of the calculation of the standard error. Using Equation 5.6 gives the same answer, but it is less susceptible to computation errors because small numbers are not squared.

$$0.1595 = \frac{(0.8401)(0.5690)\sqrt{(5.319^2 + 3.629^2)}}{(5.319)(3.629)}$$

The 95% normal theory confidence limits for the $\hat{a}_1\hat{b}_1$ mediated effect are equal to

Lower confidence limit (LCL) = $0.4781 - 1.96\ (0.1595) = 0.1655$

Upper confidence limit (UCL) = $0.4781 + 1.96\ (0.1595) = 0.7907$

Corresponding asymmetric confidence limits based on the distribution of the product yielded confidence limits of 0.1986 and 0.8213. Applying the normal theory computations to the $\hat{a}_2\hat{b}_2$ mediated effect, the upper confidence limit was 0.2862 and the lower confidence limit was −0.0511. Using the distribution of the product method critical values, the confidence limits were 0.3106 and −0.0261. The $\hat{a}_1\hat{b}_1$ mediated effect ($s_{\hat{a}_1\hat{b}_1}$ = 0.1595) was statistically significant ($t_{\hat{a}_1\hat{b}_1}$ = 2.9975) and the $\hat{a}_2\hat{b}_2$ mediated effect ($s_{\hat{a}_2\hat{b}_2}$ = 0.0860) was not ($t_{\hat{a}_2\hat{b}_2}$ = 1.3663).

The standard error of the total mediated effect using Equation 5.8 is equal to 0.1892, yielding a z statistic of 3.1486 and lower and upper confidence limits of 0.2405 and 0.9507, respectively:

$$0.1892 = \sqrt{0.1595^2 + 0.0860^2 + 2(0.8401)(0.2219)(0.0079)}$$

The solution for the standard error of the total mediated effect estimator, $\hat{c} - \hat{c}'$ in Equation 5.9, is close to the standard error for the total mediated effect:

$$0.1777 = \sqrt{0.1734^2 + 0.2073^2 - \frac{(2)(8.3879^2)}{(40)(84.8487)}}$$

Using formula 5.10 or 5.11 for the standard error of the difference between two mediated effects, the difference between the two mediated effects is equal to 0.3605 with a standard error of 0.1729 yielding a z statistic of 2.0850 and leading to the conclusion that the two mediated effects were significantly different.

The EQS (Bentler, 1997) and LISREL (Jöreskog & Sörbom, 2001) covariance structure modeling programs include routines to compute the total mediated effect and the total direct effects and their standard errors. Procedures to test specific mediated effects are now available in the Mplus (Muthén & Muthén, 2004) program, although it is not difficult to compute these effects by hand using the methods described in this chapter. Bollen (1987) gives matrix routines to compute these quantities. Procedures to compute specific mediated effects in models with multiple independent, mediating, and dependent variables are described in chapter 6.

5.12 Assumptions

The assumptions outlined for the single mediator model also apply to the multiple mediator model. The multiple mediator model addresses some omitted variable limitations of the single mediator model because it explicitly includes additional mediating variables. It is still possible that some important mediating variables have been omitted or that the ordering of relations among variables is incorrect. For example, it is assumed that there are no interactions between the independent variable and each of the mediators. These interactions can be tested statistically, but a problem arises if there are many mediators because the number of possible interactions among the mediators and the independent variable can be very large. For example, with eight mediators and one independent variable, there are eight possible two-way interactions with the mediator and the independent variable alone and this does not include interactions among mediators or higher-way interactions. With so many possible relations among the variables, theory or prior research is often used to limit the number of interactions tested.

5.13 Summary

The purpose of this chapter was to describe mediation analysis for the multiple mediator model, which was a straightforward extension of methods to investigate the single mediator model. The causal steps approach to identifying mediators breaks down somewhat in the multiple mediator case, primarily because more than one mediated effect is present. There are specific mediated effects through each mediator, and there is a total mediated effect composed of all the mediated effects. The multiple mediator model is extended to more complicated models in later chapters in this book. In the next chapter, mediation analysis for path analysis models that incorporate multiple mediators, multiple independent variables, and multiple dependent variables is described. The ordinary least-squares approach to mediation described in chapters 3, 4, and 5 will no longer provide accurate estimation of coefficients and standard errors. With these more complex models, ordinary least squares will be replaced with the very general method of maximum likelihood estimation and related methods.

5.14 Exercises

5.1   The following estimates were obtained from a hypothetical study of the effects of exposure to a social influences based prevention program on subsequent alcohol use among 300 high school students. The data were simulated on the basis of a study by Hansen and Graham (1991). Each subject received a different number of sessions (X) of a social influences prevention program. After the program was delivered, subjects were measured on the perceived social norms regarding alcohol use (M1) and skills learned to resist drug use (M2). The variance of X was equal to 125.5616, the mean square error was equal to 10.1913 for Model 5.2 and the covariance between $\hat{b}_1$ and $\hat{b}_2$ was 0.0040.

Equation 5.1: $Y = i_1 + cX + e_1$
$$\hat{Y} = 40.4269 - 0.0014X$$
$$(0.0603)$$

Equation 5.2: $Y = i_2 + c'X + b_1M_1 + b_2M_2 + e_2$
$$\hat{Y} = 45.8271 + 0.0044\,X - 0.4830\,M1 + 0.3365\,M2$$
$$(0.0635)\quad\ (0.0647)\qquad\ (0.0562)$$

Equation 5.3: $M_1 = i_3 + a_1X + e_3$
$$\hat{M}_1 = 125.9704 + 0.3441X$$
$$(0.0471)$$

Equation 5.4: $M_2 = i_4 + a_2X + e_4$
$$\hat{M}_2 = 21.2260 + 0.0542X$$
$$(0.0129)$$

a.   Compute each mediated effect and standard error.
b.   Evaluate each step in the causal steps approach to establishing mediation. Describe the discrepancy between the conclusions of

applying the causal step approach and the approach described in part a.

c. What are the 95% confidence intervals for the mediated effects?

d. What is your conclusion about the effect of the program? What study would you do next?

5.2. Find a research article in which multiple mediators were addressed (several articles are described in the first three chapters of this book). Summarize how mediation was tested.

5.3. The following SAS computer output was obtained from a simulation of the Harris and Rosenthal (1985) results using coefficients for the four-mediator model described on p. 377 in figure 2 of their article. The four mediators were social climate (MED1), feedback (MED2), input (MED3), and output (MED4) as described at the beginning of this chapter.

a. Calculate each specific mediated effect and the total mediated effect.

b. Test the significance of each mediated effect and compute the confidence limits of each mediated effect using one of the formulas for the standard error of each effect.

c. Pick two mediated effects and test whether they are significantly different from each other.

```
Model: MODEL1
Dependent Variable: Y
```

Analysis of Variance

Source	DF	Sum of Squares	Mean Square	F Value	Prob>F
Model	1	4.07554	4.07554	3.239	0.0726
Error	398	500.72745	1.25811		
C Total	399	504.80299			

Root MSE	1.12165	R-square	0.0081	
Dep Mean	0.06019	Adj R-sq	0.0056	
C.V.	1863.56579			

Parameter Estimates

Variable	DF	Parameter Estimate	Standard Error	T for H0: Parameter=0	Prob > |T|
INTERCEP	1	0.061165	0.05608535	1.091	0.2761
X	1	-0.095112	0.05284463	-1.800	0.0726

```
Model: MODEL2
Dependent Variable: Y
```

Analysis of Variance

Source	DF	Sum of Squares	Mean Square	F Value	Prob>F
Model	5	80.09383	16.01877	14.861	0.0001
Error	394	424.70917	1.07794		
C Total	399	504.80299			

```
       Root MSE       1.03824     R-square     0.1587
       Dep Mean       0.06019     Adj R-sq     0.1480
       C.V.        1724.97684
```

Parameter Estimates

Variable	DF	Parameter Estimate	Standard Error	T for H0: Parameter=0	Prob > |T|
INTERCEP	1	0.045016	0.05208877	0.864	0.3880
X	1	-0.279107	0.05449605	-5.122	0.0001
MED1	1	0.281868	0.05323348	5.295	0.0001
MED2	1	0.059703	0.05495897	1.086	0.2780
MED3	1	0.335794	0.05427165	6.187	0.0001
MED4	1	0.114041	0.05350677	2.131	0.0337

```
Model: MODEL3
Dependent Variable: MED1
```

Analysis of Variance

Source	DF	Sum of Squares	Mean Square	F Value	Prob>F
Model	1	25.33725	25.33725	26.329	0.0001
Error	398	383.01093	0.96234		
C Total	399	408.34818			

```
       Root MSE       0.98099     R-square     0.0620
       Dep Mean       0.06380     Adj R-sq     0.0597
       C.V.        1537.58471
```

Parameter Estimates

Variable	DF	Parameter Estimate	Standard Error	T for H0: Parameter=0	Prob > |T|
INTERCEP	1	0.061367	0.04905173	1.251	0.2116
X	1	0.237149	0.04621743	5.131	0.0001

```
Model: MODEL4
Dependent Variable: MED2

                        Analysis of Variance

                        Sum of         Mean
        Source      DF   Squares       Square      F Value    Prob>F

        Model        1    7.74522      7.74522       8.573     0.0036
        Error      398  359.56140      0.90342
        C Total    399  367.30662

            Root MSE        0.95048    R-square     0.0211
            Dep Mean        0.01789    Adj R-sq     0.0186
            C.V.         5314.34360


                        Parameter Estimates

                    Parameter      Standard     T for H0:
      Variable  DF   Estimate         Error   Parameter=0    Prob > |T|

      INTERCEP   1   0.016540    0.04752644        0.348        0.7280
      X          1   0.131117    0.04478027        2.928        0.0036

Model: MODEL5
Dependent Variable: MED3

                        Analysis of Variance

                        Sum of         Mean
        Source      DF   Squares       Square      F Value    Prob>F

        Model        1   26.58042     26.58042      28.789     0.0001
        Error      398  367.46580      0.92328
        C Total    399  394.04622

            Root MSE        0.96088    R-square     0.0675
            Dep Mean        0.01191    Adj R-sq     0.0651
            C.V.         8065.58439


                        Parameter Estimates

                    Parameter      Standard     T for H0:
      Variable  DF   Estimate         Error   Parameter=0    Prob > |T|

      INTERCEP   1   0.009421    0.04804600        0.196        0.8447
      X          1   0.242897    0.04526981        5.366        0.0001
```

```
Model: MODEL6
Dependent Variable: MED4
```

Analysis of Variance

Source	DF	Sum of Squares	Mean Square	F Value	Prob>F
Model	1	26.69263	26.69263	28.123	0.0001
Error	398	377.75293	0.94913		
C Total	399	404.44556			

Root MSE	0.97423	R-square	0.0660
Dep Mean	-0.04397	Adj R-sq	0.0637
C.V.	-2215.64527		

Parameter Estimates

Variable	DF	Parameter Estimate	Standard Error	T for H0: Parameter=0	Prob > |T|
INTERCEP	1	-0.046468	0.04871388	-0.954	0.3407
X	1	0.243409	0.04589909	5.303	0.0001

6

Path Analysis
Mediation Models

> Obviously, we believe it is important to interpret patterns of direct and indirect causation in path models and other structural equation models. Such interpretations help us answer questions of the form, "How does variable X affect variable Y?," or "How much does mechanism Z contribute to the effect of X on Y?," or "Does mechanism Z contribute as much to explaining the effect of X on Y in the population A as in population B?" At the same time, we should be disappointed if our efforts to elucidate such causal interpretations were to lead researchers to generate vast quantities of uninteresting or meaningless components. Sometimes a detailed interpretation will speak to an important research question, and at other times it will not. We offer no substitute for the thoughtful interpretation of social data.
>
> **—Duane Alwin & Robert Hauser, 1975, p. 47**

6.1 Overview

This chapter extends the mediation model described in earlier chapters to more complex models. These models may have more than one independent variable, mediating variable, or dependent variable and are commonly called path analysis models. First, the matrix methods required for the specification of mediation in path analysis are described and illustrated using the two-mediator model from chapter 5. Matrix calculations for the mediated effects and their standard errors are described. Second, the mediation models are extended to include more than one mediator, more than one independent variable, and more than one dependent variable. With more than one dependent variable, ordinary least squares regression approaches are no longer appropriate because the correlations among the dependent variables cannot be simultaneously estimated and a new method must be used. As will be shown, however, the extensions of the general mediation model can be considered as a system of regression models whose parameters and standard errors are estimated simultaneously. An example from sociology is used to illustrate the programming of these models with the LISREL (Jöreskog & Sörbom, 2001), Mplus (Muthén & Muthén, 2004), and EQS (Bentler, 1997) covariance structure analysis computer programs.

The material covered in this chapter is not easy, although the chapter should not be difficult for persons already familiar with matrix algebra and covariance structure analysis. Persons not familiar with these topics may wish to review material in one of several textbooks on covariance structure analysis such as Bollen (1989), Kaplan (2000), or Kline (1998). Several other regression and multivariate statistics books such as Cohen, Cohen, West, and Aiken (2003) and Tatsuoka (1988) provide presentations of matrix algebra. The return on your investment in learning the material in this chapter is substantial. With the methods in this and related chapters, several assumptions of the simple mediation model can be investigated, including the influence of omitted variables, reliability of measures, and longitudinal relations.

6.2 The Structural Model and the Measurement Model

Covariance structure analysis is a general method to estimate and evaluate hypothesized models, in which the accuracy of the model is judged by the similarity of the predicted covariance matrix among the variables to the observed covariance matrix among the variables. There are two types of models in covariance structure analysis, the measurement model and the structural model. The structural model contains information on the relations among constructs. The measurement model describes how each measured variable is related to a latent or unobserved construct. The construct is called a latent construct or latent variable because it is not observed directly but must be inferred from variables that are measured. Measurement models typically include two or more observed variables hypothesized to measure a latent construct so that the part of each variable that is related to the construct can be separated from the error, the part of the variable that is unrelated to the construct. Models in which one observed variable is used to measure one latent variable are called manifest variable models. In this case, it is often assumed that the single variable is a perfect measure of the latent construct. Latent variable models and the measurement model used to define the latent variable are described in the next chapter. This chapter focuses on manifest variables and how they are related in the structural model. Once the structural model is understood, the general model incorporating both structural and measurement models is straightforward, as will be discussed in chapter 7.

Path analysis is another common name for analysis of relations among variables where each construct is measured by one variable. Path analysis is a method of estimating coefficients in the structural model that was originally invented by Sewall Wright (Wright, 1921, 1934). In the original articles and subsequent developments, path analysis focused on the decomposition of effects based on correlations or standardized variables. More recently, path analysis has come to describe the analysis of any structural model containing only manifest variables and no latent variables. Either the correlation matrix or the covariance matrix is analyzed. In this book, path analysis refers to the analysis of any manifest variable model.

6.3 Matrix Representation of Mediation Models

As models become more complex with multiple mediators, independent, and dependent variables, it becomes difficult to keep track of all the parameters in the regression equations. Matrices are commonly used to organize the information contained in complex models. Once the matrices are specified, matrix equations can be used to estimate important model effects, including mediation effects and their standard errors. Learning how to write mediation models in matrix form is complicated, but it makes the computation of more complex models much simpler. The use of matrix equations also makes it easier to understand the basis of the calculations.

The following structural model summarizes the matrix calculations in the general manifest variable mediator model using Greek symbols to represent matrices and parameters:

$$\eta = B\eta + \Gamma\xi + \zeta \tag{6.1}$$

where η is a vector of dependent variables, ξ is a vector of independent variables and ζ is a vector representing estimates of residuals. The B matrix codes the coefficients among the dependent variables and the Γ matrix codes the coefficients relating independent variables to dependent variables. Mediating variable coefficients are represented in both the B and Γ matrices because a mediating variable is both a dependent variable in the regression relating the independent variable to the mediator and an independent variable in the regression relating the mediator to the dependent variable. In Equation 6.1, there can be more than one independent and dependent variable so this model represents a system of equations rather than single equations as discussed in chapters 3, 4, and 5. In addition to the B and Γ matrices, two additional matrices, Ψ and Φ, are used to represent variances and covariances. The elements in each matrix are represented by Greek letters and subscripts to uniquely identify each parameter. Four more matrices will be added in chapter 7 to incorporate measurement models and another four matrices will be included to model mean structure in chapter 8. The Greek notation used in this book is one of the most widely used notational method for specifying matrices in covariance structure analysis.

By specifying the mediation relations in matrix form, a matrix equation for the predicted covariance matrix is obtained. An iterative procedure, usually maximum likelihood, is used to estimate the parameters of the equation that make the predicted covariance matrix closest to the observed covariance matrix. Several measures of model fit or closeness of the predicted and observed covariance matrix are available. One of these tests is the χ^2 test of model fit. If the χ^2 test is statistically significant, the model is rejected as an adequate representation of the observed covariance matrix. The χ^2 test is based on the parameters estimated in the model. All of the parameters specified in the matrix equations represent free parameters to be estimated by the model. The total number of possible parameters is equal to the number of variances and covariances among the variables in the model. The difference between the number of free variances and covariances among variables in the model and the number of parameters estimated in the model provides the degrees of freedom for the χ^2 test. The statistical significance of the χ^2 test of model fit is included in the output of covariance structure computer programs.

One problem with the χ^2 test is that it is a function of sample size so that very highly significant χ^2 values may be obtained simply because the sample size is large. Several alternative measures of fit have been proposed (Hu & Bentler, 1999). To conserve space in this book only the root mean square error of approximation (RMSEA) (square root of $((\chi^2/\text{degrees of freedom}-1)/(\text{sample size}-1)))$ will be used. The RMSEA provides a measure of the extent to which the deviations from predicted and observed elements of the covariance matrix are large or small, adjusted for sample size. Generally models with a RMSEA of ≤ 0.05 are good models and models with a RMSEA > 0.1 represent poor fit. Confidence limits for the RMSEA are also available and provide more information on the fit of the model.

Models are specified in covariance structure analysis computer programs in two general ways. The first method specifies the equations that comprise the model along with the variances and covariances among the error terms in the model. This approach to specifying models is the one that we have used in the book so far. This method is used in the CALIS LINEQS program, Mplus (Muthén & Muthén, 2004), and in EQS (Bentler, 1997). The second method is to specify the matrices and parameters of these matrices in the program. This matrix specification method is the method used by LISREL (Jöreskog & Sörbom, 2001) and other programs. These programs are described in this chapter and additional programs are included on the CD that comes with this book.

6.4 Matrix Representation of the Two-Mediator Model

The regression coefficients and standard errors from the two-mediator model analysis described in chapter 5 are used to illustrate the matrix formulas for the calculation of indirect effects (mediated effects) and their standard errors. The new symbols and notation simplify the organization and computation of indirect effects for more complex models. In Equation 6.1, the η vector contains the dependent variables, Y, M_1, and M_2, the ξ vector contains the X variable, and the ζ vector contains the errors, e, described in chapter 5. To make these differences more concrete, the matrix form of the structural equation for the two-mediator model discussed in chapter 5 and defined by Equations 5.2, through 5.4 is shown in matrix form in Equation 6.2:

$$\begin{bmatrix} M_1 \\ M_2 \\ Y \end{bmatrix} = \begin{bmatrix} 0 & 0 & 0 \\ 0 & 0 & 0 \\ b_1 & b_2 & 0 \end{bmatrix} \begin{bmatrix} M_1 \\ M_2 \\ Y \end{bmatrix} + \begin{bmatrix} a_1 \\ a_2 \\ c' \end{bmatrix} X + \begin{bmatrix} e_1 \\ e_2 \\ e_3 \end{bmatrix} \tag{6.2}$$

The matrix equation using Greek letters to code parameters is shown in Equation 6.3 and Figure 6.1 shows the path diagram.

$$\begin{bmatrix} \eta_1 \\ \eta_2 \\ \eta_3 \end{bmatrix} = \begin{bmatrix} 0 & 0 & 0 \\ 0 & 0 & 0 \\ \beta_{31} & \beta_{32} & 0 \end{bmatrix} \begin{bmatrix} \eta_1 \\ \eta_2 \\ \eta_3 \end{bmatrix} + \begin{bmatrix} \gamma_1 \\ \gamma_2 \\ \gamma_3 \end{bmatrix} \xi + \begin{bmatrix} \zeta_1 \\ \zeta_2 \\ \zeta_3 \end{bmatrix} \tag{6.3}$$

The matrix equation from Equation 6.3 corresponds to Equations 6.4 through 6.6, which represent the same information as Equations 5.3, 5.4, and 5.2, respectively.

$$\eta_1 = \gamma_1 \xi + \zeta_1 \tag{6.4}$$

$$\eta_2 = \gamma_2 \xi + \zeta_2 \tag{6.5}$$

$$\eta_3 = \beta_{31} \eta_1 + \beta_{32} \eta_2 + \gamma_3 \xi + \zeta_3 \tag{6.6}$$

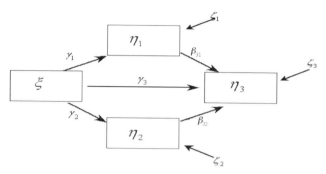

Figure 6.1. Two mediator model with Greek notation.

There are two more specifications in the covariance structure analysis model that must be made for the accurate estimation of the two-mediator model. The variances of each variable and the covariance between the mediators must be specified for the estimation of the two-mediator model, but this is not reflected in Equation 6.3. A Ψ matrix specifies the covariances among the dependent variables. In this example, the Ψ matrix is a 3×3 matrix, with variances of the η variables along the diagonal, that is, $\psi_{11} = \text{Var}(\eta_1)$. Note that the two mediators η_1 and η_2, are dependent as well as independent variables in this model. The ψ_{21} element of the matrix codes the covariance between the two mediators. The second specification is the Φ matrix which is a 1×1 matrix containing the variance of the single ξ variable, ϕ_{11}.

$$\Psi = \begin{bmatrix} \psi_{11} & 0 & 0 \\ \psi_{21} & \psi_{22} & 0 \\ 0 & 0 & \psi_{33} \end{bmatrix}, \quad \Phi = [\phi_{11}]$$

Once specified in this way, the parameters of the model can be estimated with ordinary least squares regression as described in chapter 5 or by other more general approaches including maximum likelihood. The maximum likelihood (ML) estimation procedure is a general method that can be used to estimate the parameters for a large number of models. The method uses an iterative procedure to estimate the parameters of the model that have the greatest likelihood of generating the observed covariance matrix among the variables in the model. In the two-mediator model, there are 10 estimated parameters, γ_1, γ_2, γ_3, β_{31}, β_{32}, ψ_{11}, ψ_{22}, ψ_{33}, ψ_{21}, and ϕ_{11}. There are 10 free variances and covariances in the covariance matrix among the four variables (number of variables times number of variables plus 1 divided by 2:4(4 + 1))/2 = 10). Because the number of estimated parameters equals the number of free variances and covariances, the model is called a saturated model and there are no degrees of freedom so the χ^2 measure of fit equals zero. If the direct effect coefficient, γ_3 (corresponding to the c' coefficient in chapter 5), was set to zero then the χ^2 test would have 1 degree of freedom. Because there are positive degrees of freedom, the χ^2 test of significance tests whether the complete mediation model is an adequate representation of the data. A general approach to comparing models is also available based on the difference in χ^2 values between two nested models where the smaller model contains fewer parameters than the larger model. The difference between the χ^2 for the two models provides a statistical test of whether the additional parameters in the larger model are equal to zero. More on these approaches can be found in Bollen (1989), Kaplan (2000), and Kline (1998).

6.5 EQS Code for the Two-Mediator Model

The EQS program for the two-mediator model for the data from chapter 5 is shown in Table 6.1 and the output is shown in Table 6.2. The number of cases, variables, method of estimation, and location of the raw data set (in

Table 6.1   EQS Program for the Two-Mediator Model

```
/TITLE
  CHAPTER 6 EXAMPLE EQS MEDIATION ANALYSIS
/SPECIFICATIONS
  CAS=40; VAR=5; ME=ML; DA='c:\twomed.txt'; MA=RAW;
/LABEL
  V1=S; V2=X; V3=M1; V4=M2; V5=y;
/EQUATIONS
  V3 = 1*V2 + E1;
  V4 = 1*V2 + E2;
  V5 = 1*V2 + 1*v3+ 1*v4 + E3;
/VARIANCES
  V2 = 1*;
  E1 =  2*; E2 = 2*; E3 = 2*;
/COVARIANCES
  E1,E2 = 1*;
/PRINT
EFFECTS=YES;PARAMETERS=YES;
/END
```

Table 6.2   Selected EQS Output for the Two-Mediator Model

MEASUREMENT EQUATIONS WITH STANDARD ERRORS AND TEST
STATISTICS

```
M1  = V3  = 0.840*V2 + 1.000 E1
            0.156
            5.388

M2  = V4  = 0.222*V2 + 1.000 E2
            0.144
            1.540

Y      = V5 = 0.569*V3 +   0.530*V4 +   0.112*V2 + 1.000 E3
              0.151          0.163         0.199
              3.777          3.250         0.563
```

MAXIMUM LIKELIHOOD SOLUTION (NORMAL DISTRIBUTION THEORY)
VARIANCES OF INDEPENDENT VARIABLES

```
V             F
V2 - X        84.849*
              19.214
              04.416
```

MAXIMUM LIKELIHOOD SOLUTION (NORMAL DISTRIBUTION THEORY)
VARIANCES OF INDEPENDENT VARIABLES

```
E             D
E1 - M1       80.447*
              18.218
              04.416

E2 - M2       68.742*
              15.567
              04.416

              I
E3 - Y        64.944*
              14.707
              04.416
```

MAXIMUM LIKELIHOOD SOLUTION (NORMAL DISTRIBUTION THEORY)
COVARIANCES AMONG INDEPENDENT VARIABLES

```
E             D
E2 - M2       -22.067*
E1 - M1        12.421
              -1.777
```

an external file on the c: directory) is specified in the SPECIFICATIONS section. The EQUATIONS section contains the equations for the two-mediator model. The VARIANCES section specifies the variances of X along with the error variances in each of the regression equations. The COVARIANCES section specifies that the covariance between the two mediators is free to vary. The PRINT section requests that an effect decomposition, EFFECTS, is included in the output and the correlations among the estimates are requested with the PARAMETERS=YES command. The use of this optional output will be described later in this chapter.

The EQS output for the regression estimates, standard errors, and t statistics are shown in Table 6.2. The estimated variances and covariance between the two mediators are also given. Note that the estimates are comparable to the results for ordinary least squares regression analysis.

A statistical test of complete mediation can also be conducted by estimating a model with γ_3 fixed to zero and comparing the χ^2 from this model with the χ^2 from the saturated model. The difference between the two χ^2 values, 0.324, is nonsignificant with 1 degree of freedom so the complete mediation model cannot be rejected. Note that because the saturated model χ^2 is equal to 0, the test of the difference between the saturated model and the model with γ_3 fixed to zero is the same as the model fit χ^2 for the model with γ_3 fixed to zero. The RMSEA for this model, .000, also suggests excellent fit for the complete mediation model. Note that relations in the model could be further investigated with χ^2 difference tests; for example, a test of whether the relation from η_2 to η_3, $\hat{\beta}_{32}$, is statistically significant.

The results from EQS can also be put into matrix format as shown in the following:

$$\hat{\Gamma} = \begin{bmatrix} 0.8401 \\ 0.2219 \\ 0.1122 \end{bmatrix} \quad \hat{\beta} = \begin{bmatrix} 0 & 0 & 0 \\ 0 & 0 & 0 \\ 0.5690 & 0.5297 & 0 \end{bmatrix}$$

$$\hat{\Psi} = \begin{bmatrix} 80.4470 & -22.0670 & 0 \\ -22.0670 & 68.7425 & 0 \\ 0 & 0 & 64.9442 \end{bmatrix} \quad \hat{\Phi} = [84.8487]$$

6.6 LISREL Program for the Two-Mediator Model

The EQS program specified the regression equations comprising the relations in the model. The LISREL program instead specifies the matrices as described earlier in this chapter. The LISREL program in Table 6.3 specifies each matrix in the analysis. These matrices are the B, Γ, Ψ,

Table 6.3 LISREL Program for the Two-Mediator Model

```
Two-Mediator Model
DA NI=5 NO=40 MA=CM
RA FI=c:\twomed.txt
LA
'obs' 'x' 'M1' 'M2' 'Y'
se
3 4 5 2 1
MO NY=3 NX=1 BE=FU,FI GA=FR PS=FU,FI
FR BE 3 1 BE 3 2
FR PS 1 1 PS 2 2 PS 3 3 PS 2 1
OU ef se tv pc ef ss   nd=4
```

and Φ matrices, which are given by two-letter keywords in LISREL: BE, GA, PS, and PH, respectively. The GA matrix is 3×1 with the following parameters, γ_1, γ_2, and γ_3. In the 3×3 BE matrix, the β_{31} and β_{32} parameters are free. The 3×3 PS matrix includes ψ_{11}, ψ_{22}, ψ_{33}, and ψ_{21}. ϕ_{11} is the single element in the 1×1 PH matrix. The output from the LISREL analysis is shown in Table 6.4.

6.7 Decomposition of Effects

Alwin and Hauser (1975) described a general conceptual and statistical approach for the decomposition of total effects into direct and indirect effects for the path analysis model. They integrated their own prior work and earlier work by others (Duncan, Featherman, & Duncan, 1972) and focused on understanding the complex relations among variables. Fox (1980) clarified this earlier work by showing that the total effects (T) among the variables for models such as the two-mediator model example in chapter 5, is equal to:

$$T = \sum_{k=1}^{\infty} \mathbf{B}^{*k}$$

(6.7)

where k is equal to powers of the direct effects in the model, and B* is a matrix of direct effects among the variables. T is defined if the infinite sum converges. To describe this method, assume that the two-mediator model described in chapter 5 is reparameterized so that B and Γ matrices are included in a 4×4 matrix, B*, which represents all the direct effects in the model.

Table 6.4   Selected LISREL Output for the Two-Mediator Model

LISREL Estimates (Maximum Likelihood)

BETA

	M1	M2	Y
M1	—	—	—
M2	—	—	—
Y	0.5690	0.5297	—
	(0.1526)	(0.1651)	
	3.7282	3.2082	

GAMMA

	X
M1	0.8401
	(0.1580)
	5.3188
M2	0.2219
	(0.1460)
	1.5197
Y	0.1122
	(0.2018)
	0.5558

PHI

X
84.8487
(19.4656)
4.3589

PSI

	M1	M2	Y
M1	80.4470		
	(18.4558)		
	4.3589		
M2	−22.0670	68.7425	
	(12.5835)	(15.7706)	
	−1.7536	4.3589	
Y	—	—	64.9442
			(14.8992)

(*continued*)

Table 6.4 (Continued)

Covariance Matrix of Parameter Estimates

	BE 3,1	BE 3,2	GA 1,1	GA 2,1	GA 3,1	PH 1,1
BE 3,1	0.0233					
BE 3,2	0.0075	0.0273				
GA 1,1	0.0000	0.0000	0.0250			
GA 2,1	0.0000	0.0000	-0.0068	0.0213		
GA 3,1	-0.0212	-0.0123	0.0000	0.0000	0.0407	
PH 1,1	0.0000	0.0000	0.0000	0.0000	0.0000	378.9108
PS 1,1	0.0000	0.0000	0.0000	0.0000	0.0000	0.0000
PS 2,1	0.0000	0.0000	0.0000	0.0000	0.0000	0.0000
PS 2,2	0.0000	0.0000	0.0000	0.0000	0.0000	0.0000
PS 3,3	0.0000	0.0000	0.0000	0.0000	0.0000	0.0000

Covariance Matrix of Parameter Estimates

	PS 1,1	PS 2,1	PS 2,2	PS 3,3	AL 1	AL 2
PS 1,1	340.6168					
PS 2,1	-93.4329	158.3442				
PS 2,2	25.6291	-79.8390	248.7120			
PS 3,3	0.0000	0.0000	0.0000	221.9865		

Two-Mediator Model

Standardized Solution

BETA

	M1	M2	Y
M1	—	—	—
M2	—	—	—
Y	0.5708	0.3830	—

GAMMA

	X
M1	0.6533
M2	0.2394
Y	0.0875

Correlation Matrix of Y and X

	M1	M2	Y	X
M1	1.0000			
M2	-0.0618	1.0000		
Y	0.6043	0.3687	1.0000	
x	0.6533	0.2394	0.5520	1.0000

PSI

	M1	M2	Y
M1	0.5732		
M2	-0.2181	0.9427	
Y	—	—	0.4656

$$B^* = \begin{bmatrix} 0 & 0 & 0 & 0 \\ \gamma_1 & 0 & 0 & 0 \\ \gamma_2 & 0 & 0 & 0 \\ \gamma_3 & \beta_{31} & \beta_{32} & 0 \end{bmatrix}$$

Applying Equation 6.7 yields the following matrix of total effects:

$$T = B^* + B^{*2} + B^{*3} + \cdots = \begin{bmatrix} 0 & 0 & 0 & 0 \\ \gamma_1 & 0 & 0 & 0 \\ \gamma_2 & 0 & 0 & 0 \\ \gamma_3 + \gamma_1\beta_{31} + \gamma_2\beta_{32} & \beta_{31} & \beta_{32} & 0 \end{bmatrix}$$

Note that the B^{*3} or higher powered matrix is zero so that only the B^* and B^{*2} matrix are combined to form the total effects matrix. The total indirect effects, I, can then be calculated from the difference of the total effects and the direct effects.

$$I = T - B^* \tag{6.8}$$

$$I = \begin{bmatrix} 0 & 0 & 0 & 0 \\ \gamma_1 & 0 & 0 & 0 \\ \gamma_2 & 0 & 0 & 0 \\ \gamma_3 + \gamma_1\beta_{31} + \gamma_2\beta_{32} & \beta_{31} & \beta_{32} & 0 \end{bmatrix} - \begin{bmatrix} 0 & 0 & 0 & 0 \\ \gamma_1 & 0 & 0 & 0 \\ \gamma_2 & 0 & 0 & 0 \\ \gamma_3 & \beta_{31} & \beta_{32} & 0 \end{bmatrix}$$

$$= \begin{bmatrix} 0 & 0 & 0 & 0 \\ 0 & 0 & 0 & 0 \\ 0 & 0 & 0 & 0 \\ \gamma_1\beta_{31} + \gamma_2\beta_{32} & 0 & 0 & 0 \end{bmatrix}$$

Using the two-mediator model from chapter 5 as an example, the following matrices illustrate that the total effects minus the direct effects yields the total indirect effects. In this case, there is one total indirect effect, which equals 0.5956. Note that this method does not provide information on the specific indirect effect through M1 and the specific indirect effect through M2. The general effect decomposition methods do not yield specific indirect effects, only the total indirect effects.

$$\hat{I} = \begin{bmatrix} 0 & 0 & 0 & 0 \\ 0.8401 & 0 & 0 & 0 \\ 0.2219 & 0 & 0 & 0 \\ 0.7078 & 0.5690 & 0.5297 & 0 \end{bmatrix} - \begin{bmatrix} 0 & 0 & 0 & 0 \\ 0.8401 & 0 & 0 & 0 \\ 0.2219 & 0 & 0 & 0 \\ 0.1122 & 0.5690 & 0.5297 & 0 \end{bmatrix}$$

$$= \begin{bmatrix} 0 & 0 & 0 & 0 \\ 0 & 0 & 0 & 0 \\ 0 & 0 & 0 & 0 \\ 0.5956 & 0 & 0 & 0 \end{bmatrix}$$

This matrix formulation can be applied in a straightforward manner for many models. However, the matrix formulation must be expanded to incorporate models that can handle more than one independent variable and more than one dependent variable. The general matrix equations for the total effects, $T_{\eta\eta}$, and total indirect effects, $I_{\eta\eta}$, of η on η that include the different specification of B and Γ matrices as described in Equation 6.1 are shown in Equations 6.9 and 6.10, where I is an identify matrix with the same dimensions as matrix B.

$$T_{\eta\eta} = (I - B)^{-1} - I \tag{6.9}$$

$$I_{\eta\eta} = (I - B)^{-1} - I - B \tag{6.10}$$

The total effects, $T_{\eta\xi}$, and total indirect effects, $I_{\eta\xi}$, of ξ on η are shown in Equations 6.11 and 6.12, respectively.

$$T_{\eta\xi} = (I - B)^{-1}\Gamma \tag{6.11}$$

$$I_{\eta\xi} = (I - B)^{-1}\Gamma - \Gamma \tag{6.12}$$

The values for B and Γ when substituted in these equations yield the same estimate of the total indirect effect of 0.5956 for the two-mediator model in $I_{\eta\xi}$.

6.8 Standard Errors of Indirect Effects

In one of the most important papers on mediation, Sobel (1982) derived the large sample standard errors of the matrix of total indirect effects. Sobel used the multivariate delta method to find these standard errors, which requires a matrix of partial derivatives of the indirect effects and the covariance matrix among coefficients estimates in the model as described in chapter 4. Matrix calculus methods were used to derive the matrix of partial derivatives necessary for pre- and post-multiplying the covariance matrix among the parameter estimates to obtain the standard errors of indirect effects.

The general equation for matrices of partial derivatives is described here first. After that a method that is generally easier to use for the calculation of indirect effect standard errors derived later by Sobel (1986) is given.

The variance of the indirect effects is obtained by pre- and post-multiplying the covariance matrix among the parameter estimates by the matrix of partial derivatives of the matrices of indirect effects, as shown in Equation 6.13:

$$VAR = N^{-1}(\partial F / \partial \hat{\theta}) \, \Sigma(\hat{\theta}) \, (\partial F / \partial \hat{\theta})' \qquad (6.13)$$

where VAR is the matrix of variances (along the diagonal) and covariances of the indirect effects, $\Sigma(\hat{\theta})$ is the covariance matrix among the parameter estimates, $(\partial F / \partial \hat{\theta})$ is the vector (or matrix) of partial derivatives of the effects, and N is sample size. Sobel (1986) presented general matrix equations for the partial derivatives of indirect effects that use specialized matrices to select partial derivatives indicated by V_β and V_Γ. As described in Sobel (1986, pp. 170–171), the partial derivatives for each indirect effect matrix $I_{\eta\eta}$ and $I_{\eta\xi}$ are given in Equations 6.14 and 6.15, respectively.

$$\partial \text{vec} \, I_{\eta\eta} / \partial \hat{\theta} = V_B'((I-B)^{-1} \otimes ((I-B)^{-1})' - I_m \otimes I_m) \qquad (6.14)$$

$$\partial \text{vec} \, I_{\eta\xi} / \partial \hat{\theta} = V_B'((I-B)^{-1} \, \Gamma \otimes ((I-B)^{-1})') + V_\Gamma'(I_n \otimes ((I-B)^{-1} - I)') \qquad (6.15)$$

In Equations 6.14 and 6.15, vec indicates that the elements in the indirect effect matrices are reshaped into a column vector and $\otimes$ is the Kronecker or tensor product. The dimensions of the matrices are given by the number of η variables, m, the number of ξ variables, n, the number of Y variables, p, and the number of X variables, q. The dimension values are used to construct identity and output matrices necessary for the matrix derivatives. The V_β and V_Γ matrices select partial derivatives for each parameter estimated. For most applications these matrices consist of 0s and 1s. The number of columns of V_β and V_Γ are equal to the number of direct effect parameters estimated. The number of rows is equal to the number of elements in each subscripted matrix, for example, V_β has m^2 rows for elements in the B matrix and V_Γ has m times n rows for elements in the Γ matrix.

6.9 Standard Errors of Indirect Effects for the Two-Mediator Model

The V_β and V_Γ matrices for the two-mediator model are shown. For the two-mediator model, the number of columns corresponds to the five direct effect parameters in the following order: β_{31}, β_{32}, γ_1, γ_2, and γ_3. V_β has m² rows (0, 0, β_{31}, 0, 0, β_{32}, 0, 0, and 0) and V_Γ has m times n equals three rows, which is equal to the number of parameters estimated (γ_1, γ_2, and γ_3). For the two-mediator model V_β is 9×5 and V_Γ is 3×5. In each matrix there is a one where the same element is in the column and the row; for example, the 3,1 element of V_β is one because the first column and third row corresponds to the β_{31} parameter and the 2,4 element of the V_Γ matrix is one because the second row and fourth column correspond to the γ_2 parameter.

$$V_B = \begin{bmatrix} 0 & 0 & 0 & 0 & 0 \\ 0 & 0 & 0 & 0 & 0 \\ 1 & 0 & 0 & 0 & 0 \\ 0 & 0 & 0 & 0 & 0 \\ 0 & 0 & 0 & 0 & 0 \\ 0 & 1 & 0 & 0 & 0 \\ 0 & 0 & 0 & 0 & 0 \\ 0 & 0 & 0 & 0 & 0 \\ 0 & 0 & 0 & 0 & 0 \end{bmatrix} \quad V_\Gamma = \begin{bmatrix} 0 & 0 & 1 & 0 & 0 \\ 0 & 0 & 0 & 1 & 0 \\ 0 & 0 & 0 & 0 & 1 \end{bmatrix}$$

The vector of estimates, $\hat{\theta}$, and covariance matrix among these five estimates are shown. The estimated direct effect parameters of the model are $\hat{\beta}_{31}$, $\hat{\beta}_{32}$, $\hat{\gamma}_1$, $\hat{\gamma}_2$, and $\hat{\gamma}_3$, and are contained in $\hat{\theta}$. Note that covariances among these five estimates are zero with four exceptions; the covariances between $\hat{\beta}_{31}$ and $\hat{\beta}_{32}$, $\hat{\beta}_{31}$ and $\hat{\gamma}_3$, $\hat{\beta}_{32}$ and $\hat{\gamma}_3$, and $\hat{\gamma}_1$ and $\hat{\gamma}_2$ are all nonzero. Furthermore, $\hat{\gamma}_1$ and $\hat{\gamma}_2$ are uncorrelated with $\hat{\beta}_{31}$ and $\hat{\beta}_{32}$.

$$\hat{\Sigma}_\theta = \begin{bmatrix} 0.0233 & 0.0075 & 0.0000 & 0.0000 & -0.0212 \\ 0.0075 & 0.0273 & 0.0000 & 0.0000 & -0.0123 \\ 0.0000 & 0.0000 & 0.0250 & -0.0068 & 0.0000 \\ 0.0000 & 0.0000 & -0.0068 & 0.0213 & 0.0000 \\ -0.0212 & -0.0123 & 0.0000 & 0.0000 & 0.0407 \end{bmatrix} \quad \hat{\theta} = \begin{bmatrix} 0.5690 \\ 0.5297 \\ 0.8401 \\ 0.2219 \\ 0.1122 \end{bmatrix}$$

For the two-mediator model, there are no indirect effects of η on η so the indirect effect equation is not necessary for this model. There are indirect effects of ξ on η. Using LISREL estimates, applying Equations 6.12 and 6.15 for the derivatives and the covariance matrix among the estimates yields the following matrix of indirect effects and standard errors of the indirect effects. In this case the matrices include one indirect effect and one standard error of the indirect effect:

$$\hat{I}_{\xi\eta} = \begin{bmatrix} 0 \\ 0 \\ 0.5956 \end{bmatrix} \quad \hat{V}_{\xi\eta} = \begin{bmatrix} 0 \\ 0 \\ 0.175 \end{bmatrix}$$

The total indirect effect has the same value as for ordinary least squares regression described in chapter 5. The standard error is also close. Note that there is only one total indirect effect that includes all indirect effects, which in this case corresponds to the sum of the indirect effect through M1 and the indirect effect through M2.

6.10 Effect Decomposition in EQS

In the EQS program in Table 6.1, the code EFFECTS=YES is included. This EQS option prints out the total indirect effects and their standard errors. Because of the small sample size, estimates from EQS, LISREL, and Mplus differ somewhat. The total indirect effect from EQS was equal to 0.596 with a standard error of 0.172 as shown in Table 6.5. The effect decomposition for standardized regression coefficients are also given.

6.11 Effect Decomposition in LISREL

In the LISREL OU line, the EF keyword was included so that effect decomposition results are printed out. The same type of output described earlier for EQS is given in the LISREL output and is shown in Table 6.6.

Table 6.5   EQS Effect Decomposition Output for the Two-Mediator Model

Decomposition of Effects with Nonstandardized Values			
Parameter Total Effects			
M1	=V3 =	.840*V2	+ 1.000 E1
M2	=V4 =	.222*V2	+ 1.000 E2
Y	=V5 =	.569*V3	+ .530*V4 + .708*V2 +
		.569 E1	+ .530 E2 + 1.000 E3

Decomposition of Effects with Nonstandardized Values			
Parameter Indirect Effects			
Y	=V5 =	0.596*V2	+ 0.569 E1	+ 0.530 E2
		0.172	0.151	0.163
		3.455	3.777	3.250

Table 6.6   LISREL Effect Decomposition
Output for the Two-Mediator Model

Total and Indirect Effects

```
Total Effects of X on Y

              X
M1        0.8401
         (0.1580)
          5.3188
M2        0.2219
          0.1460)
          1.5197
Y         0.7078
         (0.1734)
          4.0810

Indirect Effects of X on Y

              X
M1        —
M2        —
Y         0.5956
         (0.1747)
          3.4099

Total Effects of Y on Y

              M1        M2         Y
M1        —         —          —
M2        —         —          —
Y         0.5690    0.5297      —
         (0.1526)  (0.1651)
          3.7282    3.2082
```

6.12 Specific Indirect Effects

As you probably noticed, the aforementioned indirect effect and standard error formulas are for the standard errors of total indirect effects. The standard error of the total indirect effect is included in the output of both the LISREL and EQS programs. For complex models, the total indirect effect may contain several indirect effects, and only one or a few of them may be of substantive interest. The current versions of EQS, LISREL, and AMOS do not print out specific indirect effects and their standard errors.

As shown in Table 6.7 for the two-mediator model, the total indirect effect can be decomposed into two specific indirect effects. The results

Table 6.7 Specific Indirect Effects and Standard Errors
for the Two-Mediator Model

Effect	Parameters	Estimate	Standard Error
X→M1→Y	$\gamma_1\beta_{31}$	0.4780	0.1566
X→M2→Y	$\gamma_2\beta_{32}$	0.1175	0.0860

for specific indirect effects are often summarized in tables that contain the specific indirect effects and their standard errors. Table 6.7 shows this type of table for the two-mediator model. The Effect column contains the specific indirect effect of interest, for example, X→M1→Y, corresponding to the specific indirect effect of X to M1 to Y. Note that the specific indirect effect through social climate (M1) is 3.05 (0.4780/0.1566) times larger than its standard error, and the indirect effect through amount of information input (M2) is only 1.37 (0.1175/0.0860) times its standard error, leading to the conclusion that only the social climate mediator was statistically significant. Table 6.7 could also be enhanced to include confidence limits such as LCL = .0604 and UCL = .3197 product distribution confidence limits for X to M1 to Y. As the models become more complex, tables of specific indirect effects can be quite large, illustrating the number of indirect effects in more complex models.

The estimates of specific indirect effects can be obtained by setting the B and Γ coefficients not involved in the indirect effect to 0 and calculating the indirect effects using Equations 6.10 and 6.12. The standard errors of these specific indirect effects can be obtained by changing the V_β matrix and the V_Γ matrix to correspond to the parameters of interest. For the two-mediator model, this is done by altering the V_β matrix so that the partial derivatives for certain parameters are not included in the calculation of the standard error. For example, to get the indirect effect through M1, include only the relevant estimates in the B and Γ matrices; that is, β_{32}, γ_2, and γ_3 are set to zero. Set element 6,2 of the V_β matrix to zero and elements 2,4 and 3,5 to zero in the V_Γ matrix. When this is done, the indirect effect through M1 equals 0.4780, and its standard error is 0.1566. The indirect effect through M2 is obtained by setting β_{31}, γ_1, and γ_3 equal to 0, setting element 3,1 of the V_β matrix to zero, and elements 1,3 and 3,5 in the V_Γ matrix equal to zero. Applying Equations 6.11 and 6.12 gives an indirect effect estimate of 0.1175 and a standard error of 0.0860. For more complex mediation models, the computation of specific indirect effects still follows these procedures, but calculation of the standard errors of specific indirect effects requires more detailed use of the V matrices and the covariance matrix among the estimates.

6.13 Hand Calculations for the Standard Error of Indirect Effects

Often researchers are interested in specific indirect effects but altering the B, Γ, V_β, and V_Γ matrices to calculate the specific indirect effect and standard error using a matrix programming language can be cumbersome. Another method can be used in many situations based on the formulas described earlier in this book for the variance of a function of random variables. Like the matrix equation method described earlier, this method uses the coefficients and the covariance matrix among the coefficients for the indirect effect of interest. The coefficients and standard errors are included in the output of all covariance structure analysis programs. The covariance matrix among parameter estimates requires a keyword for it to be printed out as part of analysis, for example, PARAMETERS=YES in the output statement for EQS, PC for LISREL, PCOVES for CALIS, TECH3 for Mplus, and $covest for AMOS. The covariance among parameter estimates is required for the calculation of standard errors of indirect effects. In some situations, especially with very large samples, the covariance matrix contains very small values, which can cause rounding errors in the calculations. In this and other situations, calculations are more accurate if the correlation among parameters and the standard errors of the coefficients are used to obtain the covariance matrix by pre- and post-multiplying the correlation matrix by the vector of standard errors of the parameters.

The standard error for any two-path indirect effect, $\hat{\gamma}\hat{\beta}$, can be obtained using Equation 6.16, but here $\hat{\beta}$ is used in place of the $\hat{b}$ coefficient and $\hat{\gamma}$ is used in place of the $\hat{a}$ coefficient:

$$\sigma^2_{\hat{\beta}\hat{\gamma}} = \hat{\gamma}^2\sigma^2_{\hat{\beta}} + \hat{\beta}^2\sigma^2_{\hat{\gamma}} + 2\hat{\gamma}\hat{\beta}\sigma_{\hat{\gamma}\hat{\beta}} \tag{6.16}$$

If there is a zero covariance term between $\hat{\gamma}$ and $\hat{\beta}$, $\sigma_{\hat{\gamma}\hat{\beta}}$, in this equation, the equation for this standard error is the same as Equation 3.6. If the covariance between $\hat{\gamma}$ and $\hat{\beta}$ is nonzero, then the following term should be added as in the formula, $2\hat{\gamma}\hat{\beta}\sigma_{\hat{\gamma}\hat{\beta}}$, where $\sigma_{\hat{\gamma}\hat{\beta}}$ is the covariance between $\hat{\gamma}$ and $\hat{\beta}$. If the covariance matrix among the estimates is not available, the correlation among the estimates and the standard errors of the coefficients can be used to compute the covariance between $\hat{\gamma}$ and $\hat{\beta}$, $\sigma_{\hat{\gamma}\hat{\beta}}$, which equals $r_{\hat{\gamma}\hat{\beta}}\sigma_{\hat{\gamma}}\sigma_{\hat{\beta}}$, where $r_{\hat{\gamma}\hat{\beta}}$ is the correlation between $\hat{\gamma}$ and $\hat{\beta}$, and $\sigma_{\hat{\gamma}}$ and $\sigma_{\hat{\beta}}$ are the standard errors of $\hat{\gamma}$ and $\hat{\beta}$, respectively.

For more complex tests of the indirect effect, a similar approach may be used, but it requires careful incorporation of coefficients, standard errors, and covariances among the parameters of interest. Each test requires obtaining information from the covariance matrix among the estimates, or, alternatively, the correlations among the estimates and the standard errors of the estimates. In terms of the two-mediator model, it may be useful to test whether the indirect effect through $\hat{\gamma}_1\hat{\beta}_{31}$ is equal to the indirect effect $\hat{\gamma}_2\hat{\beta}_{32}$. The general covariance matrix among the four parameters in the two-mediator model is shown:

$$\Sigma = \begin{bmatrix} \sigma_{\beta_{31}\beta_{31}} & \sigma_{\beta_{32}\beta_{31}} & \sigma_{\gamma_1\beta_{31}} & \sigma_{\gamma_2\beta_{31}} \\ \sigma_{\beta_{31}\beta_{32}} & \sigma_{\beta_{32}\beta_{32}} & \sigma_{\gamma_1\beta_{32}} & \sigma_{\gamma_2\beta_{32}} \\ \sigma_{\beta_{31}\gamma_1} & \sigma_{\beta_{32}\gamma_1} & \sigma_{\gamma_1\gamma_1} & \sigma_{\gamma_2\gamma_1} \\ \sigma_{\beta_{31}\gamma_2} & \sigma_{\beta_{32}\gamma_2} & \sigma_{\gamma_1\gamma_2} & \sigma_{\gamma_2\gamma_2} \end{bmatrix}$$

The observed covariance among the four parameter estimates is shown in the following matrix:

$$\hat{\Sigma}_\theta = \begin{bmatrix} 0.023300 & 0.007500 & 0.000000 & 0.000000 \\ 0.007500 & 0.027300 & 0.000000 & 0.000000 \\ 0.000000 & 0.000000 & 0.025000 & -0.006800 \\ 0.000000 & 0.000000 & -0.006800 & 0.040700 \end{bmatrix}$$

The vector of partial derivatives for the function, $\hat{\gamma}_1\hat{\beta}_{31} - \hat{\gamma}_2\hat{\beta}_{32}$, is equal to $[\hat{\gamma}_1, -\hat{\gamma}_2, \hat{\beta}_{31}, -\hat{\beta}_{32}]$, which yields the following sample coefficients for the partial derivatives: $[0.8401, -0.2219, 0.5690, -0.5297]$. The covariance matrix among the parameter estimates is pre- and post-multiplied by the vector of partial derivatives in order to give the variance of $\hat{\gamma}_1\hat{\beta}_{31} - \hat{\gamma}_2\hat{\beta}_{32}$. The square root of this variance equals 0.1820 which is the standard error of $\hat{\gamma}_1\hat{\beta}_{31} - \hat{\gamma}_2\hat{\beta}_{32}$ that can be used to construct confidence limits for this difference.

The difference between the two indirect effects can also be computed by hand using the following general formula for the difference between two indirect effects. The covariances among the coefficients are used in the following formula for the variance of the difference between two indirect effects:

$$\sigma^2_{\hat{\gamma}_1\hat{\beta}_{31}-\hat{\gamma}_2\hat{\beta}_{32}} = \hat{\gamma}_1^2\sigma^2_{\hat{\beta}_{31}} + \hat{\beta}_{31}^2\sigma^2_{\hat{\gamma}_1} + \hat{\gamma}_2^2\sigma^2_{\hat{\beta}_{32}} + \hat{\beta}_{32}^2\sigma^2_{\hat{\gamma}_2} - 2\hat{\gamma}_1\hat{\gamma}_2\sigma_{\hat{\beta}_{31}\hat{\beta}_{32}} - 2\hat{\beta}_{31}\hat{\beta}_{32}\sigma_{\hat{\gamma}_1\hat{\gamma}_2}$$
$$+ 2\hat{\gamma}_1\hat{\beta}_{31}\sigma_{\hat{\beta}_{31}\hat{\gamma}_1} - 2\hat{\gamma}_1\hat{\beta}_{32}\sigma_{\hat{\beta}_{31}\hat{\gamma}_2} + 2\hat{\beta}_{32}\hat{\gamma}_2\sigma_{\hat{\beta}_{32}\hat{\gamma}_2} - 2\hat{\beta}_{31}\hat{\gamma}_2\sigma_{\hat{\beta}_{32}\hat{\gamma}_1} \tag{6.17}$$

The formula can be simplified somewhat by using the variances of the two indirect effects as shown in Equation 6.18:

$$\sigma^2_{\hat{\gamma}_1\hat{\beta}_{31}-\hat{\gamma}_2\hat{\beta}_{32}} = \sigma^2_{\hat{\gamma}_1\hat{\beta}_{31}} + \sigma^2_{\hat{\gamma}_2\hat{\beta}_{32}} - 2\hat{\gamma}_1\hat{\gamma}_2\sigma_{\hat{\beta}_{31}\hat{\beta}_{32}} - 2\hat{\beta}_{31}\hat{\beta}_{32}\sigma_{\hat{\gamma}_1\hat{\gamma}_2} + 2\hat{\gamma}_1\hat{\beta}_{31}\sigma_{\hat{\beta}_{31}\hat{\gamma}_1}$$
$$- 2\hat{\gamma}_1\hat{\beta}_{32}\sigma_{\hat{\beta}_{31}\hat{\gamma}_2} - 2\hat{\beta}_{32}\hat{\gamma}_2\sigma_{\hat{\beta}_{32}\hat{\gamma}_2} - 2\hat{\beta}_{31}\hat{\gamma}_2\sigma_{\hat{\beta}_{32}\gamma_1}$$

$$(6.18)$$

In many cases, including testing the equality of the two mediators in the two-mediator model, this formula is simplified considerably because several covariances are zero; $\sigma_{\hat{\beta}_{31}\hat{\gamma}_1}$, $\sigma_{\hat{\beta}_{31}\hat{\gamma}_2}$, $\sigma_{\hat{\beta}_{32}\hat{\gamma}_2}$, and $\sigma_{\hat{\beta}_{32}\hat{\gamma}_1}$ are zero here. Note that this formula is very similar to the standard error of the difference between the two indirect effects (Equation 5.10) described in chapter 5 for the ordinary regression model except that Equation 6.17 includes more covariance terms that are not available in ordinary least squares regression analysis, that is, $\sigma_{\hat{\gamma}_1\hat{\gamma}_2}$. These additional covariances are typically small. Nevertheless Equation 6.17 should be more accurate than assuming these covariances are equal to zero. Using the estimates from the two-mediator model in Equation 6.17 results in a value of 0.1820 for the standard error as shown in the following:

$$\sigma^2_{\hat{\gamma}_1\hat{\beta}_{31}-\hat{\gamma}_2\hat{\beta}_{32}} = (0.1566)^2 + (0.0860)^2 - 2(0.5690)(0.5297)(-0.0068)$$

$$- 2(0.8401)(0.2219)(0.0075) + 0 - 0 + 0 - 0$$

$$= 0.0331 = (0.1820)^2$$

The difference between the two indirect effects, $0.4780 - 0.1175 = 0.3605$, is 1.98 times larger than its standard error, suggesting that the difference between the two indirect effects is statistically significant.

The standard errors of many indirect effects and functions of indirect effects can be obtained using matrix methods or inserting sample estimates in formulas for different tests of indirect effects. The researcher must specify the function to be tested and the partial derivatives of the function. The covariance among parameter estimates is obtained from the output of a covariance structure analysis program. The calculation of the standard error is obtained by pre- and post-multiplying the covariance matrix among parameters by the vector of partial derivatives. Alternatively, sample estimates can be inserted in equations for the indirect effects. In most cases, many of the covariances in the formulas are zero, which simplifies the calculation.

More on contrasts among indirect effects in a mediation model can be obtained in MacKinnon (2000) and Williams and MacKinnon (in press). The standard error of several contrasts are described, and Williams and MacKinnon report the results of a statistical simulation, suggesting that these contrasts are generally accurate.

6.14 Mplus Code for Specific Indirect Effects in the Two-Mediator Model

The Mplus program includes commands for the estimation of specific indirect effects. The Mplus code to estimate the two-mediator model and output is shown in Table 6.8 along with the INDIRECT command line where the specification of indirect effects occurs. The specification in Mplus uses the ON command to indicate which variables have effects on other variables; for example, Y ON M1 M2 X, indicates that M1, M2, and X have effects on Y. The MODEL INDIRECT command is used to indicate which specific indirect effects are to be estimated. The Mplus results lead to the same research conclusions described earlier.

6.15 Path Analysis Models for More Than One Dependent, Independent, or Mediating Variable

Path analysis models provide a way to model comprehensive relations among variables including indirect or mediated effects. These specific mediated effects can be estimated and their standard errors determined using the multivariate delta method. Computer programs such as Mplus may also be used to estimate and compute the standard errors. The two-mediator model outlined in chapter 5 illustrated the methods.

The matrix approach in Equation 6.1 can also be extended to models with more than one independent variable, more than one mediator, and more than one dependent variable. The dimensions of matrix equations are increased to incorporate the additional variables. As for the earlier models, these more complex models can be represented by equations or by matrices. In the next section, the general approach to investigating mediation covariance structure models is illustrated for a model with three independent variables, two mediating variables, and one dependent variable.

6.16 Socioeconomic Status and Achievement

An example from sociology is used to illustrate the general manifest variable mediation model. Duncan et al. (1972, p. 38) presented data from a process model of achievement for data from 3,214, 35- to 44-year-old men measured during March 1962 who had nonfarm backgrounds and were in the experienced civilian labor force. The data were based on responses to the Occupational Changes in a Generation (OCG) questionnaire. The OCG data were collected in conjunction with the 1962 Current Population Survey of the Bureau of the Census. Several books on occupational

Table 6.8 Mplus Program and Selected Output for the Two-Mediator Model

```
TITLE: Two Mediator Example;

DATA:
NOBS = 40;
NGROUPS = 1;
FILE IS c:\MyFiles\twomed.dat.txt;

VARIABLE:
NAMES ARE ID X M1 M2 Y;
USEVARIABLES ARE X M1 M2 Y;

ANALYSIS:
TYPE IS GENERAL;
ESTIMATOR IS ML;
ITERATIONS=1000;
CONVERGENCE = 0.000001;

MODEL:
Y ON M1 M2 X;
M1 ON X;
M2 ON X;
M1 WITH M2;
MODEL INDIRECT:
Y IND X;

OUTPUT:  SAMPSTAT RESIDUAL STANDARDIZED CINTERVAL TECH1
TECH2 TECH3 TECH4 TECH5; TOTAL, TOTAL INDIRECT, SPECIFIC
INDIRECT, AND DIRECT EFFECTS
```

Estimates	S.E.	Est./S.E.	Std	StdYX
Effects from X to Y				
Total	0.708	0.169	4.187	0.708	0.552
Total indirect	0.596	0.170	3.499	0.596	0.465
Specific indirect				
Y				
M1				
X	0.478	0.153	3.132	0.478	0.373
Y				
M2				
X	0.118	0.083	1.409	0.118	0.092
Direct				
Y				
X	0.112	0.197	0.570	0.112	0.087

(continued)

Table 6.8 (Continued)

TOTAL, TOTAL INDIRECT, SPECIFIC INDIRECT, AND DIRECT
EFFECTS

	Lower .5%	Lower 2.5%	Estimates	Upper 2.5%	Upper .5%
Effects from X to Y					
Total	0.272	0.376	0.708	1.039	1.143
Total indirect	0.157	0.262	0.596	0.929	1.034
Specific indirect					
Y					
M1					
X	0.085	0.179	0.478	0.777	0.871
Y					
M2					
X	−0.097	−0.046	0.118	0.281	0.332
Direct					
Y					
X	−0.394	−0.273	0.112	0.498	0.619

achievement have used the OCG data (Blau & Duncan, 1967; Duncan et al., 1972). These data have also been widely used for illustration of new developments in the analysis of covariance structure models and the estimation of indirect effects and their standard errors, at least in part because of the large sample size (N = 3,214) and interesting effects. Alwin and Hauser (1975) used these data to describe the decomposition of effects in path analysis. Sobel (1982) used this example to illustrate the computation of the standard errors of indirect effects and Sobel (1986) used the data to illustrate general matrix equations for partial derivatives of indirect effects. Sobel (1987) used the example to provide a simpler description of the computation of indirect effects and their standard errors. Stone and Sobel (1990) used the model to generate data to evaluate the statistical properties of the method described by Sobel (1982, 1986) to obtain standard errors in a simulation study. Bollen (1987) used the model as one example of the computation of different types of indirect effects including specific indirect effects. In this section, I describe the estimation of the model, calculation of total indirect effects, and specific indirect effects. Estimation of the model in EQS, LISREL, and Mplus programs are described, and the relevant output is used to estimate indirect effects and their standard errors. There are six variables: X1, father's education;

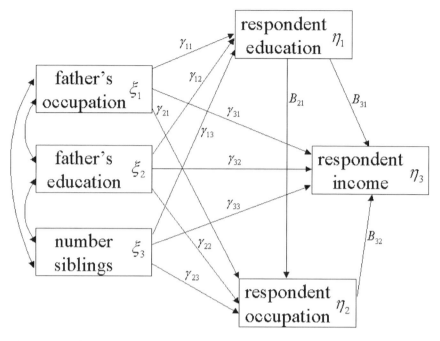

Figure 6.2. Socioeconomic status and achievement.

X2, father's occupation; X3, number of siblings in the respondent's family; Y1, respondent's education; Y2, respondent's occupational status; and Y3, respondent's income. A diagram of the model is shown in figure 6.2 and the equations corresponding to figure 6.2 are the following:

$$\eta_1 = \gamma_{11}\xi_1 + \gamma_{12}\xi_2 + \gamma_{13}\xi_3 + \zeta_1 \tag{6.19}$$

$$\eta_2 = \beta_{21}\eta_1 + \gamma_{21}\xi_1 + \gamma_{22}\xi_2 + \gamma_{23}\xi_3 + \zeta_2 \tag{6.20}$$

$$\eta_3 = \beta_{31}\eta_1 + \beta_{32}\eta_2 + \gamma_{31}\xi_1 + \gamma_{32}\xi_2 + \gamma_{33}\xi_3 + \zeta_3 \tag{6.21}$$

In matrix form, the equations are

$$
\begin{bmatrix} \eta_1 \\ \eta_2 \\ \eta_3 \end{bmatrix} =
\begin{bmatrix} 0 & 0 & 0 \\ \beta_{21} & 0 & 0 \\ \beta_{31} & \beta_{32} & 0 \end{bmatrix}
\begin{bmatrix} \eta_1 \\ \eta_2 \\ \eta_3 \end{bmatrix} +
\begin{bmatrix} \gamma_{11} & \gamma_{12} & \gamma_{13} \\ \gamma_{21} & \gamma_{22} & \gamma_{23} \\ \gamma_{31} & \gamma_{32} & \gamma_{33} \end{bmatrix}
\begin{bmatrix} \xi_1 \\ \xi_2 \\ \xi_3 \end{bmatrix} +
\begin{bmatrix} \zeta_1 \\ \zeta_2 \\ \zeta_3 \end{bmatrix} \tag{6.22}
$$

6.17 EQS Code for the Achievement Example

The EQS code shown in Table 6.9 for the achievement model is very similar to the two-mediator model described earlier. There are six variables in the model, and the correlation matrix and standard deviations serve as input to the program. The three equations are specified in the EQUATIONS section, and the variances and residuals are specified in the VARIANCES section. Note that E1, E2, and E3 represent residuals for respondent's income, occupation, and education, respectively. The covariances among the independent variables, X1, X2, and X3 are specified in the COVARIANCES section. Decomposition of effects, EFFECTS=YES, and correlation matrix among estimates, PARAMETERS=YES, are selected in the PRINT section. The EQS output for the achievement model is shown in Table 6.10.

Table 6.9 EQS Program for the Achievement Model

```
/TITLE
  MULTIPLE MEDIATOR MODEL PATH ANALYSIS
/SPECIFICATIONS
  CASES=3214; VARIABLES=6; ME=ML; ANALYSIS=COVARIANCE;
  MATRIX=CORRELATION;
/LABEL
  V1=INC1961; V2=OCC1962; V3=EDUC; V4=NUMSIB; V5=FATHOCC;
  V6=FATHEDUC;
/EQUATIONS
  V1 =   1*V2 + 1*V3 +1*V6 + 1*V5 + 1*V4 +E1;
  V2 =   1*V3 + 1*V5 +1*V4 + 1*V6 + E2;
  V3 =   1*V4 +1*V5 + 1*V6 +  E3;
/VARIANCES
  V4=9*; V5=423*; V6=36*;
  E1=25*; E2=525*; E3=9.2*;
/COVARIANCES
  V6,V5=45*;V6,V4=-3*; V5,V4= -16*;
/PRINT
EFFECTS=YES; PARAMETERS=YES;
/MATRIX=KM
  1.000
  0.4418 1.000
  0.3759 0.6426  1.000
  -0.1752-0.2751 -0.3311 1.000
  0.2587 0.3899  0.4341  -0.2476        1.000
  0.2332 0.3194  0.4048  -0.2871 0.5300 1.000
/STANDARD DEVIATIONS
  5.36 24.71 3.20 2.88 23.14 3.72
/END
```

Table 6.10   Selected EQS Output for the Achievement Model

MEASUREMENT EQUATIONS WITH STANDARD ERRORS AND TEST
STATISTICS

```
INC1961 =V1   = .070*V2 +   .200*V3 + -.037*V4 +  .011*V5
                .004         .036         .031        .004
               15.682        5.493      -1.186       2.534
                .071*V6 + 1.000 E1
                .028
                2.585
OCC1962 =V2 = 4.377*V3 + -.463*V4 +   .135*V5 +  .049*V6
                .120         .123         .017        .108
               36.408       -3.761      724          .453
               1.000 E2
EDUC   =V3 =    -.228*V4 +  .038*V5 + .171*V6 + 1.000 E3
                .018         .002        .016
               -12.945     15.526     10.956
```

MAXIMUM LIKELIHOOD SOLUTION (NORMAL DISTRIBUTION THEORY)
VARIANCES OF INDEPENDENT VARIABLES

V	F
V4 -NUMSIB	8.294*
	0.207
	40.081
V5 -FATHOCC	535.460*I
	13.359
	40.081
V6 -FATHEDUC	13.838*
	0.345
	40.081

MAXIMUM LIKELIHOOD SOLUTION (NORMAL DISTRIBUTION THEORY)
VARIANCES OF INDEPENDENT VARIABLES

E	D
E1 -INC1961	22.523*
	0.562
	40.081
E2 -OCC1962	347.556*
	8.671
	40.081
E3 -EDUC	7.485*
	0.187
	40.081

Table 6.10 (Continued)

```
MAXIMUM LIKELIHOOD SOLUTION (NORMAL DISTRIBUTION THEORY)
COVARIANCES AMONG INDEPENDENT VARIABLES
V                     F
V5 -FATHOCC       -16.501*
V4 -NUMSIB          1.211
                  -13.623
V6 -FATHEDUC       -3.076*
V4 -NUMSIB          0.197
                  -15.642
V6 -FATHEDUC       45.623*
V5 -FATHOCC         1.719
                   26.544

DECOMPOSITION OF EFFECTS WITH NONSTANDARDIZED
VALUES MAXIMUM LIKELIHOOD SOLUTION (NORMAL
DISTRIBUTION THEORY)

STANDARDIZED SOLUTION:
INC1961 =V1  = 0.325*V2 + 0.119*V3 + -0.020*V4 + 0.049*V5
               0.049*V6 + 0.885 E1
 OCC1962 =V2  = 0.567*V3 + -0.054*V4 + 0.127*V5 + 0.007*V6
               0.754 E2
EDUC    =V3  =  -0.205*V4 + 0.278*V5 + 0.198*V6 + 0.855 E3

MAXIMUM LIKELIHOOD SOLUTION (NORMAL DISTRIBUTION
THEORY)CORRELATIONS AMONG INDEPENDENT VARIABLES
V                     F
V5 -FATHOCC        -0.248*
V4 -NUMSIB

V6 -FATHEDUC       -0.287*
V4 -NUMSIB

V6 -FATHEDUC        0.530*
V5 -FATHOCC
```

6.18 LISREL Analysis of the Achievement Model

The program in Table 6.11 will estimate the same achievement model with LISREL. Most of this program is straightforward, and you will notice that the matrix specifications are directly related to the matrix equations, but there are variances and covariances among parameters that are specified as well. Output from the program is shown in Table 6.12.

Table 6.11   LISREL Program for the Achievement Model

```
Family Characteristics Effects on Child Achievement
DA NI=6 NO=3214 MA=cm ME=ML
KM
1
.4418 1
.3759 .6426 1
-.1752 -.2751 -.3311 1
.2587 .3899 .4341 -.2476 1
.2332 .3194 .4048 -.2871 .5300 1
SD
5.36 24.71 3.20 2.88 23.14 3.72
LA
'INC1961' 'OCC1962' 'EDUC' 'NUMSIB' 'FATHOCC'
 'FATHEDUC'
se
3 2 1 5 6 4
MO NY=3 NX=3 BE=sd GA=FR
OU ef se tv pc ef ss ND=4
```

Putting the estimates from the LISREL output in each matrix gives the following matrices:

$$\hat{\Gamma} = \begin{bmatrix} 0.038 & 0.171 & -0.228 \\ 0.135 & 0.049 & -0.463 \\ 0.011 & 0.071 & -0.037 \end{bmatrix} \quad \hat{\beta} = \begin{bmatrix} 0 & 0 & 0 \\ 4.377 & 0 & 0 \\ 0.200 & 0.070 & 0 \end{bmatrix}$$

$$\hat{\Psi} = \begin{bmatrix} 7.4852 & 0 & 0 \\ 0 & 347.5564 & 0 \\ 0 & 0 & 22.5230 \end{bmatrix}$$

$$\hat{\Phi} = \begin{bmatrix} 535.4596 & 0 & 0 \\ 46.6228 & 13.8384 & 0 \\ -16.5009 & -3.0759 & 8.2994 \end{bmatrix}$$

Table 6.12 LISREL Output for the Achievement Model

```
LISREL Estimates (Maximum Likelihood)
```

BETA

	EDUC	OCC1962	INC1961
EDUC	—	—	—
OCC1962	4.3767	—	—
	(0.1203)		
	36.3906		
INC1961	0.1998	0.0704	—
	(0.0364)	(0.0045)	
	5.4905	15.6751	

GAMMA

	FATHOCC	FATHEDUC	NUMSIB
EDUC	0.0385	0.1707	-0.2281
	(0.0025)	(0.0156)	(0.0176)
	15.5183	10.9514	-12.9393
OCC1962	0.1352	0.0490	-0.4631
	(0.0175)	(0.1082)	(0.1232)
	7.7205	0.4529	-3.7590
INC1961	0.0114	0.0712	-0.0373
	(0.0045)	(0.0275)	(0.0314)
	2.5331	2.5835	-1.1858

PHI

	FATHOCC	FATHEDUC	NUMSIB
FATHOCC	535.4596		
	(13.3656)		
	40.0625		
FATHEDUC	45.6228	13.8384	
	(1.7195)	(0.3454)	
	26.5320	40.0625	
NUMSIB	-16.5009	-3.0759	8.2944
	(1.2118)	(0.1967)	(0.2070)
	-13.6170	-15.6346	40.0625

PSI

Note: This matrix is diagonal.

EDUC	OCC1962	INC1961
7.4852	347.5564	22.5230
(0.1868)	(8.6754)	(0.5622)
40.0625	40.0625	40.0625

(*continued*)

Table 6.12 (Continued)

Squared Multiple Correlations for Structural Equations

	EDUC	OCC1962	INC1961
	0.2690	0.4308	0.2160

Covariance Matrix of Parameter Estimates

	BE 2,1	BE 3,1	BE 3,2	GA 1,1	GA 1,3
BE 2,1	0.0145				
BE 3,1	0.0000	0.0013			
BE 3,2	0.0000	-0.0001	0.0000		
GA 1,1	0.0000	0.0000	0.0000	0.0000	
GA 1,2	0.0000	0.0000	0.0000	0.0000	
GA 1,3	0.0000	0.0000	0.0000	0.0000	0.0003
GA 2,1	-0.0006	0.0000	0.0000	0.0000	0.0000
GA 2,2	-0.0025	0.0000	0.0000	0.0000	0.0000
GA 2,3	0.0033	0.0000	0.0000	0.0000	0.0000
GA 3,1	0.0000	0.0000	0.0000	0.0000	0.0000
GA 3,2	0.0000	-0.0002	0.0000	0.0000	0.0000
GA 3,3	0.0000	0.0002	0.0000	0.0000	0.0000
PH 1,1	0.0000	0.0000	0.0000	0.0000	0.0000
PH 2,1	0.0000	0.0000	0.0000	0.0000	0.0000
PH 2,2	0.0000	0.0000	0.0000	0.0000	0.0000
PH 3,1	0.0000	0.0000	0.0000	0.0000	0.0000
PH 3,2	0.0000	0.0000	0.0000	0.0000	0.0000
PH 3,3	0.0000	0.0000	0.0000	0.0000	0.0000
PS 1,1	0.0000	0.0000	0.0000	0.0000	0.0000
PS 2,2	0.0000	0.0000	0.0000	0.0000	0.0000
PS 3,3	0.0000	0.0000	0.0000	0.0000	0.0000

Covariance Matrix of Parameter Estimates

	GA 2,1	GA 2,2	GA 2,3	GA 3,1	GA 3,3
GA 2,1	0.0003				
GA 2,2	-0.0008	0.0117			
GA 2,3	0.0001	0.0019	0.0152		
GA 3,1	0.0000	0.0000	0.0000	0.0000	
GA 3,2	0.0000	0.0000	0.0000	-0.0001	
GA 3,3	0.0000	0.0000	0.0000	0.0000	0.0010
PH 1,1	0.0000	0.0000	0.0000	0.0000	0.0000
PH 2,1	0.0000	0.0000	0.0000	0.0000	0.0000
PH 2,2	0.0000	0.0000	0.0000	0.0000	0.0000
PH 3,1	0.0000	0.0000	0.0000	0.0000	0.0000
PH 3,2	0.0000	0.0000	0.0000	0.0000	0.0000

Table 6.12 (Continued)

PH 3,3	0.0000	0.0000	0.0000	0.0000	0.0000
PS 1,1	0.0000	0.0000	0.0000	0.0000	0.0000
PS 2,2	0.0000	0.0000	0.0000	0.0000	0.0000
PS 3,3	0.0000	0.0000	0.0000	0.0000	0.0000

Covariance Matrix of Parameter Estimates

	PH 1,1	PH 2,1	PH 2,2	PH 3,1	PH 3,3
PH 1,1	178.6399				
PH 2,1	15.2207	2.9568			
PH 2,2	1.2968	0.3934	0.1193		
PH 3,1	-5.5050	-0.7476	-0.0874	1.4684	
PH 3,2	-0.4690	-0.1149	-0.0265	0.1337	
PH 3,3	0.1696	0.0316	0.0059	-0.0853	0.0429
PS 1,1	0.0000	0.0000	0.0000	0.0000	0.0000
PS 2,2	0.0000	0.0000	0.0000	0.0000	0.0000
PS 3,3	0.0000	0.0000	0.0000	0.0000	0.0000

Covariance Matrix of Parameter Estimates

	PS 1,1	PS 2,2	PS 3,3
PS 1,1	0.0349		
PS 2,2	0.0000	75.2620	
PS 3,3	0.0000	0.0000	0.3161

6.19 Total Indirect Effects and Standard Errors for the Achievement Example

The total indirect effects are calculated by LISREL and EQS using Equations 6.10 and 6.12. These total indirect effects are shown for both the EQS (Table 6.13) and LISREL (Table 6.14) output. Note that each total indirect effect is statistically significant at least in part because of the large sample size. For example, the indirect effect of the number of siblings on respondent's occupation in 1962 was −0.9982 with a standard error of 0.0819. The total indirect effect of father's occupation on respondent's income in 1961 was equal to 0.0291 with a standard error of 0.0022. The total indirect effect of father's occupation on respondent's income is actually composed of three indirect effects: (a) father's occupation to respondent's education to respondent's income, $\xi_1 \rightarrow \eta_1 \rightarrow \eta_2$, (b) father's occupation to respondent's education to respondent's occupation to respondent's income, $\xi_1 \rightarrow \eta_1 \rightarrow \eta_2 \rightarrow \eta_3$, and (c) father's occupation to respondents' occupation to respondent's

Table 6.13   EQS Effect Decomposition for the Achievement Model

```
PARAMETER TOTAL EFFECTS

INC1961 =V1 =  0.070*V2 +  0.508*V3 + -0.186*V4 + 0.040*V5 +
               0.161*V6 +  1.000 E1 +  0.070 E2  +  0.508 E3
OCC1962 =V2 =  4.377*V3 + -1.461*V4 +  0.303*V5 + 0.796*V6 +
               1.000 E2 +  4.377 E3
EDUC =V3 = -0.228*V4 +  0.038*V5 +  0.171*V6 + 1.000 E3

DECOMPOSITION OF EFFECTS WITH NONSTANDARDIZED VALUES
PARAMETER INDIRECT EFFECTS

INC1961 =V1 =  0.308*V3 + -0.148*V4 + 0.029*V5 + 0.090*V6
               0.021         0.014       0.002       0.012
              14.403       -10.286      13.186       7.413
               0.070 E2 +  0.508 E3
               0.004        0.031
              15.682       16.601
OCC1962 =V2 = -0.998*V4 +  0.168*V5 + 0.747*V6 + 4.377 E3
               0.082         0.012       0.071       0.120
             -12.197        14.281      10.492      36.402
```

income $\xi_1 \to \eta_2 \to \eta_3$. Note that there are both two-path and three-path indirect effects in the total indirect effect of father's education on respondent's income. The EQS (Version 6.0) and LISREL (Version 8.8) programs do not include the calculation of these specific indirect effects and their standard errors. Other methods are required for computing these effects, as will be described later.

The matrices of total indirect effects and standard errors in EQS and LISREL were calculated using Equations 6.14 and 6.15 just as for the two-mediator model. The V_β and V_Γ matrices for the total indirect effects for this model are given in Sobel (1986), and also in Sobel (1987), but the V_β and V_Γ matrices are different in each article to correspond to the different ordering of the model parameters in the covariance matrix among the parameter estimates. The V_β and V_Γ matrices shown later are different from the V_β and V_Γ matrices in these two publications as well, but are consistent with the order of the parameters in the covariance matrix among parameter estimates in the LISREL output described in this chapter. Here the order of the columns corresponds to the estimated elements of the B matrix first, followed by the estimated elements of the Γ matrix. The order of the parameters in the columns for the achievement model is, $\beta_{21}, \beta_{31}, \beta_{32}, \gamma_{11}, \gamma_{12}, \gamma_{13}, \gamma_{21}, \gamma_{22}, \gamma_{23}, \gamma_{31}, \gamma_{32},$ and γ_{33}. The subscripts for the rows are 11, 21, 31, 12, 22, 32, 13, 23, and 33, so for the V_Γ matrix the rows correspond to $\gamma_{11}, \gamma_{21}, \gamma_{31}, \gamma_{12}, \gamma_{22}, \gamma_{32}, \gamma_{13}, \gamma_{23},$ and γ_{33}. The

Table 6.14   LISREL Effect Decomposition for the Achievement Model

Total and Indirect Effects

Total Effects of X on Y

	FATHOCC	FATHEDUC	NUMSIB
EDUC	0.0385	0.1707	-0.2281
	(0.0025)	(0.0156)	(0.0176)
	15.5183	10.9514	-12.9393
OCC1962	0.3035	0.7963	-1.4613
	(0.0201)	(0.1263)	(0.1427)
	15.1217	6.3065	-10.2369
INC1961	0.0405	0.1614	-0.1858
	(0.0046)	(0.0292)	(0.0330)
	8.7286	5.5342	-5.6352

Indirect Effects of X on Y

	FATHOCC	FATHEDUC	NUMSIB
EDUC	—	—	—
OCC1962	0.1683	0.7473	-0.9982
	(0.0118)	(0.0713)	(0.0819)
	14.2746	10.4868	-12.1916
INC1961	0.0291	0.0902	-0.1485
	(0.0022)	(0.0121)	(0.0143)
	13.3260	7.4621	-10.3749

Total Effects of Y on Y

	EDUC	OCC1962	INC1961
EDUC	—	—	—
OCC1962	4.3767	—	—
	(0.1203)		
	36.3906		
INC1961	0.5080	0.0704	—
	(0.0318)	(0.0045)	
	15.9928	15.6751	

Indirect Effects of Y on Y

	EDUC	OCC1962	INC1961
EDUC	—	—	—
OCC1962	—	—	—
INC1961	0.3083	—	—
	(0.0214)		
	14.3963		

corresponding V_β and V_Γ matrices for the order of the covariances among the parameters are shown in the following. The construction of the V_β and V_Γ matrices can be confusing because the order of the subscripts for the rows, 11, 21, 31, 12, 22, 32, 13, 23, and 33 differs from the order of subscripts for the columns 11, 12, 13, 21, 22, 23, 31, 32, and 33. And the order of the columns will differ depending on the order of the estimates in the covariance matrix among the estimates. Many different V_β and V_Γ matrix setups are possible that can be used to test indirect effects. It is critical that the order of the variables in the columns of the V_β and V_Γ matrices is the same as the order of the variables in the covariance matrix among the estimates for these calculations to be accurate.

$$V_\beta = \begin{bmatrix} 0 & 0 & 0 & 0 & 0 & 0 & 0 & 0 & 0 & 0 & 0 & 0 \\ 1 & 0 & 0 & 0 & 0 & 0 & 0 & 0 & 0 & 0 & 0 & 0 \\ 0 & 1 & 0 & 0 & 0 & 0 & 0 & 0 & 0 & 0 & 0 & 0 \\ 0 & 0 & 0 & 0 & 0 & 0 & 0 & 0 & 0 & 0 & 0 & 0 \\ 0 & 0 & 0 & 0 & 0 & 0 & 0 & 0 & 0 & 0 & 0 & 0 \\ 0 & 0 & 1 & 0 & 0 & 0 & 0 & 0 & 0 & 0 & 0 & 0 \\ 0 & 0 & 0 & 0 & 0 & 0 & 0 & 0 & 0 & 0 & 0 & 0 \\ 0 & 0 & 0 & 0 & 0 & 0 & 0 & 0 & 0 & 0 & 0 & 0 \\ 0 & 0 & 0 & 0 & 0 & 0 & 0 & 0 & 0 & 0 & 0 & 0 \end{bmatrix}$$

$$V_\Gamma = \begin{bmatrix} 0 & 0 & 0 & 1 & 0 & 0 & 0 & 0 & 0 & 0 & 0 & 0 \\ 0 & 0 & 0 & 0 & 0 & 0 & 1 & 0 & 0 & 0 & 0 & 0 \\ 0 & 0 & 0 & 0 & 0 & 0 & 0 & 0 & 0 & 1 & 0 & 0 \\ 0 & 0 & 0 & 0 & 1 & 0 & 0 & 0 & 0 & 0 & 0 & 0 \\ 0 & 0 & 0 & 0 & 0 & 0 & 0 & 1 & 0 & 0 & 0 & 0 \\ 0 & 0 & 0 & 0 & 0 & 0 & 0 & 0 & 0 & 0 & 1 & 0 \\ 0 & 0 & 0 & 0 & 0 & 1 & 0 & 0 & 0 & 0 & 0 & 0 \\ 0 & 0 & 0 & 0 & 0 & 0 & 0 & 0 & 1 & 0 & 0 & 0 \\ 0 & 0 & 0 & 0 & 0 & 0 & 0 & 0 & 0 & 0 & 0 & 1 \end{bmatrix}$$

6.20 Specific Indirect Effects and Standard Errors for the Achievement Example

The 13 specific indirect effects and their standard errors for the achievement model are shown in Table 6.15. Four of the specific indirect effects

Table 6.15   Specific Indirect Effects and Standard Errors
for the Achievement Model

Effect	Parameter	Estimate	Standard Error
$\xi_1\rightarrow\eta_1\rightarrow\eta_2$	$\gamma_{11}\beta_{21}$	0.1685	0.0118
$\xi_1\rightarrow\eta_2\rightarrow\eta_3$	$\gamma_{21}\beta_{32}$	0.0095	0.0014
$\xi_1\rightarrow\eta_1\rightarrow\eta_3$	$\gamma_{11}\beta_{31}$	0.0077	0.0015
$\xi_1\rightarrow\eta_1\rightarrow\eta_2\rightarrow\eta_3$	$\gamma_{11}\beta_{21}\beta_{32}$	0.0119	0.0011
$\xi_2\rightarrow\eta_1\rightarrow\eta_2$	$\gamma_{12}\beta_{21}$	0.7471	0.0713
$\xi_2\rightarrow\eta_2\rightarrow\eta_3$	$\gamma_{22}\beta_{32}$	0.0035	0.0076
$\xi_2\rightarrow\eta_1\rightarrow\eta_3$	$\gamma_{12}\beta_{31}$	0.0341	0.0070
$\xi_2\rightarrow\eta_1\rightarrow\eta_2\rightarrow\eta_3$	$\gamma_{12}\beta_{21}\beta_{32}$	0.0526	0.0060
$\xi_3\rightarrow\eta_1\rightarrow\eta_2$	$\gamma_{13}\beta_{21}$	−0.9983	0.0818
$\xi_3\rightarrow\eta_1\rightarrow\eta_3$	$\gamma_{13}\beta_{31}$	−0.0456	0.0090
$\xi_3\rightarrow\eta_2\rightarrow\eta_3$	$\gamma_{23}\beta_{32}$	−0.0326	0.0089
$\xi_3\rightarrow\eta_1\rightarrow\eta_2\rightarrow\eta_3$	$\gamma_{13}\beta_{21}\beta_{32}$	−0.0703	0.0073
$\eta_1\rightarrow\eta_2\rightarrow\eta_3$	$\beta_{21}\beta_{32}$	0.3081	0.0214

and their standard errors are shown in the EQS and LISREL output: $\xi_3\rightarrow$ $\eta_1\rightarrow\eta_2$ = −0.9982 (se = 0.0819), $\xi_2\rightarrow\eta_1\rightarrow\eta_2$ = 0.7473 (se = 0.0713), $\xi_1\rightarrow\eta_1\rightarrow\eta_2$ = 0.1683 (se = 0.0118), and $\eta_1\rightarrow\eta_2\rightarrow\eta_3$ = 0.3083 (se = 0.0214). As described earlier, some of the total indirect effects in the LISREL and EQS output are composed of several indirect effects.

Nine of the specific indirect effects are not included in the total indirect effects in the computer output. In this section a method to calculate these specific indirect effects are described. I use $\xi_2\rightarrow\eta_1\rightarrow\eta_3$, $\hat{\gamma}_{12}\hat{\beta}_{31}$, as an example of a specific indirect effect that is not included in the total indirect effects output in LISREL or EQS. One alternative is to alter the B and Γ matrices so that only the coefficients in the specific indirect effect are included in the B and Γ matrices. Then the V_β and V_Γ matrices are altered so only the 3,2 element in the V_β matrix and element 4,5 in the V_Γ matrix equal one, and all other elements are zero. Applying formula 6.15 gives an estimate of 0.0341 with a standard error of 0.0070 for that indirect effect.

It is possible to calculate indirect effects and their standard errors separate from the program as long as the correlations among the parameter estimates, standard errors of estimates, and estimates of relevant coefficients are available. This standard error can also be estimated directly from the coefficients and standard errors of the parameter estimates using

Equation 6.16 ($\sigma_{\hat{\gamma}_{12}\hat{\beta}_{31}} = 0$) to give the same estimate and standard error as shown in the following:

$$\sigma^2_{\hat{\gamma}_{12}\hat{\beta}_{31}} = (0.1707)^2\,(0.0364^2) + (0.1998)^2 (0.0156)^2 = (0.0070)^2$$

A similar approach is used for the estimate of the standard error of the three-path indirect effect, $\xi_2 \rightarrow \eta_1 \rightarrow \eta_2 \rightarrow \eta_3$, $\hat{\gamma}_{12}\hat{\beta}_{21}\hat{\beta}_{32}$, which is also not included in the EQS or LISREL output. Again an alternative is to alter the B and Γ matrices so that only the coefficients in the indirect effect are included in these matrices before applying Equation 6.14 and 6.15. Then the V_β and V_Γ matrices are altered so the 2,1 and 6,3 elements in the V_β matrix and element 4,5 in the V_Γ matrix are one, and all other elements are zero. Applying formula 6.15 gives an estimate of .0526 with a standard error of .0060 for this three-path indirect effect.

An alternative is to compute the standard error based on the covariance matrix among the estimates. Equation 6.23 shows the formula for the standard error of a three-path indirect effect for the product of three paths where the indirect effect is represented by $\hat{\gamma}\hat{\beta}_1\hat{\beta}_2$. Note that this formula is generic for the product of three coefficients, $\hat{\gamma}\hat{\beta}_1\hat{\beta}_2$; the coefficients and standard errors for a specific indirect effect need to be specified by the researcher.

$$\sigma^2_{\hat{\gamma}\hat{\beta}_1\hat{\beta}_2} = \hat{\gamma}^2\hat{\beta}_1^2\sigma^2_{\hat{\beta}_2} + \hat{\gamma}^2\hat{\beta}_2^2\sigma^2_{\hat{\beta}_1} + \hat{\beta}_1^2\hat{\beta}_2^2\sigma^2_{\hat{\gamma}} + 2\hat{\gamma}^2\hat{\beta}_1\hat{\beta}_2\sigma_{\hat{\beta}_2\hat{\beta}_1} + 2\hat{\gamma}\hat{\beta}_1^2\hat{\beta}_2\sigma_{\hat{\gamma}\hat{\beta}_2}$$
$$+ 2\hat{\gamma}\hat{\beta}_1\hat{\beta}_2^2\sigma_{\hat{\gamma}\hat{\beta}_1} \tag{6.23}$$

Putting in estimates in Equation 6.23 for the three path indirect effect, $\xi_2 \rightarrow \eta_1 \rightarrow \eta_2 \rightarrow \eta_3$ indirect effect, $\hat{\gamma}_{12}\hat{\beta}_{21}\hat{\beta}_{32} = 0.0526$, and covariances gives a standard error of .0060. Note that all of the covariance terms are zero for this case.

$$\sigma^2_{\hat{\gamma}_{12}\hat{\beta}_{21}\hat{\beta}_{32}} = (0.1707)^2\,(4.3767)^2\,(0.0045)^2 + (0.1707)^2\,(0.0704)^2\,(0.1203)^2$$

$$+ (4.3767)^2\,(0.0704)^2\,(0.156)^2 + 0 + 0 + 0$$

$$= (0.0060)^2$$

The equality of indirect effects can be tested in this model as described earlier in this chapter. To illustrate this procedure with the achievement example, the two indirect effects for father's occupation (ξ_1) on respondent's income (η_3) are compared, one indirect effect through respondent's education (η_1) and the other indirect effect is through respondent's occupation (η_2). Equation 6.17 is used to test the equality of two indirect effects, $\xi_1 \rightarrow \eta_1 \rightarrow \eta_3 = \hat{\gamma}_{11}\hat{\beta}_{31} = 0.0077$ and $\xi_1 \rightarrow \eta_2 \rightarrow \eta_3 = \hat{\gamma}_{21}\hat{\beta}_{32} = 0.0095$. The covariance between $\hat{\beta}_{31}$ and $\hat{\beta}_{32}$ was $-.0001$ as shown in Table 6.12. The covariance between $\hat{\beta}_{31}$ and $\hat{\beta}_{32}$ could also be obtained by multiplying the correlation (not shown in Table 6.12) between $\hat{\beta}_{31}$ and $\hat{\beta}_{32}$ ($-.5404$) by $\sigma_{\hat{\beta}_{31}}$ (.0025) and $\sigma_{\hat{\beta}_{32}}$ (.0175). All other correlations were zero: $\sigma_{\hat{\gamma}_{11}\hat{\beta}_{32}} = 0$; $\sigma_{\hat{\gamma}_{21}\hat{\beta}_{31}} = 0$; $\sigma_{\hat{\gamma}_{11}\hat{\beta}_{31}} = 0$; $\sigma_{\hat{\gamma}_{21}\hat{\beta}_{32}} = 0$; $\sigma_{\hat{\gamma}_{11}\hat{\beta}_{21}} = 0$. Plugging numbers into Equation 6.17 yields the following test of the equality of the two indirect effects.

$$\sigma^2_{\hat{\gamma}_{11}\hat{\beta}_{31} - \hat{\gamma}_{21}\hat{\beta}_{32}} = (0.0385)^2 (0.0364)^2 + (0.1998)^2 (0.0025)^2$$

$$+ (0.1352)^2 (0.0045)^2 + (0.0704)^2 (0.0175)^2$$

$$- 2(0.0385)(0.1352)(-.0001)$$

$$+ 0 + 0 + 0 + 0$$

$$= (0.002)^2$$

It appears that these two indirect effects are not significantly different from each other, $\hat{\gamma}_{11}\hat{\beta}_{31} - \hat{\gamma}_{21}\hat{\beta}_{32} = 0.0077 - 0.0095 = -0.0018$, which is about the size of the standard error of .002. As a result, it appears that the two indirect effects are not significantly different from each other.

6.21 Mplus for Specific Indirect Effects and Their Standard Errors

The capabilities for calculating specific indirect effects, and their standard errors are described in this section for several of the specific indirect effects in the achievement model. Mplus code for the achievement example is shown in Table 6.16. The line "INC1961 IND EDUC FATEDUC" requests the estimates and standard errors of the three indirect effects from father's occupation on income in 1961. The line "INC1961 IND FATHOCC" requests the single indirect effect of father's education on education to 1961 income. Lines to estimate all of the indirect effects are included as a homework problem at the end of this chapter.

As shown in the Table 6.17, the indirect effects of father's occupation on 1961 income contains the indirect effect through 1962 occupation ($\xi_1 \rightarrow \eta_2 \rightarrow \eta_3 = \hat{\gamma}_{21}\hat{\beta}_{32} = 0.010$, se = 0.001, z = 6.930) education ($\xi_1 \rightarrow \eta_1 \rightarrow \eta_3 = \hat{\gamma}_{11}\hat{\beta}_{31} = 0.008$, se = 0.001, z = 5.180), and the three-path indirect effect from father's occupation to education, to 1962 occupation to 1961 income ($\xi_1 \rightarrow \eta_1 \rightarrow \eta_2 \rightarrow \eta_3 = \hat{\gamma}_{11}\hat{\beta}_{21}\hat{\beta}_{32} = .012$, se = .001, z = 10.561) are the same as shown in Table 6.17.

Table 6.16 Mplus Program for Specific Indirect Effects in the
Achievement Model

```
TITLE; ACHIEVEMENT EXAMPLE, DATA ON PAGE 38 IN DUNCAN,
FEATHERMAN, AND DUNCAN 1972
DATA:
  TYPE IS std CORRELATION;
  NGROUPS = 1;
  NOBSERVATIONS = 3214;
  FILE IS c:\myfiles\Medbook\covach2.dat;
VARIABLE:
  NAMES ARE INC1961 OCC1962 EDUC NUMSIB FATHOCC FATHEDUC;
  USEVARIABLES ARE INC1961 OCC1962 EDUC NUMSIB FATHOCC
  FATHEDUC;
ANALYSIS:
  TYPE IS GENERAL;
  ESTIMATOR IS ML;
  ITERATIONS = 1000;
  CONVERGENCE = 0.00005;
MODEL:
  INC1961 ON EDUC OCC1962 FATHEDUC NUMSIB FATHOCC;
  EDUC ON FATHOCC FATHEDUC NUMSIB ;
  OCC1962 ON FATHOCC FATHEDUC NUMSIB EDUC;
MODEL INDIRECT:
INC1961 IND EDUC FATHEDUC;
INC1961 IND FATHOCC;
OUTPUT:  SAMP MOD STAND TECH1 TECH2;
```

Note that the first effect listed is the direct effect of father's occupation to
1961 income.

6.22 Nonrecursive Models

So far in this book, recursive models have been described. Recursive models
always have unidirectional arrows between variables. In the last example,
there was a path from respondent's education to respondent's occupation
but not a path from respondent's occupation to respondent's education. If
both paths were in the model, the model is a nonrecursive model and the
relation between respondent's education and occupation would be called a
reciprocal relation. Reciprocal relations are composed of repeated mediation
effects, and the equations described in this chapter are accurate for the calculation of mediation effects and standard errors in nonrecursive models.

Table 6.17 Mplus MODEL INDIRECT Output for the Achievement Model

```
INDIRECT EFFECTS OUTPUT
 TOTAL EFFECT FROM FATHOCC TO INC1961
 TOTAL INDIRECT EFFECT FROM FATHOCC      0.029   0.002   13.334
   TO INC1961
 SPECIFIC EFFECTS FROM FATHOCC TO
 INC1961
 INC1961
 FATHOCC                                 0.029   0.002   13.334
 INC1961
 OCC1962
 FATHOCC                                 0.010   0.001    6.930
 INC1961
 EDUC
 FATHOCC                                 0.008   0.001    5.180
 INC1961
 OCC1962
 EDUC
 FATHOCC                                 0.012   0.001   10.561
 COMBINED PARTIAL INDIRECT EFFECT        0.034   0.007    4.912
   FROM FATHEDUC TO INC1961
 SPECIFIC EFFECTS FROM FATHEDUC
   TO INC1961
 INC1961
 EDUC
 FATHEDUC                                0.034   0.007    4.912
```

Nonrecursive models include reciprocal relations among variables. Using two variables, X1 and X2, for example, the two paths relating X1 to X2 and X2 to X1 represent a reciprocal relation. In these models, typically the two variables X1 and X2 are measured simultaneously. Models with reciprocal relations may more accurately reflect the true relations among variables such that both variables cause each other. For example, in a model of political party affiliation and political candidate preference, it is likely that party affiliation affects candidate preference but also candidate preference may affect party affiliation. At some time sequence, one variable causes the other variable and the two variables do not cause each other simultaneously. However, a reciprocal relation is often modeled because the timing of measurement is not sufficient to shed light on the order of the reciprocal relation.

Complications owing to nonrecursive models are described here based on the simplest reciprocal model, in which the path, β_{21}, relates X1 to X2 and

β_{12} relates X2 to X1. The total relation of X1 on X2 is complicated because the effect of X1 on X2 equals β_{21} plus the effect of X1 on X2 back to X1 and then back to X2, $\beta_{21}\beta_{12}\beta_{21,}$ plus X1 to X2 to X1 to X2 to X1 to X2, $\beta_{21}\beta_{12}\beta_{21}\beta_{12}\beta_{21}$, and so on for all possible looping through the path coefficients. Collecting terms, the 0, 1, 2, 3, 4, and 5 loop effects are β_{21}, $\beta_{21}{}^2\beta_{12}$, $\beta_{21}{}^3\beta_{12}{}^2$, $\beta_{21}{}^4\beta_{12}{}^3$, and $\beta_{21}{}^5\beta_{12}{}^4$, respectively. The effects in each loop form a geometric series that has a sum equal to the looping effect of $1/(1 - \beta_{21}\beta_{12})$ and a total relation of X1 to X2 of $\beta_{21}/(1 - \beta_{21}\beta_{12})$. The looping effects enhance or multiply direct and indirect effects (Hayduk, 1987). For the two-variable system, if the looping effect, $\beta_{21}\beta_{12}$, is negative, then the total effect of X1 on X2 is reduced. If the looping effect is positive, then the total effect of X1 on X2 is increased. The infinite looping of effects leads to the addition of multiple mediated effects.

The general matrix formulas for the calculation of indirect effects and standard errors described in this chapter also apply to these looping mediated effects and their standard errors (Hayduk, 1987). With these formulas, the indirect effects and standard errors for complicated models with combinations of reciprocal and regular relations can be obtained. These estimates of indirect effects and standard errors are calculated using covariance structure analysis programs. Regarding the matrix of indirect effects $I_{\eta\eta}$ for reciprocal models, as described by Hayduk (1987), the terms along the diagonal are composed entirely of the aforementioned looping effects. Hayduk further suggested that it may be useful to investigate the looping effect separately from other effects for the relation between two variables.

Note that the simple model for reciprocal effects of X1 and X2 is not identified because there are more unknowns than free parameters. Often the reciprocal relations are part of a larger model and sufficient degrees of freedom are available to estimate the model. However a problem arises regarding estimation of reciprocal relations. Because recursive models, by definition, have paths in only one direction, many coefficients are set to zero. In nonrecursive models, more coefficients may be included to model reciprocal relations. An option in these situations is to use instrumental variables to assist in the estimation of the model. For the simple model for X1 related to X2, a variable must be related to X1 but not to X2, and another variable must be found that is related to X2 but not to X1. Essentially the instrumental variable for X1 is used to make a new variable that is the predicted X1 variable and the analogous thing happens for X2, i.e., a new variable for X2 is obtained by its prediction from another instrumental variable. With these instrumental variables, the model is identified. A method of estimation called two-stage least squares is used to estimate the parameters of models with instrumental variables. The instrumental variable estimation comprises the first stage and the estimation of the rest of the model is the second stage.

6.23 Summary

The purpose of this chapter was to describe mediation analysis for the path analysis model. Conceptually the analysis of mediating variables in path analysis models was a straightforward extension of methods to investigate the multiple mediator model using multiple regression equations. Models with more than one independent variable, more than one mediator, and more than one dependent variable can be evaluated with these methods. A benefit of these models is that they can more clearly incorporate additional variables in a comprehensive model. The calculation of effects in these models is simplified by the use of matrices and matrix equations for the standard errors of indirect effects. The LISREL, Mplus, EQS, and AMOS covariance structure analysis programs include routines to calculate the total indirect effects. Additional calculations are necessary to compute specific indirect effects and standard errors of specific indirect effects. Although not emphasized in this chapter, confidence limits for indirect effects in path analysis models are useful to researchers and product of coefficients and resampling methods provide the most accurate confidence limits. Chapter 12 describes resampling methods for path analysis models discussed in this chapter. The Mplus program includes commands by which users can request specific indirect effects and their standard errors including resampling methods. A matrix equation for the calculation of these values and a method to calculate these values by hand were described. A classic mediation model from sociology was used to illustrate the use of the methods. In the next chapter, general covariance structure modeling approaches that incorporate latent variables are described.

There are several limitations to the structural equation modeling approach described in this chapter (see MacCallum & Austin, 2000, for discussion of the strengths and limitations of these models). The assumptions of mediation models described earlier apply here as well, including uncorrelated errors, descriptive versus causal relations, and the inclusion of important variables. A primary limitation of these models is that there are often many possible models that would fit the data as well or even better than the model tested. A prudent researcher carefully considers these alternative models and compares models on the basis of theoretical predictions. Similarly, no interactions among mediators or interactions between independent variables and mediators were included in the models in this chapter, yet in many contexts these interaction effects may be present. As the number of variables in these models increases, the number of possible relations among variables quickly becomes unwieldy. Theory and replication of previous research are a critical part of the specification and testing of structural equation models. As mentioned in the quote for this chapter, careful specification of the tests beforehand and replication of these tests with additional data in different contexts is critical.

6.24 Exercises

6.1. Write out the matrix equations for the model in Exercise 5.1.

6.2. Kerckhoff (1974) shows the correlations for 767 twelfth grade students for the following variables: X1, intelligence; X2, number of siblings; X3, father's education; X4, father's occupation; Y1, grades; Y2, educational expectation; and Y3, occupational aspiration. Kenny (1979) reanalyzed these data, and this example is described in the LISREL 8 manual on pages 159–164 (Jöreskog & Sörbom, 2001). These data have also been widely used in covariance structure analysis programs (LISREL) and also in papers on indirect effects and their standard errors. The equations are the following:

$$Y_1 = \gamma_{11}X_1 + \gamma_{12}X_2 + \gamma_{13}X_3 + \gamma_{14}X_4 + \zeta_1$$

$$Y_2 = \beta_{21}Y_1 + \gamma_{21}X_1 + \gamma_{22}X_2 + \gamma_{23}X_3 + \gamma_{24}X_4 + \zeta_2$$

$$Y_3 = \beta_{31}Y_1 + \beta_{32}Y_2 + \gamma_{31}X_1 + \gamma_{32}X_2 + \gamma_{33}X_3 + \gamma_{34}X_4 + \zeta_3$$

The correlation matrix among the seven variables is

X1	1.00						
X2	−0.100	1.000					
X3	0.277	−0.152	1.000				
X4	0.250	−0.108	0.611	1.000			
Y1	0.572	−0.105	0.294	0.248	1.000		
Y2	0.489	−0.213	0.446	0.410	0.597	1.000	
Y3	0.335	−0.153	0.303	0.331	0.478	0.651	1.000

   a. Write the equations in matrix form.

   b. Estimate the parameters of the model using a covariance structure program such as Amos, EQS, LISREL, or Mplus.

   c. Calculate several indirect effects and standard errors.

   d. Test the equality of two indirect effects.

   e. What do you conclude about the relations of ambition and attainment?

6.3. SAS CALIS can be used to specify the model either by equations or by matrices. The equations method is used in the CALIS program below. The three regression equations are listed after the LINEQS statements. The variances of each dependent variable are specified under the STD section and the covariance between M1 and M2 is specified under the COV statement. The variance of the X variable is automatically included in this program. The Method=ML specifies maximum likelihood estimation of the model parameters based on the covariance matrix (COV).

```
PROC CALIS DATA=a METHOD=ML COV;
LINEQS
M1=a1 X + E1,
M2=a2 X + E2,
Y= c X + b1 M1 + b2 M2+ E3;
STD
E1=EE1,
E2=EE2,
E3=EE3;
COV
E1 E2 = CM1M2;
```

    a. Run this program for the two-mediator model data from chapter 6.
    b. Are the parameter estimates and standard errors the same as those for EQS or LISREL? Why?

6.4   For the three indirect effects of X_3 on Y_3 in the socioeconomic achievement model studied in this chapter, compute each effect by hand using formulas in this chapter. Find the V_β and V_Γ, matrices specified in Sobel (1982) and Sobel (1987). What is the order of parameters in the columns in these two cases? Why are these matrices different across those two articles and in this chapter?

6.5   The models examined in this chapter assumed that the measures were perfect measures of latent constructs. For the socioeconomic achievement model discuss the reliability and validity of each measured variable. What suggestions do you have to improve each measure? One option to improve the measurement of the variables is to include multiple indicators of each construct. Pick at least three indicators of each of the six constructs in the model.

6.6.   The achievement data are used in many different publications. Which specific indirect effects are given in the Sobel (1982) paper? What is the sample size recommended in the Stone and Sobel (1990) simulation study for models like the achievement example. Describe in detail the results for one total indirect effect for the achievement example described in Stone and Sobel (1990).

6.7   Write the Mplus code for the MODEL INDIRECT to estimate all of the specific indirect effects in Table 6.15.

7

Latent Variable
Mediation Models

> Who has seen the wind?
>   Neither I nor you:
> But when the leaves hang trembling
>   The wind is passing thro'.
>
> Who has seen the wind?
>   Neither you nor I:
> But when the trees bow down their heads
>   The wind is passing by.
>
> **—Christina Georgina Rossetti, 1872, p. 93**

7.1 Overview

This chapter extends the mediation structural model described in chapter 6 to explicitly model measurement error. First, measurement error is described along with the influence of measurement error on the estimation of the mediation effect. Second, the use of measurement models to overcome problems with measurement error is described. Third, the general model that includes both a measurement model and a structural model is presented and methods to decompose effects are extended to measurement models for latent variables. The methods are illustrated with the analysis of data from a study of intentions to use steroids among football players.

7.2 Measurement Error

All of the prior development of the mediation model in this book has assumed that the independent variable, mediating variable, and dependent variables have been measured without error. But measurement error is common in all fields including the social sciences. Measurement error can be random owing to unsystematic chance factors or nonrandom owing to systematic factors. Measurement error can distort estimates of relations between variables. For example, in most cases an observed regression coefficient is smaller than the true regression parameter because of measurement error in the independent variable. Similarly, the largest possible correlation between a measure and any other measure is the square root of the measure's reliability. For the case of mediation, the $\hat{a}$ and $\hat{b}$ coefficients are reduced as reliability of the measures decrease so that unreliability reduces the size of the mediated effect (Hoyle & Kenny, 1999).

Measurement is the assigning of numbers to units in a systematic way as a means of representing properties of the units (Allen & Yen, 1979). Measurement may be the most overlooked aspect of research in many disciplines, at least in part because of the difficulty of doing it well. Measurement is one of the most challenging aspects of research for at least six major reasons as summarized by Crocker and Algina (1986): (a) no single approach to measurement is universally accepted, (b) measurements are usually based on a sample of behavior, (c) because behaviors are sampled, there is some error inherent in the sampling, (d) units of measurement are not often well defined in many fields, for example, a 2-point difference at low levels of an attitudes scale may have a different meaning than a difference of 2 points at high values, (e) constructs must be defined by relations to other constructs or observable phenomenon in addition to their own internal consistency, and (f) measurement may differ across time of measurement and across subgroups of persons.

There are two major aspects of measurement: validity and reliability. The first aspect of measurement is validity, which is the extent to which the measure actually measures what it is hypothesized to measure. Validity is often determined by convergent validity, the extent to which the construct is related to other measures of the same construct, and discriminant validity, the extent to which it is not related to measures of other constructs. The second aspect of measurement is reliability or the consistency with which a measure of a construct measures that construct. There are quantitative measures of reliability based on measurement on one occasion or measurement on multiple occasions. Measures of internal consistency reliability, such as coefficient alpha, are used for measurement on one occasion. A multiple occasion measure of reliability is the test–retest correlation. More information on reliability and validity can be found in psychometric texts such as Crocker and Algina (1986), Allen and Yen (1979), and Lord and Novick (1968). This chapter addresses unreliability by using latent variable models. It is assumed that a program of research has generated valid measures of constructs.

7.3 The Effect of Unreliability on Mediation Analysis

Hoyle and Kenny (1999, p. 202) demonstrated how measurement error affects mediation analysis. Specifically the $\hat{a}$ path is reduced by the unreliability of the X variable. The $\hat{b}$ path is reduced by the unreliability of the mediator with an error free independent variable partialled out. Importantly, as unreliability in the mediator increases, the $\hat{c}'$ path is overestimated, and the $\hat{b}$ path is underestimated so that unreliability in the mediator reduces the size of the mediated effect and increases the size of the direct effect. Hoyle and Kenny (1999) found that the use of latent variable models removed the effects of unreliability in the mediators compared with using a single measure of the mediator with less than perfect reliability. The point is that the mediators are often not measured perfectly, which leads to underestimation of true mediation effects. The use of latent variable models improves the accuracy of mediated effect measurement.

One of the most serious effects of measurement error on regression results occurs when covariates have considerable measurement error (Darlington, 1990). Substantial error in covariates affects regression coefficients in an unpredictable manner, sometimes increasing coefficients and other times reducing or even reversing regression coefficients. For regular mediation analysis and analyses including covariates, reliable measures of constructs are critical.

7.4 Latent Variable Models

One way to reduce the effect of measurement error is to specify a model for how individual measures are related to the hypothetical or latent constructs of interest. These measurement models use multiple indicators of a latent construct to model the relation between each indicator and the latent construct into two parts, the true relation and error. The latent variable is specified as the true measure of the construct. To use the water consumption example from chapter 3, thirst could be conceptualized as a latent measure indicated by three observed measures of (a) self-reported thirst, (b) blood volume, and (c) saliva levels. Here the three measures are hypothesized to be indicators of a latent construct of thirst.

Latent variables are also called hypothetical, unmeasurable, or unobservable variables. Bollen (2002) reviewed latent variables and identified the following four formal definitions of latent variables: (a) local independence—the requirement that once a latent variable is held constant the indicators of that latent construct are independent, (b) expected value—

the average of an infinite number of measures of the same latent construct will equal the true score on the construct, (c) nondeterministic function of observed variables—a latent variable is a variable that cannot be completely determined by measured variables, and (d) no sample value—a latent variable is a variable for which there is no value for at least some observations in a sample. Definitions a and b are most relevant here as they refer to multiple indicators of a latent variable.

7.5 *The Measurement Model*

The measurement model represents how observed measures are related to a latent construct. These latent constructs are indicated by η for latent variables that are endogenous (variables affected by other variables, Y) and ξ for latent exogenous (variables not affected by other variables, X) variables. There are measurement models for endogenous and exogenous latent variables, where m is the number of endogenous variables, n is the number of exogenous variables, q is the number of X variables, and p is the number of Y variables. Matrices for the measurement of exogenous latent variables are described in the lambda X, Λ_x, (q × n) matrix that codes the relation between each observed measure and the latent variable, and the theta delta, Θ_δ, (q × q) matrix that codes the covariance matrix among the errors δ, for the X variables. For endogenous latent variables, lambda Y, Λ_y, (p × m) codes the relation between the observed measures and the latent endogenous variable, and the theta epsilon, Θ_ε, (p × p) matrix codes the covariance matrix among the error variances ε, among the Y variables. It is possible to specify an entire model in what is called an all-Y model so that the Λ_x and Θ_δ matrices are not required. This all-Y model often makes it easier to specify models, but the more complete model is described here to be consistent with most papers on indirect effects with latent variables.

For latent variable models, and unlike in chapter 6, the vectors of η and ξ variables are latent and not directly observed but are measured with multiple indicators as specified in the measurement model matrices, Λ_y, Θ_δ, Λ_x, and Θ_ε. The measurement model is specified in Equations 7.1 for the Y variables and 7.2 for the X variables:

$$y = \Lambda_y \eta + \varepsilon \qquad (7.1)$$

$$x = \Lambda_x \xi + \delta \qquad (7.2)$$

where Λ_x represents the relations between the observed X variables and latent ξ variables and Λ_y represents the relations between the observed Y variables and the latent η variables. Examples of the specification of measurement models will be given later in this chapter.

7.6 The Structural Model

The following equation describes the structural model relating independent variables, mediating variables, and dependent variables as described in chapter 6:

$$\eta = B\eta + \Gamma\xi + \zeta \tag{7.3}$$

where η is a vector of endogenous variables, ξ is a vector of exogenous variables, and ζ is a vector representing unexplained variability. The B (m $\times$ m) matrix codes the coefficients among the endogenous variables, and Γ (m $\times$ n) codes the coefficients relating exogenous variables to endogenous variables. The covariance matrix among the ξs is specified in the Φ (n $\times$ n) matrix, and the covariance matrix among the ηs is specified in the Ψ (m $\times$ m) matrix. Note that these are the same matrices in the structural model equation described in chapter 6. In fact, the only difference between the models in this chapter and those in chapter 6 is the addition of measurement models. As will be shown later, the matrix equations for the indirect effects and their standard errors are now expanded to include measurement models.

7.7 Indirect Effects in Latent Variable Models

With the addition of measurement models, there are two more types of total indirect effects in addition to $I_{\eta\eta}$ and $I_{\eta\xi}$ in Equations 6.10 and 6.12, respectively. There are total indirect effects of η variables on Y variables and total indirect effects of ξ variables on Y variables as shown in Equations 7.4 and 7.5. An indirect effect of a ξ variable on a Y variable is the effect of a ξ variable on an η variable, which is then is related to a Y variable for $I_{y\xi}$. An example of an η variable on a Y variable is the effect of an η variable to another η variable to a Y variable for $I_{y\eta}$. Often these mediated effects $I_{y\xi}$ and $I_{y\eta}$ are not central to a research hypothesis, because mediational hypothesis typically focus on latent variables in the $I_{\eta\eta}$ and $I_{\eta\xi}$ matrices.

$$I_{y\eta} = \Lambda_y(I - B)^{-1} - \Lambda_y \tag{7.4}$$

$$I_{y\xi} = \Lambda_y(I - B)^{-1}\Gamma \tag{7.5}$$

As shown in Equation 6.13, the standard errors of the indirect effects in $I_{y\eta}$ and $I_{y\xi}$ require their respective matrices of partial derivatives. The two additional equations for the partial derivatives of the $I_{y\eta}$ and $I_{y\xi}$ total indirect effect matrices are shown in Equations 7.6 and 7.7 respectively.

$$\partial \mathrm{vecI}_{y\eta} / \partial \hat{\theta} = V'_{\Lambda y}(((I-B)^{-1}-I) \otimes I_P) + V'_B((I-B)^{-1} \otimes (\Lambda_y(I-B)^{-1})') \tag{7.6}$$

$$\partial \mathrm{vecI}_{y\xi} / \partial \hat{\theta} = V'_B((I-B)^{-1}\Gamma \otimes (\Lambda_y(I-B)^{-1})')$$

$$+V'_\Gamma(I_n \otimes (\Lambda_y(I-B)^{-1})') + V'_{\Lambda y}((I-B)^{-1}\Gamma \otimes I_p) \tag{7.7}$$

The elements in these equations are the same as those described in chapter 6 with a few additions. The $V_{\Lambda y}$ matrix selects the variables for which partial derivatives are calculated from the Λ_y matrix. Note that X variables are not part of the indirect effect calculations or partial derivatives because there are no indirect effects on these variables. The number of η variables (m), the number of ξ variables (n), the number of Y variables (p), and the number of X variables (q) are used to construct identity and output matrices.

As described in detail in chapter 6, the matrices V_β, V_Γ, and $V_{\Lambda y}$, select partial derivatives. For most applications, these matrices consist of zeroes and ones. For each matrix, the number of columns is equal to the number of parameters estimated. The number of rows is equal to the number of elements in each subscripted matrix. For example, the $V_{\Lambda y}$ matrix has rows equal to m times p.

7.8 Matrix Representation of a Three-Indicator Latent Variable Mediation Model

The manifest variable model described in earlier chapters assumed that each measure was measured without error or, in other words, had reliability of 1. If reliability is less than 1, these models can be improved by specifying a measurement model for each construct. As discussed earlier, the extension of manifest variable models to include measurement models for each construct requires four more matrices corresponding to the coefficients relating each indicator to each latent factor and the unexplained variability for each indicator. The eight matrices for a three factor latent variable model with three indicators of each factor are shown. Note that Λ_x is a 3×1 matrix with a coefficient for each observed variable and the latent variable ξ and Λ_y is a 6×2 matrix with coefficients relating three observed variables to η_1 and three observed variables to η_2. There is a 3×3 matrix of errors among the δ, Θ_δ, and a 6×6 matrix of errors among the ε in Θ_ε. Both of these error matrices have only nonzero diagonal elements. The other matrices are the same as for the path analysis model described in chapter 6.

$$\begin{bmatrix} \lambda_{x1} \\ \lambda_{x2} \\ \lambda_{x3} \end{bmatrix} = \Lambda x \qquad \begin{bmatrix} \delta_{11} & 0 & 0 \\ 0 & \delta_{22} & 0 \\ 0 & 0 & \delta_{33} \end{bmatrix} = \Theta_\delta \qquad \begin{bmatrix} \lambda_{y11} & 0 \\ \lambda_{y21} & 0 \\ \lambda_{y31} & 0 \\ 0 & \lambda_{y42} \\ 0 & \lambda_{y52} \\ 0 & \lambda_{y62} \end{bmatrix} = \Lambda y$$

$$\begin{bmatrix} \varepsilon_{11} & 0 & 0 & 0 & 0 & 0 \\ 0 & \varepsilon_{22} & 0 & 0 & 0 & 0 \\ 0 & 0 & \varepsilon_{33} & 0 & 0 & 0 \\ 0 & 0 & 0 & \varepsilon_{44} & 0 & 0 \\ 0 & 0 & 0 & 0 & \varepsilon_{55} & 0 \\ 0 & 0 & 0 & 0 & 0 & \varepsilon_{66} \end{bmatrix} = \Theta_\varepsilon$$

$$\begin{bmatrix} \gamma_1 \\ \gamma_2 \end{bmatrix} = \Gamma \qquad \begin{bmatrix} 0 & 0 \\ \beta_{21} & 0 \end{bmatrix} = B \qquad \begin{bmatrix} \psi_{11} & 0 \\ 0 & \psi_{22} \end{bmatrix} = \Psi \qquad \begin{bmatrix} \phi_{11} \end{bmatrix} = \Phi$$

The matrix equations in 7.8 and 7.9 correspond to Equations 6.5, and 6.6.

$$\eta_1 = \gamma_1 \xi + \zeta_1 \tag{7.8}$$

$$\eta_2 = \gamma_2 \xi + \beta_{21} \eta_1 + \zeta_2 \tag{7.9}$$

The three-factor, three-indicator latent variable model is shown in figure 7.1. Note that latent variables are represented by circles, and measured variables are represented by rectangles. Pointed arrows represent a hypothesized direction of influence.

Once matrices (or a figure for some programs such as Amos) are specified in this way, the parameters of the model can be estimated with maximum likelihood or other approaches. It is important to note that when described in the aforementioned matrices, the models are not statistically identified. The need for identification stems from the use of latent variables that are not measured and have no original scale of measurement. Methods to identify measurement models include fixing one path of each latent variable to equal one or fixing the variance of the latent variables

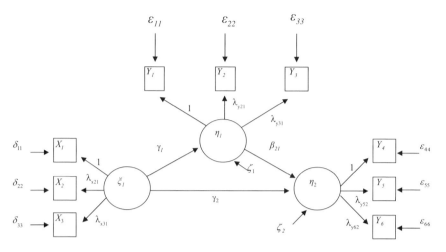

Figure 7.1. Three-factor, three-indicator latent variable model.

to equal one. As shown in figure 7.1, one path for each latent variable was fixed to equal one.

In this model there are 21 estimated parameters, λ_{x21}, λ_{x31}, λ_{y21}, λ_{y31}, λ_{y52}, λ_{y62}, γ_1, γ_2, β_1, δ_{11}, δ_{22}, δ_{33}, ε_{11}, ε_{22}, ε_{33}, ε_{44}, ε_{55}, ε_{66}, ψ_{11}, ψ_{22}, and ϕ_{11}. There are 45 free variances and covariances in the covariance matrix among the nine variables, that is, $(9(9 + 1))/2 = 45$ free parameters, so this model has $45 - 21 = 24$ degrees of freedom. With nonzero degrees of freedom it is possible to obtain a χ^2 test with 24 degrees of freedom of whether the model is consistent with the observed data.

7.9 Hypothetical Three-Variable Mediation Model With Latent Factors

A real data example from 547 high school football players is used to illustrate the three-factor three-indicator latent variable (Goldberg et al., 1996). The football players were measured before the football season, immediately after the season, and several months after the end of the season. For this illustration, the data will be used to investigate the extent to which coaches' tolerance of steroids affect players perceptions about the severity of steroid use that then affects intentions to use steroids. Although these three variables were measured at all three time points, for this example each measure was taken at a different time point consistent with the temporal ordering of the mediation hypothesis. The measure at the first time was coaches' tolerance measured by three questionnaire items:

coach1—I have talked with at least one of my coaches about different ways to get stronger instead of using steroids, coach2—On my team there are rules against using steroids, and coach3—If I were caught using steroids, I would be in trouble with my coaches. Three questionnaire items assessing perceived severity of steroid use were measured immediately after the season: severe1—The bad effects of anabolic steroids go away as soon as you stop using them, severe2—Only a few people who use anabolic steroids ever have any harmful or unpleasant side effects, and severe3—Anabolic steroids are not dangerous if you use them only a few months each year. Intentions to use steroids were measured at the last wave: intent1—I intend to try or use anabolic steroids, intent2—I would be willing to use anabolic steroids to know how it feels, and intent3—I am curious to try anabolic steroids. Although the raw data from the 547 participants could be used for analysis, the covariance matrix is used in these examples and will yield equivalent answers to the analysis of raw data for the model estimated. The covariance matrix among these nine variables is the data input into a covariance structure program to estimate the parameters of the three-factor latent variable model.

There are two matrices of indirect effects and standard errors in this model. First, $I_{\eta\xi}$ was described in chapter 6 and codes the effects of ξ to η_2, $\gamma_1\beta_{21}$. Second, $I_{y\eta}$ corresponds to the effects of η_1 on Y4, η_1 on Y5, and η_1 on Y6. There are no examples of the $I_{y\xi}$ indirect effect matrix in the LISREL output, but these indirect effects are given in the EQS output.

7.10 LISREL Model for the Three-Factor Latent Variable Model

The LISREL Program for the three-latent variable model is shown in Table 7.1. The correlation matrix and the list of standard deviations are used to enter the covariance matrix for analysis. Note that the specification of the LISREL program exactly corresponds to the matrix representation of the three-factor, three-indicator model described earlier. There are additional keywords for the additional matrices required for latent variable models: LY, LX, TE, and TD matrices. One indicator on each latent variable is fixed at 1, LX(1,1), LY(1,1), and LY (4,2). LISREL expects the order of variables in the analysis to start with the Y variables and then the X variables. The SE command changes the ordering of the variables so that the Y variables come first. The EF command on the output, OU, line requests decomposition of effects as described in chapter 6.

Selected LISREL output is shown in Table 7.2. The null hypothesis that the model fits the data cannot be rejected with a χ^2 of 29.11 with 24 degrees of freedom and probability of 0.22. The root mean squared error of approximation was 0.018, indicating very good fit. As a result, the model is an

Table 7.1 LISREL Program for the Latent Variable Mediation Model

```
THREE FACTOR MODEL
DA NI=9 NO=547
KM
 1.00000
 0.26471    1.00000
 0.28632    0.62004    1.00000
-0.16839   -0.16309   -0.13774   1.00000
-0.14364   -0.18831   -0.17279   0.53254   1.00000
-0.12833   -0.20156   -0.17097   0.59639   0.67350   1.00000
-0.11335   -0.06592   -0.11003   0.15927   0.19443   0.21261   1.00000
-0.04452   -0.03775   -0.06406   0.16619   0.23220   0.23696   0.70284   1.00000
-0.07918   -0.03466   -0.06772   0.11044   0.22294   0.21583   0.65218   0.82221   1.00000
SD
*
1.932 1.534 1.294 1.440 1.485 1.448 1.197 1.397 1.536
LA
coach1 coach2 coach3 severe1 severe2 severe3 intent1 intent2 intent3
SE
4 5 6 7 8 9 1 2 3
MO NX=3 NK=1 NY=6 NE=2 PS=SY,FI GA=FU,FI PH=FU,FI TE=DI,FR LX=FU,FI LY=FU,FI
 BE=FU,FI
FR LX(2) LX(3)
FR LY(2,1) LY(3,1)
FR LY(5,2) LY(6,2)
VA 1 LX(1) LY(1,1) LY(4,2)
FR BE(2,1)
FR GA(1) GA(2)
FR PS(1,1) PS(2,2)
FR PH(1,1)
OU MI RS EF MR SS SC
```

excellent fit to the data. The estimated direct effect parameters among the latent variables are $\hat{\beta}_{21}$ in the B matrix and $\hat{\gamma}_1, \hat{\gamma}_2$, in the Γ matrix. The effect from ξ to $\eta_1, \hat{\gamma}_1$, was -0.41 ($s_{\hat{\gamma}_1} = 0.09$) and from η_1 to $\eta_2, \hat{\beta}_{21}$, was 0.27 ($s_{\hat{\beta}_{21}} = 0.05$), which yields the estimator of the mediated effect $\hat{\beta}_{21}$ times $\hat{\gamma}_1$ equal to -0.11 with a standard error of 0.03 so the estimate was -3.56 times larger than the standard error. Note that for some latent variable models such as this one, there is a nonzero covariance between $\hat{\beta}_{21}$ and $\hat{\gamma}_1$ so Equation 6.16 with $2\hat{\gamma}\hat{\beta}\sigma_{\hat{\gamma}\hat{\beta}}$ for the indirect effect standard error should be used ($\sigma_{\hat{\gamma},\hat{\beta}21} = .0002$ for the example). The product distribution confidence limits (LCL $= -.176$, UCL $= -.055$) also incorporate the correlation ($r_{\gamma,\hat{\beta}21} = .0515$). The identical value of the mediated effect and standard error are shown in the Indirect Effects of KSI on ETA section of the LISREL output. The data appear to be consistent with mediation whereby perceived coach tolerance of anabolic steroid use affects perceived severity of anabolic steroid use that affects intentions to use steroids. Of course, there are alternative interpretations of these results, including one that the measures do not reflect true temporal ordering because they are not based on change in variables. More on mediation methods with longitudinal data is described in chapter 8.

Table 7.2   Selected LISREL Output for the Latent Variable Mediation Model

```
LISREL Estimates (Maximum Likelihood)
        LAMBDA-Y
                ETA 1         ETA 2
                --------      --------
 severe1         1.00          - -
 severe2         1.18          - -
                (0.08)
                15.30
 severe3         1.27          - -
                (0.08)
                15.44
 intent1         - -           1.00
 intent2         - -           1.47
                              (0.07)
                              21.41
 intent3         - -           1.50
                              (0.07)
                              20.97
        LAMBDA-X
                KSI 1
                --------
 coach1          1.00
 coach2          1.75
                (0.25)
                 6.96
 coach3          1.48
                (0.21)
                 6.94
        BETA
                ETA 1         ETA 2
                --------      --------
 ETA 1           - -           - -
 ETA 2           0.27          - -
                (0.05)
                 5.53
        GAMMA
                KSI 1
                --------
 ETA 1          -0.41
                (0.09)
                -4.46
 ETA 2           0.00
                (0.07)
                 0.02
```

(*continued*)

Table 7.2 (Continued)

```
          PHI
               KSI 1
               --------
                 0.47
                (0.13)
                 3.78
          PSI
          Note: This matrix is diagonal.
               ETA 1      ETA 2
               --------   --------
                 0.89       0.73
                (0.11)     (0.07)
                 8.29       9.84
          THETA-EPS
          severe1  severe2  severe3  intent1  intent2  intent3
          -------  -------  -------  -------  -------  -------
           1.10      0.86     0.53     0.63     0.22     0.56
          (0.08)    (0.08)   (0.08)   (0.04)   (0.05)   (0.06)
          13.57     10.64     6.78    14.47     4.76     9.73
          THETA-DELTA
               coach1     coach2     coach3
               --------   --------   --------
                 3.26       0.91       0.63
                (0.21)     (0.16)     (0.12)
                15.81       5.65       5.49
          Indirect Effects of KSI on ETA
               KSI 1
               --------
   ETA 1        - -
   ETA 2       -0.11
              (0.03)
              -3.56
          Indirect Effects of ETA on Y
               ETA 1      ETA 2
               --------   --------
severe1         - -        - -
severe2         - -        - -
severe3         - -        - -
intent1        0.27        - -
              (0.05)
               5.53
intent2        0.39        - -
              (0.07)
               5.66
intent3        0.40        - -
              (0.07)
               5.61
```

The indirect effect of ETA on Y matrix is one of the new indirect effect matrices for the latent variable model. These indirect effects represent the effects of ETA on the individual Y measures. For example, the indirect effect of η_1 to η_2 to Y_1 is given in the product of $\hat{\beta}_{21}$, coefficient of 0.27, and the LY(4,1) coefficient of 1.0, which yields an indirect effect of 0.27 and standard error equal to 0.05, which is identical to these values for $\hat{\beta}_{21}$ because LY(4,1) is fixed at 1.0. The indirect effect of η_1 to η_2 to Y_2 is given in the product of the $\hat{\beta}_{21}$ coefficient of 0.27, and the LY(5,2) coefficient of 1.47, which yields an indirect effect of 0.39 and standard error equal to 0.07. The indirect effect of η_1 to η_2 to Y_3 is given in the product of the $\hat{\beta}_{21}$ coefficient of 0.27, and the LY(6,2) coefficient of 1.50, which yields an indirect effect of 0.40 and standard error equal to 0.07.

7.11 EQS Code for the Latent Variable Mediation Model

The EQS code for the latent variable model is shown in Table 7.3. The model is identical to the models in chapter 6 except that three latent factors, F1, F2, and F3, are specified. Additional statements are required to specify the relations among the factors. As described in chapter 6, the EQS program specifies models using an equation format. The input matrix is specified as a correlation matrix, but the analysis is requested for the covariance matrix, ANALYSIS=COVARIANCE. The Print line with EFFECTS=YES requests decomposition of effects as described in chapter 6.

The same estimates and standard errors were obtained in the EQS analysis of the latent variable mediation model as for the LISREL output (Table 7.4). The estimates and standard errors are shown in equation form. The indirect effect of most interest is listed in the Indirect Effects output section, in which the indirect effects for intent or F3 are shown. Note that there are additional indirect effect estimates and standard errors in the EQS output, which would have also been present if the LISREL program had been set up as an all-Y model. The same indirect effects and standard errors in LISREL for the effect of ETA on Y are shown in the PARAM-ETER INDIRECT EFFECTS section of the output in the first coefficients of F2 for intent1 ($0.266 \times 1 = 0.266$), intent2 ($0.266 \times 1.470 = .391$), and intent3 ($0.266 \times 1.499 = .394$).

The indirect effects and standard errors of F1 on SEVERE1 (Y1) ($-0.415 \times 1 = -0.415$), F1 on SEVERE2 (Y2) ($-0.415 \times 1.175 = -0.487$), and F1 on SEVERE3 (Y3) ($-0.415 \times 1.269 = -0.526$) are included in the output. These effects correspond to the $I_{y\eta}$ matrix in the LISREL output. More detailed indirect effects are given in the EQS output. To use INTENT1 (Y4) as an example, the indirect effect of F2 (η_1) ($0.266 \times 1 = 0.266$), F1 (ξ_1) ($-0.415 \times 0.266 \times 1 = -0.109$), D2 (residual for the severity latent variable $1 \times 0.266 \times 1 = 0.266$, and D3 (residual for the intentions latent variable ($1 \times 1 = 1$) are shown. The same

Table 7.3   EQS Program for the Latent Variable Mediation Model

```
/TITLE
 Three Factor Latent Variable
/SPECIFICATIONS
 VARIABLES=9; CASES=547;
 METHOD=ML; MATRIX=CORRELATON; ANALYSIS=COVARIANCE;
/LABELS
 V1=COACH1; v2=COACH2; v3=COACH3; v4=SEVERE1; v5=SEVERE2; v6=SEVERE3;
 v7=INTENT1; v8=INTENT2; v9=INTENT3;
 F1=COACHTOL; F2=SEVERE; F3=INTENT;
/EQUATIONS
 V1   =    1 F1   + E1;
 V2   =    *F1   + E2;
 V3   =    *F1   + E3;
 V4   =    1  F2   + E4;
 V5   =    *F2   + E5;
 V6   =    *F2 + E6;
 V7   =    1  F3 + E7;
 V8   =    *F3 + E8;
 V9   =    *F3 + E9;
 F2   =    *F1 + D2;
 F3   =    *F1 + *F2 + D3;
/VARIANCES
 F1 = *; D2 TO D3=*;E1 TO E9=*;
/MATRIX
 1.00000
 0.26471    1.00000
 0.28632    0.62004    1.00000
-0.16839   -0.16309   -0.13774    1.00000
-0.14364   -0.18831   -0.17279    0.53254    1.00000
-0.12833   -0.20156   -0.17097    0.59639    0.67350    1.00000
-0.11335   -0.06592   -0.11003    0.15927    0.19443    0.21261    1.00000
-0.04452   -0.03775   -0.06406    0.16619    0.23220    0.23696    0.70284    1.00000
-0.07918   -0.03466   -0.06772    0.11044    0.22294    0.21583    0.65218    0.82221    1.00000
/STANDARD DEVIATIONS
 1.932 1.534 1.294 1.440 1.485 1.448 1.197 1.397 1.536
/PRINT
EFFECTS=YES;
/END
```

effects are present for INTENT2 (Y5) and INTENT3 (Y6). For most research questions, many of the indirect effects are not relevant.

7.12 Adjusting for Reliability in Manifest Variable Models

There are research situations in which it is not possible or unrealistic to obtain multiple indicators of a latent variable. One approach in this situation is to adjust for unreliability of measures in a manifest variable model. For a construct with a single indicator, the manifest variable models described in this book assume that the error variance is zero and the single indicator is a perfect measure of the latent construct. As described in this chapter, this may not be true in many research areas. One adjustment

Table 7.4 Selected EQS Output for the Latent Variable Mediation Model

```
MEASUREMENT EQUATIONS WITH STANDARD ERRORS AND TEST
STATISTICS
 STATISTICS SIGNIFICANT AT THE 5% LEVEL ARE MARKED WITH @.
 COACH1  =V1  =   1.000 F1    + 1.000 E1
 COACH2  =V2  =   1.746*F1    + 1.000 E2
                  .251
                 6.956@
 COACH3  =V3  =   1.482*F1    + 1.000 E3
                  .214
                 6.936@
 SEVERE1 =V4  =   1.000 F2    + 1.000 E4
 SEVERE2 =V5  =   1.175*F2    + 1.000 E5
                  .077
                15.296@
 SEVERE3 =V6  =   1.269*F2    + 1.000 E6
                  .082
                15.441@
 INTENT1 =V7  =   1.000 F3    + 1.000 E7
 INTENT2 =V8  =   1.470*F3    + 1.000 E8
                  .069
                21.409@
 INTENT3 =V9  =   1.499*F3    + 1.000 E9
                  .071
                20.971@
 SEVERE  =F2  =  -.415*F1     + 1.000 D2
                  .093
                -4.458@
 INTENT  =F3  =   .266*F2   +   .001*F1    + 1.000 D3
                  .048          .068
                 5.534@         .020
 VARIANCES OF INDEPENDENT VARIABLES
 ---------------------------------
 STATISTICS SIGNIFICANT AT THE 5% LEVEL ARE MARKED WITH @.
                  V                           F
                  ---                         ---
                              F1  -COACHTOL        .474*
                                                   .125
                                                 3.784@


                  E                           D
                  ---                         ---
 E1  -COACH1          3.258* D2  -SEVERE           .892*
                      .206                         .108

                    15.814@                      8.286@
```

(continued)

Table 7.4 (Continued)

```
E2   -COACH2             .907*  D3   -INTENT           .732*
                         .161                          .074
                        5.649@                        9.839@


E3   -COACH3             .633*
                         .115
                        5.492@


E4   -SEVERE1           1.100*
                         .081
                       13.566@


E5   -SEVERE2            .860*
                         .081
                       10.641@


E6   -SEVERE3            .529*
                         .078
                        6.778@


E7   -INTENT1            .632*
                         .044
                       14.469@


E8   -INTENT2            .222*
                         .047
                        4.760@


E9   -INTENT3            .561*
                         .058
                        9.728@


    DECOMPOSITION OF EFFECTS WITH NONSTANDARDIZED VALUES
    STATISTICS SIGNIFICANT AT THE 5% LEVEL ARE MARKED WITH @.

    PARAMETER INDIRECT EFFECTS
    --------------------------
SEVERE1 =V4  =    -.415 F1  + 1.000 D2
                   .093
                  -4.458@
SEVERE2 =V5  =    -.487 F1  + 1.175 D2
                   .108          .077
                  -4.499@      15.296@
```

Table 7.4 (Continued)

```
SEVERE3 =V6   =    -.526 F1  + 1.269 D2
                    .116         .082
                  -4.542@      15.441@
INTENT1 =V7   =     .266 F2  -  .109 F1 +  .266 D2 + 1.000 D3
                    .048         .067       .048
                   5.534@      -1.622      5.534@
INTENT2 =V8   =     .391 F2  -  .160 F1 +  .391 D2 + 1.470 D3
                    .069         .099       .069       .069
                   5.656@      -1.625      5.656@     21.409@
INTENT3 =V9   =     .399 F2  -  .163 F1 +  .399 D2 + 1.499 D3
                    .071         .101       .071       .071
                   5.608@      -1.624      5.608@     20.971@
INTENT  =F3   =    -.110*F1     +.266 D2
                    .031         .048
                  -3.563@       5.534@
```

for manifest variable models is to use an estimate of reliability from prior research and fix the error variance of the single measure equal to one minus the reliability of the measure times the variance of the measure (and fix the loading to 1). The resulting model is then estimated, and the new model coefficients are adjusted for unreliability. If the data for the construct are actually a composite of the sum of many items, then the reliability of that scale is used as the reliability measure and the single composite measure is used in the covariance structure analysis model. Generally this method is better than ignoring unreliability but not as good as estimating a latent variable model (Stephenson & Holbert, 2003). Some of the limitations of this method include the extent to which the reliability estimate is accurate; the method may conceal measures that are actually composed of more than one factor, and the relation of these factors may have important relations with other variables in the model that will be ignored (Bagozzi & Heatherton, 1994). Nevertheless, this approach provides some adjustment for unreliability in manifest variable models. If the reliability of the measures is high to begin with this adjustment does not affect results substantially.

7.13 Summary

The purpose of this chapter was to describe mediation analysis for models that include a measurement model for latent constructs. Measurement error is important because it can reduce mediation relations and can either increase or decrease coefficients when unreliable covariates are used. At a minimum, reliability coefficients should be reported for constructs used in a mediation analysis. Latent variable measurement models require the addition of matrices or equations specifying how individual items are related to latent constructs. Once the measurement models are specified, the usual tests for indirect effects can be based on more reliable measures of latent constructs. There are two additional types of indirect effects for these models with corresponding matrices of partial derivatives for the computation of their standard errors. Distribution of the product and resampling methods (chapter 12) are useful for latent variable mediation models. Practical limitations of latent variable models are the computational difficulty of simultaneously estimating complex structural and measurement models and ambiguity regarding obtaining an actual score for an individual on an unobserved latent variable. Although measurement error is directly addressed in latent variable models, other assumptions regarding mediation still apply including timing of measurement, omitted variables, and inference regarding causal relations. The latent variable model as described in this chapter does not explicitly include temporal relations. As temporal priority is an important aspect of mediation, longitudinal mediation models are the focus of the next chapter. The latent growth curve longitudinal model described in the next chapter requires specifying latent variables to model change over time.

7.14 Exercises

7.1   Write out the matrices and computer programs for a three-variable latent variable model with four indicators for each latent variable.

7.2   Write out the matrices for the two-mediator model described in the last chapter but include three indicators of each latent factor.

7.3   Describe the additional indirect effect matrices when latent variables are added to a model.

7.4   Do you think that using indicators of latent variables improve the measurement of these constructs? Why?

7.5   Rerun the three-factor latent variable example in the book, but reverse the order of the variables such that intent at wave 3 is first, followed by severity, followed by coach tolerance at wave 1, for example, SE 1 2 3 4 5 6 7 8 9. What is your conclusion about the mediated effect of intentions to perceived severity to coach tolerance using the data in reverse order? What data would help you interpret these results?

7.6   Write out the matrices for a model with a single binary X variable, four indicators of the mediator and four indicators of the dependent variable. Describe the meaning of each indirect effect matrix.

7.7   The reliability of a covariate may increase or decrease an observed correlation. The following SAS program, based on formulas in Cohen and Cohen (1983, pp. 406–412), calculates the observed partial correlation, obsr, and true partial correlation, truer, as a function of ry1—the correlation between X1 and Y, ry2—the correlation between X2 and Y, r12—the correlation between X1 and X2, ryy—the reliability of Y, r11—the reliability of X1, and r22—the reliability of X2. Vary the values of ry1 and ry2 and compare the true partial correlation to the observed partial correlation. What do you conclude about how the reliability of X1 affects the observed partial correlation?

```
data a;
input ry2 ry1 r12 r11 ryy r22;
obsr=(ry2-(ry1*r12))/(sqrt((1-ry1**2)*(1-r12**2)));
truer=(r11*ry2-(ry1*r12))/
(sqrt((r11-ry1**2)*(r11-r12**2)));
cards;
.3  .5 .6 .7 1 1
;
```

8

Longitudinal Mediation Models

A "correctly specified model" is, always has been, and always will be a fiction. A more realistic view of models is that they are simplifications of extremely complicated behavior. It is a mistake to assume that any model actually represents the underlying processes absolutely correctly, even after certain obvious faults have been corrected. All that can be hoped is that a model captures some reasonable approximation to the truth, serving perhaps as a descriptive device or summarizing tool

—Robert Cudeck, 1991, p. 261

8.1 Overview

None of the mediation models described so far have included measurement of the same variable on repeated occasions. For a variety of reasons, repeated measurement improves interpretation of mediational processes because change within individuals can be examined in addition to differences among individuals. This chapter provides an overview of the additional information available for mediation models applied to longitudinal data. Mediation models for unconditional and conditional two-wave mediation models are described followed by autoregressive, latent growth curve, and latent difference score models for three waves of data. A person-oriented model requiring longitudinal binary data is also described. Finally, a data example is used to illustrate the models, and the model parameters are estimated with covariance structure analysis programs.

8.2 Cross-Sectional Versus Longitudinal Data

Several aspects of longitudinal data elucidate mediating processes. First, longitudinal data provide more information regarding the temporal precedence of X, M, and Y. In the single mediator model in which all variables are measured at the same occasion, the time ordering among the variables is based on theoretical or other grounds. If the X variable represents random assignment to conditions, then X precedes both M and Y in the cross-sectional model. However, the temporal relation between M and Y must be based on theory or prior research. Longitudinal data allow for the examination of whether changes in M are more likely to precede changes in Y. If a variable is measured at time 1, it is more likely that it will cause the time 2 variable than vice versa. Although it is unlikely that the time 2 variable can cause the time 1 variable, it is possible to think of situations in which a third variable causes both time 1 and time 2 effects. Three or more waves of data generally provide more accurate representations of the temporal order of change over time that lead to more accurate conclusions about mediation.

The second benefit of longitudinal data is that both changes within individuals and cross-sectional relations can be investigated. For cross-sectional data, estimates of effects are based on differences among individuals. Longitudinal relations are based on changes within individuals. Longitudinal data with two waves, for example, allow for examination of cross-sectional relations at each wave in addition to the examination of change between the two waves. This capability is important because changes within an individual can be different from changes among individuals. For example, the predictors of why one person has a higher score on a dependent variable than others at one time may be quite different from the predictors of why the change in the score for one person was greater than that for the others. Although longitudinal relations are generally of most interest, there are situations in which cross-sectional relations are more important than longitudinal relations. Students are more appropriately assigned to classrooms on the basis of aptitude or achievement rather than changes in these measures. Similarly, legislators may more appropriately fund counties on the basis of cross-sectional differences in population, rather than the percent growth in county population. The percent change in population may be less important than static population levels.

A third benefit of longitudinal data is that the data address some alternative explanations of cross-sectional mediated effects. One alternative explanation of an observed cross-sectional relation is the existence of an omitted variable that explains the relation. Longitudinal data remove some omitted variable explanations because the participant's own scores control for extraneous variables. Change within an individual removes alternative explanations of effects that are due to static differences among individuals because each individual serves as a control for himself or herself. For example, biological factors such as genetics are unlikely explanations for longitudinal relations because these variables are not likely to have changed across waves of measurement.

Gollob and Reichardt (1991) described three related limitations of using cross-sectional data to investigate longitudinal relations. First, it takes time for variables to exert their effects. If variables are measured at the same time, there may not be enough time for X to affect M or M to affect Y. Second, variables have effects on themselves, for example, M is related to M at a later time. Third, the size of the effect depends on the time lag. The indirect effect of X on Y may be quite different if the measurement of the variables differs in seconds compared with decades. Gollob and Reichardt argued that these limitations of cross-sectional data lead to biased estimates of effects.

To clarify the limitations of cross-sectional data, Gollob and Reichardt (1991) specified a latent longitudinal model for cross-sectional data in which measures at an earlier time point are specified as latent variables. They are latent in the sense that they are not measured. In this model, there are many more unknown parameters than data values so some assumptions regarding relations must be made. Gollob and Reichardt suggested that the number of unknown parameters could be reduced by assuming that longitudinal relations among variables are known and variances at each time are equal. With this model and its (often unrealistic) assumptions, it may be possible to estimate longitudinal relations with cross-sectional data. However, Gollob and Reichardt used this example to illustrate the difficulty of assessing true relations with cross-sectional data and suggested alternative longitudinal models such as those described in this chapter. In general, cross-sectional data provide a snapshot of the relations among a system of variables at one time, under the assumption that the system has reached equilibrium so that the snapshot accurately reflects relations that would be obtained at other time points.

8.3 Additional Information From Longitudinal Data: Stability, Stationarity and Equilibrium

The introduction of repeated measurements of variables introduces several new concepts unique to longitudinal data. The first concept, stability, is the extent to which the mean of a measure is the same across time as described by Kenny (1979). Other definitions of stability relax the requirement of stable means but instead require stable trends or periodic stability of a process (see the six different types of stability outlined by Wohlwill, 1973). Similarly, Burr and Nesselroade (1990) described additional definitions of stability including strict stability for which individuals do not change over time, linear stability for which there is a linear trend over time that differs across persons, and monotonic stability reflecting the fact that persons maintain the same rank order over time. Statistical tests of nested models of stability are described in Tisak and Meredith (1990). Dwyer (1983) used the term temporal inertia, the tendency for an entity to remain stable over time, to describe stability. The tendency for temporal stability is affected by entropic decay, which refers to the tendency for a variable to change over time because of random error. The characteristics of stability and random error lead to the regression to the mean phenomenon (Campbell & Kenny, 1999) whereby persons high (or low) on a score at time one tend to regress to the mean at time two. The extent to which a person regresses to the mean is related to the amount of random error in the measures. Campbell and Kenny (1999) described artifactual effects in longitudinal analyses, owing to the regression to the mean phenomenon, especially when data are obtained from an observational study. Information on stability from longitudinal data is assessed by measuring dependency across measurement occasions.

Second is a related concept called stationarity which is the extent to which the relations among variables are the same over time (Kenny, 1979). The assumption is that the process generating the data does not change over time. Unfortunately, with real processes it is likely that relations among variables do change over time, especially for long duration studies. Consider the relation among positive body image, nutrition behaviors, and socioeconomic status at age 10 compared with the same measures at age 70. Information on stationarity can be obtained from longitudinal data by assessing the invariance of relations across measurement occasions. Researchers have identified several types of stationarity including mean and variance stationarity. However, it is possible that a process generating data is stationary, yet variance and means may change over time.

The third important concept for longitudinal data is equilibrium, which is related to stationarity and stability. Dwyer (1983) has called a system at equilibrium when there is temporal stability in the patterns of covariance and variance among variables. For mediation, the point is that the relations among X, M, and Y must have reached some equilibrium during the period of data collection for accurate estimation of their relations. For cross-sectional data, it must be assumed that equilibrium has been reached when the variables have been measured. Experimental designs seek to disturb equilibrium by creating differences among groups. The disturbance may lead to a new equilibrium or the relation among variables may return to the original equilibrium. With longitudinal data, the researcher must consider whether a system has come to equilibrium in its relations among variables. Some information about equilibrium can be obtained from longitudinal data by examining the similarity of relations in the model across multiple waves.

8.4 Difference Score Versus Analysis of Covariance Controversy

One of the recurring controversies in the analysis of longitudinal data is the preference for analysis by difference scores or analysis of covariance. For example with two waves of observation a researcher can analyze the difference between the first and second measure of X, M, and Y, and use these difference scores as the variables in the mediation equations described in earlier chapters. MacKinnon et al. (1991) used this procedure in a mediation analysis of a drug prevention program. An alternative method is analysis of covariance, in which the baseline value of each variable is included as a covariate in the analysis. Dwyer (1983) noted that these two analyses actually specify two separate hypotheses regarding how scores would change over time, an unconditional model for the difference score method and a conditional model for the analysis of covariance method. The difference score method assumes that without an effect of an independent variable, differences among individuals at baseline would be maintained at the follow-up measurement. The analysis of covariance model assumes that each individual's score would tend to regress to the mean of scores if unexposed to an independent variable. The rapidity that scores regress to the mean is a function of the amount of error in the measure. More error yields greater regression to the mean.

At least part of the controversy with difference scores was the demonstration that the difference score was unreliable in many situations (Cronbach & Furby, 1970). For example, if both the pre- and the post-test are reliable then the difference score will be less reliable because any difference between the two scores is probably due to error. Rogosa (1988) and others (see Burr & Nesselroade, 1990) demonstrated that the difference score was not always unreliable. Rogosa pointed out that the unreliability of the difference score may merely reflect that there is not substantial individual differences in growth (or change) over time. When the correlation between measurements is high, individual growth rates tend to be almost the same, so there is little variability in the growth. The difference score is more reliable when the reliability of each test is high and the correlation between tests is low (assuming the same reliability across time and equal variances across time).

Table 8.1, including values from Rogosa (1988) and some additional values, demonstrates how the reliability of the difference score is a function of the reliability of the measure and the correlation between the measures. The reliability of the difference score is 0 when both the reliability of the measure and the correlation between occasions is 0.7. Overall, if the correlation between occasions is low, then the reliability of the difference score is higher.

Table 8.2, also from Rogosa (1988), gives the ratio of the reliability of the difference score to the average reliability of the measures as a function of

Table 8.1 Difference Score Reliability as a Function of Test Reliability and Correlation Between Tests (Rogosa, 1988)

R between Tests	0.6	0.7	0.8	0.9
0.4	0.33	0.50	0.67	0.83
0.5	0.20	0.40	0.60	0.80
0.6	0.00	0.25	0.50	0.75
0.7		0.00	0.33	0.67

reliability at time 1 and the true correlation between occasions. Reliability at time 2 is 0.9. As shown in table entries greater than 1, the reliability of the difference score can be more reliable than the average reliability of the two tests. If the true correlation between tests is 0.4 and the reliability at time 1 is 0.6 and reliability at time 2 is 0.9, then the difference score is 1.06 times more reliable than the average of the reliabilities.

In summary, if the correlation between a measure at two occasions is 0.5 or less and the measure is generally reliable, the difference score has acceptable reliability. Often the correlation between adjacent waves with actual data is 0.5 or less. If you think of the reliability of the difference score as a measure of true change over time, it is not surprising that the difference is not so reliable when all people are changing the same way, yielding a high correlation between occasions.

Similar points were made by Singer and Willett (2003, pp. 42–44), in the context of precision of measuring change and reliability of change. Reliability in the change score is the proportion of population variance in observed change that is due to the true population change. High reliability of change means that the variance of the observed change score is very close to the variance of the true rate of change. If all persons have the same true rate of change, then the reliability of the change score will be low because variability in the change is low. The reliability of observed change

Table 8.2 Ratio of Difference Score Reliability to Average Reliability of Two Waves (Rogosa, 1988; Table 5.4)

	Reliability at Time 1		
R True Correlation	0.6	0.7	0.8
0.4	1.06	1.03	1.00
0.6	0.86	0.88	0.90
0.8	0.53	0.60	0.67

is affected by the size of change and also the reliability of true change. Singer and Willett (2003) conclude that reliability of change should not be the sole criterion for measurement of change.

The residualized change score is often used as an alternative to the difference score and analysis of covariance, at least in part because it adjusts for baseline differences and avoids some of the problems with the reliability of difference scores. The first step in the calculation of the residualized change score is to obtain predicted values of the wave 2 measure using the wave 1 measure. These predicted scores for wave 2, Y_2', are subtracted from the actual wave 2 score, Y_2, to form the residualized change score $Y_2 - Y_2'$. The residualized change score is then the difference between the observed score at wave 2 and the predicted score at wave 2, where the wave 1 measure is used to predict wave 2. The residualized change removes the relation between the two measures across time (Lord, 1963). Often the conclusions based on the residualized change score are indistinguishable from the analysis of covariance because both measures adjust for baseline measurement. For the mediation case, the residualized change scores would be obtained separately for X, M, and Y, and then X, M, and Y would be analyzed as if there was a single measure of each variable. One advantage of residualized change scores (and difference scores) is that the number of variables in the mediation model is reduced because the wave 1 measure is no longer needed in the analysis. For large models with multiple X, M, and Y variables, this can greatly simplify the estimation and presentation of a model. The residualized change score does not solve the limitations of other two-wave analysis methods as it can be susceptible to low reliability and it assumes regression to the mean over time, which may not be appropriate in some situations (Rogosa, 1988).

Several alternatives to change scores have been proposed. One alternative is to investigate relative change such as the natural logarithm of the time 2 to time 1 measure or the percent change relative to baseline (Törnqvist, Vartia, & Vartia, 1985). The appropriateness of these and other approaches to measuring change depend on the substantive question (Bonate, 2000).

8.5 Two-Wave Regression Models

One option with two waves of data is to analyze the difference between the pre- and post-test measures. If X does not code an experimental manipulation, then the difference scores of X, M, and Y would be entered in Equations 3.1 through 3.3, and mediation would be assessed as described in chapter 3. The interpretation of coefficients is different, as now the relation between change in X and change in M is reflected in the *a* parameter. The *b* parameter codes the relation between change in M and change in Y after adjustment for change in X. If X codes exposure to an experimental manipulation, then change in X reflects group membership. Ideally the manipulation occurs between the pre- and post-test, as this model would then be in terms of the change in M and Y before versus after the experimental manipulation. A second option is to analyze residualized change scores for X, M, and Y. For each variable a predicted score is obtained using the time 1 score on that variable as a predictor. The analysis is then conducted on the residualized scores for X, M, and Y. The interpretation of the results would consist of the change in X, M, and Y with the time 1 score removed. As for the change score as the dependent variable, there is a single mediated effect estimated relating residualized change in X to residualized change in M which is related to residualized change in Y.

An alternative to the change score method is to use the time 1 measures as covariates in an analysis of covariance model for the two-wave data as shown in Equations 8.1 and 8.2. As in previous equations, e_1 and e_2 represent residuals, and the intercepts are i_1 and i_2. This model is also called a conditional model as the scores at the second time are conditioned on the scores on the first time. Equation 8.1 represents the relation of both X measures, both M measures, and Y_1 on Y_2. In this model, the coefficient s_1 represents the stability of the Y variable over time, after adjustment for other relations in the model. In Equation 8.1, the b_1 coefficient codes the relation between M_1 and Y_2, b_2 codes the relation between M_2 and Y_2, c_1' codes the relation between X_1 and Y_2, and c_2' codes the relation between X_2 and Y_2. In Equation 8.2, a_1 codes the relation between X_1 and M_2, and a_2 codes the relation between X_2 and M_2.

There are several possible estimators of the mediated effect in this two-wave regression design, $\hat{a}_1\hat{b}_1$, an estimator representing across time relations, and $\hat{a}_2\hat{b}_2$, a contemporaneous estimator reflecting relations of measures at the second measurement. As argued by Cole and Maxwell (2003), the $\hat{a}_1\hat{b}_1$ estimator may be a better measure of the mediated effect because $\hat{a}_1$ represents the temporal relation between X and M and $\hat{b}_1$ represents the temporal relation between M and Y. The standard error formulas described in chapters 3 and 4 can be applied to test the significance and compute confidence intervals for either mediated effect.

$$Y_2 = i_1 + c_1'X_1 + c_2'X_2 + b_1M_1 + b_2M_2 + s_1Y_1 + e_1 \tag{8.1}$$

$$M_2 = i_2 + a_1X_1 + a_2X_2 + s_2M_1 + e_2 \tag{8.2}$$

If the X variable codes an experimental manipulation between waves of measurement, then there will be a single X variable in the equations and correspondingly, there will be one a_1 and one c_1' coefficient. Again there will be estimators of the mediated effect, $\hat{a}_1\hat{b}_1$, which reflects longitudinal time relations, and $\hat{a}_1\hat{b}_2$, which reflects an across time relation for $\hat{a}_1$, but a within time relation for $\hat{b}_2$. The $\hat{a}_1\hat{b}_1$ estimator may be preferable as it reflects change across time. It will also be important to assess whether $\hat{b}_1$ and $\hat{b}_2$ differ across groups as the intervention may change the relation between M and Y (see chapter 10 for more on moderator models).

A third alternative model for two-wave longitudinal data is an autoregressive mediation model. Autoregressive means regressed on itself, so in this model each variable is predicted by the same variable at an early wave. This model would not include contemporaneous relations among the variables, that is, the b_2, c'_2, and a_2 parameters in Equations 8.1 to 8.2. As in the first wave, the errors in the variables at the second wave would be allowed to covary reflecting the fact that there are contemporaneous relations among variables, but the direction of the relations are not known.

Although a statistically significant longitudinal mediation relation is a convincing demonstration of a mediation relation, not all mediation relations may be captured in the longitudinal relations. One way that the longitudinal mediation estimator may miss true mediation is if the time of measurement differs from the timing of the mediated effect. On the other hand, the contemporaneous mediated effect may be inflated by correlated errors introduced by measuring variables at the same wave. However, contemporaneous mediation may be important in some research contexts. It is important to realize that longitudinal data provide more information about longitudinal mediation effects but alternative explanations of the results remain. For example, say that Y actually causes M, which then causes X. It is possible that the mediation relation occurred between measurements of X, M, and Y, so a model of longitudinal relations may find longitudinal mediation consistent with X causes M which causes Y, when in fact the opposite relation exists. As stated many times in this book, theory, prior research, and randomized experimental designs are critical in judging the adequacy of a mediation hypothesis.

8.6 Three-Wave Models

As you might expect given the complexity of two-wave models, there are many additional complexities for models with three or more waves. Assumptions regarding stability, stationarity, equilibrium, and timing are now important across three waves. Although these models are complex, they provide potentially more accurate information regarding the relations among variables. This section begins with the discussion of the longitudinal mediation models described in Cole and Maxwell (2003) and MacKinnon (1994) and then describes a general autoregressive mediation model described earlier (Jöreskog, 1979). An alternative longitudinal model based on growth in variables is then described. The complexity of these models requires a covariance structure analysis program as described in chapters 6 and 7 to accurately estimate the parameters and standard errors of the model parameters.

Autoregressive Model I. The first longitudinal three-wave mediation model is an extension of the autoregressive mediation model described in Gollob and Reichardt (1991) and elaborated by Cole and Maxwell (2003). The model is specified in Equations 8.3 through 8.8 (intercepts and residuals are not shown to simplify presentation) and shown in figure 8.1. There are several important aspects of this model. First, relations one lag apart are specified. With three waves it is possible to consider lag two effects or effects two waves apart, but these effects are not included in these equations. Second, the stability of the measures is assessed with the relation between the same variable over time; coefficient s_1 for X, s_2 for M, and s_3 for Y. Third, only longitudinal relations consistent with longitudinal mediation are present among the variables, i.e., X_1 is related to M_2 and M_2 is related to Y_3. Fourth, covariances among the variables at the first wave are included, as are the covariances among the residual variances of X, M, and Y at each wave. Note that these covariances among residuals at each wave are not shown in the figure 8.1. In this model, the covariances among X, M, and Y at the same wave of measurement reflect that the causal order of these measures is unknown.

The longitudinal relations between X_1 and M_2, coefficient a_1, and between X_2 and M_3, coefficient a_2, both represent the relation between X and M. Similarly, the longitudinal relations between M_1 and Y_2, coefficient b_1, and between M_2 and Y_3, coefficient b_2, represent the relation between

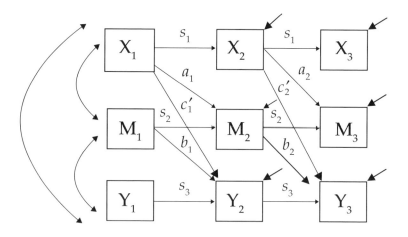

Figure 8.1. Autoregressive mediation model I.

M and Y. There are several options for the mediated effect, a_1b_1 for the first lag, a_2b_2 for the second lag, and a_1b_2 reflecting the temporal ordering of the mediated effect. The mediated effect standard errors and formulas for the confidence limits described earlier in this book can be applied to each mediated effect. The direct effect coefficients c_1' and c_2' reflect longitudinal effects between adjacent waves from X_1 to Y_2 and X_2 to Y_3, respectively. Covariance structure computer programs allow for the test of the equality of paths, such as a_1 and a_2, to evaluate whether these relations are the same at the different waves.

$$X_2 = s_1X_1 \tag{8.3}$$

$$X_3 = s_1X_2 \tag{8.4}$$

$$M_2 = a_1X_1 + s_2M_1 \tag{8.5}$$

$$M_3 = a_2X_2 + s_2M_2 \tag{8.6}$$

$$Y_2 = b_1M_1 + c_1'X_1 + s_3Y_1 \tag{8.7}$$

$$Y_3 = b_2M_2 + c_2'X_2 + s_3Y_2 \tag{8.8}$$

As described in chapter 6, the parameters of this model can be estimated by first specifying the free and fixed parameters and then estimating the parameters and standard errors using a covariance structure analysis program. Often the covariance between residual variances at adjacent waves is included in longitudinal models. These covariances between adjacent measurement errors are added because the same measure taken over repeated occasions often has similar memory or retesting effects. It is also possible that there are lag 2 autoregressive relations among variables, which refer to the relation of a variable at one time to the same variable two waves later, for example, X_1 on X_3. Similar lag 2 relations may exist between different variables, such as the effect of X_1 on M_3 and Y_3.

Autoregressive Model II. Another form of the autoregressive mediation model specified in Equations 8.9 through 8.14 (intercepts and residuals not shown in the equations) includes contemporaneous mediation relations among X, M, and Y, as well as the longitudinal mediation effect described earlier and is shown in figure 8.2. Note that within each wave, except for the first wave, the relations of X to M and M to Y are estimated. Contemporaneous estimates of mediated effects are then $\hat{a}_3\hat{b}_3$ at time 2 and $\hat{a}_4\hat{b}_4$ at time 3. Longitudinal autoregressive mediated effects include $\hat{a}_4\hat{b}_1$, $\hat{a}_2\hat{b}_2$, and the longitudinal mediated effect $\hat{a}_1\hat{b}_2$. The standard error of each mediated effect and combinations of these mediated effects can be found using the multivariate delta method described in chapter 4. It is possible

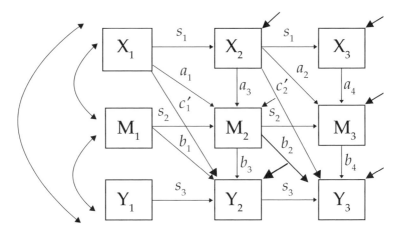

Figure 8.2. Autoregressive mediation model II with longitudinal and contemporaneous mediation.

that the contemporaneous mediated effects are small or are opposite in sign from the longitudinal mediation effects when the true model may contain longitudinal mediation. It is also possible that the contemporaneous mediation relations may more closely match the true temporal relations in the mediation model so that the cross-sectional relation is more accurate than the longitudinal relation. The contemporaneous mediation relations may also be equivalent to correlated residuals at each measurement. For example, for variables that have rapid temporal relations, a long time between measurements may lead to missing real relations.

$$X_2 = s_1 X_1 \tag{8.9}$$

$$X_3 = s_1 X_2 \tag{8.10}$$

$$M_2 = a_1 X_1 + s_2 M_1 + a_3 X_2 \tag{8.11}$$

$$M_3 = a_2 X_2 + s_2 M_2 + a_4 X_3 \tag{8.12}$$

$$Y_2 = b_1 M_1 + c_1' X_1 + s_3 Y_1 + b_3 M_2 \tag{8.13}$$

$$Y_3 = b_2 M_2 + c_2' X_2 + s_3 Y_2 + b_4 M_3 \tag{8.14}$$

Autoregressive Model III. A third type of autoregressive longitudinal mediation model allows for cross-lagged relations among variables as specified in Equations 8.15 through 8.20, for example, M_1 to X_2 and Y_2 to X_3 and is shown in figure 8.3. In this model, the direction of relations among

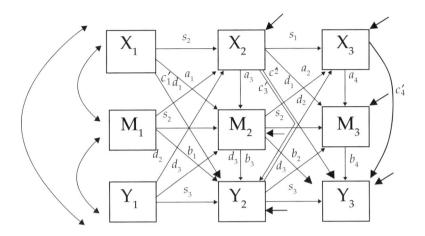

Figure 8.3. Autoregressive mediation model III with longitudinal mediation.

X, M, and Y are all free to vary. The model violates the temporal precedence of X to M to Y specified by the mediation model because paths in the reverse direction are estimated such as M to X and Y to M. However, the model could be used to assess the possibility of cross-lagged relations among variables (d_1, d_2, and d_3). Because it allows for these cross-lagged relations, it is probably a more reasonable model than assuming that these relations are zero. It is possible that the level of M at the second wave is predicted by the level of Y at the first wave because M was related to Y at earlier time points. This relation of M to Y before the study is not observed because these variables were not measured at the earlier time. From this perspective, a nonzero relation between Y to M may be expected in a longitudinal study. There are many different potential mediated effects in this model, some of which are opposite to the hypothesized temporal order of the mediation relations.

$$X_2 = s_1 X_1 + d_1 M_1 + d_2 Y_1 \tag{8.15}$$

$$X_3 = s_1 X_2 + d_1 M_2 + d_2 Y_2 \tag{8.16}$$

$$M_2 = a_1 X_1 + a_3 X_2 + s_2 M_1 + d_3 Y_1 \tag{8.17}$$

$$M_3 = a_2 X_2 + a_4 X_3 + s_2 M_2 + d_3 Y_2 \tag{8.18}$$

$$Y_2 = c_1' X_1 + c_3' X_2 + b_1 M_1 + b_3 M_2 + s_3 Y_1 \tag{8.19}$$

$$Y_3 = c_2' X_2 + c_4' X_3 + b_2 M_2 + b_4 M_3 + s_3 Y_2 \tag{8.20}$$

If X codes exposure to an intervention, then X is a single measure simplifying the model. Ideally the experimental manipulation would occur after the first or second wave of data collection so that change after the manipulation could be examined. With many repeated measures, more accurate modeling of growth over time can be assessed before and after the intervention.

8.7 Mplus Longitudinal Autoregressive Mediation Model III

The Mplus program code for the autoregressive mediation model III closely follows Equations 8.15 through 8.20 listed earlier and is shown in Table 8.3. Covariances among the measures at each wave are specified using the WITH command. The program can be easily changed to run the second and third type of autoregressive model described in this chapter by fixing certain parameters to be zero.

Table 8.3 Mplus Program for the Longitudinal Autoregressive Mediation Model III

```
TITLE:
   AUTOREGRESSIVE MEDIATION MODEL III;
DATA:
   FILE IS c:\data;
VARIABLE:
   Names = X1 X2 X3 M1 M2 M3 Y1 Y2 Y3;
   Usevariables X1 X2 X3 M1 M2 M3 Y1 Y2 Y3;
ANALYSIS:
   TYPE IS meanstructure;
MODEL:
   X2 on X1 M1 Y1;
   X2 on X2 M2 Y2;
   M2 on X1 X2 M1 Y1;
   M3 on X2 X3 M2 Y2;
   Y2 on X1 X2 M1 M2 Y1;
   Y3 on X2 X3 M2 M3 Y2;
   M1 with X1 Y1;
   X1 with Y1;
OUTPUT:
```

8.8 LISREL Longitudinal Autoregressive Mediation Model III

The program code for LISREL has the matrix specifications described in chapters 6 and 7 and is shown in Table 8.4 (assumes N = 100 and data from a file called c:\data). It is possible to specify what is called an all-Y model, which requires four matrices rather than eight matrices. An all-Y model is specified here. The matrix for BE is also listed in the table. Note that each of the paths in the BE matrix correspond to effects in the autoregressive model where the columns represent X_1, X_2, X_3, M_1, M_2, M_3, Y_1, Y_2, and Y_3 as predictor and rows represent them as dependent variables. In the second row of the BE matrix, for example, relations from X_1 to X_2, M_1 to X_2, and Y_1 to X_2 are freely estimated, as indicated by a 1 in the corresponding elements of the matrix.

Additional Autoregressive Models. A series of nested model can be used to test hypotheses regarding autoregressive mediation models. For example, the autoregressive model III can serve as the base model for several additional models such as a model that constrains all relations inconsistent with

Table 8.4   LISREL Program for the Longitudinal Autoregressive
Mediation Model III

```
LONGITUDINAL AUTOREGRESSIVE MEDIATION MODEL III
DA NI=9 NO=100 MA=cm ME=ML
RA FI=c:\data
KM
SD
LA
'X1' 'X2' 'X3' 'M1' 'M2' 'M3' 'Y1' 'Y2' 'Y3'
MO NY=9 NE=9 LY=ID BE=FU,FI PS=SY,FI TE=DI,FI
FR PS(1,1) PS(2,2) PS(3,3) PS(4,4) PS(5,5) PS(6,6) PS(7,7)
 PS(8,8) PS(9,9)
FR PS(1,4) PS(1,7) PS(4,7)
PA BE
0 0 0 0 0 0 0 0 0
1 0 0 1 0 0 1 0 0
0 1 0 0 1 0 0 1 0
0 0 0 0 0 0 0 0 0
1 1 0 1 0 0 1 0 0
0 1 1 0 1 0 0 1 0
0 0 0 0 0 0 0 0 0
1 1 0 1 1 0 1 0 0
0 1 1 0 1 1 0 1 0
OU EF
```

the temporal ordering of mediation to zero, that is, all paths from M to X, from Y to M, and from Y to X. A χ^2 difference test can be used to test this hypothesis of any paths inconsistent with the temporal ordering of mediation. Other models include a test of an equal action theory (paths from X to M) effect that would compare a model with and without the $\hat{a}$ paths constrained to be equal. Corresponding tests of the equality of the stability coefficient (path from each variable to the same variable at the next wave), and the equality of the conceptual theory paths (M to Y) can also be made using this same approach. The covariances among adjacent error terms could be added to the model and an incremental χ^2 test of adding these covariances could be used to assess the addition of these parameters. It may also be sensible in some cases to include lag 2 or higher relations among the same variables measured at one time and two times later. These models would suggest that the lag 1 relation is not sufficient and there remain dependencies between the first wave and third wave of measurement, for example. Similarly, correlated residual coefficients could replace the contemporaneous mediation effects as a way to incorporate nonspecific relations that may occur at each wave of measurement. Tests of these and other hypotheses may be conducted, starting with a complete model and making constraints to test hypotheses, or a simple model could be used with comparison of nested models used to decide the parameters to include in the longitudinal mediation model. These different types of models are more easily assessed with more waves of data. Some models cannot be estimated with three or even four waves of data. In this case, a set of nested model comparisons can be used to obtain a satisfactory model.

Finally it is very important to note that the aforementioned models (and those described later in this chapter) were based on a single measure at each occasion. As described in chapter 7, measurement models for the measures can be incorporated in these models by including multiple indicators of latent variables, and these latent variables serve as the primary constructs in the longitudinal mediation model. With all of the models described earlier, it may be useful to allow errors in the same variable to be correlated across time to reflect that the measures were collected in the same way across the measurement occasions. The addition of measurement models also increases the number of alternative models that can be tested because the additional measures generally result in more degrees of freedom.

8.9 Strengths and Limitations of Autoregressive Mediation Models

There are many possible mediated effects in autoregressive mediation models including longitudinal and contemporaneous mediated effects.

The total mediated effects can be computed as the sum of the many different longitudinal and contemporaneous mediated effects in the model. For example, the sum of the longitudinal mediated effects is the addition of each individual longitudinal mediated effect. The multivariate delta standard error can be derived for these complicated effects as described in chapter 4. However, at small samples, these estimates of the standard errors may be inaccurate because the delta method is based on asymptotic theory.

Several limitations of autoregressive models are important. In particular the cross-lagged relations among the variables can be inaccurate. In fact, many different types of models may yield the same cross-lagged coefficients. Furthermore, a true model will produce different cross-lagged coefficients. For more on the limitations of these models see Dwyer (1983) and Rogosa (1988). Rogosa (1988) recommended growth curve models, which are described in the next section.

One way to improve the interpretability of autoregressive models is to improve measurement of variables either by specifying latent variables or increasing the reliability of measures. As described in chapter 7, latent variables can be specified for the measured constructs, which addresses some of the limitations of these models.

8.10 Latent Growth Curve (LGC) Models

The autoregressive models described earlier have been criticized for several reasons. The most important criticisms are that growth or change in the measures over time and individual differences in growth are not explicitly modeled. Autoregressive models focus on the stability of the rank order of subjects on variables across time rather than trajectories of change across time. For the two-wave case, the difference score approach is the growth curve approach. With more than two waves, there are many interesting ways to proceed. The covariance structure analysis computer programs can be easily adapted to estimate the parameters of growth curve models.

When there are repeated measures for the independent variable, mediator, and dependent variables, mediation models can be tested with the latent growth curve (LGC) modeling framework (Duncan, Duncan, Strycker, Li, & Alpert, 1999; Muthén & Curran, 1997; Singer & Willet, 2003). One way that mediation effects can be investigated is with a parallel process model, in which three sets of latent growth factors are specified, one set for the independent variable, one set for the mediator, and the other set for the dependent variable. In general, there are two parts of growth models that are represented by latent factors: (a) the intercept factor, representing the starting point of the growth trajectory at time 1, and (b) the slope factor, defining the shape of the developmental growth trajectory over time. The simplest form of the slope factor codes linear change across time, but more complicated forms of growth can be specified including logistic, quadratic, cubic, and higher order growth. The latent growth curve mediation model includes the relations among the slope factor of the independent variable, the slope factor of the mediating variable, and the slope factor of the dependent variable. In this way mediation is assessed by investigating the relations among the growth in X, M, and Y.

The basic mediation LGC model examines whether the relation between an independent variable and a dependent variable is fully or partially accounted for by a mediating variable. Thus, the independent measure affects the mediating variable which, in turn, affects the dependent variable. Extending this concept to the latent growth modeling framework, the mediation model examines whether the growth in the independent variable affects the growth trajectory of the mediating variable which, in turn, affects the growth trajectory of the dependent variable. The relation between the growth of the independent variable and the growth of the dependent variable is through two sources: the indirect or mediated effect via the growth of the mediator (*ab*) and the direct effect (*c′*). Equations 8.21 through 8.29 specify these relations assuming *t* waves of measurement and individuals are represented by the *i* subscript.

Independent Variable Process:

$$X_{it} = I_{Xi} + S_{Xi}*t + \varepsilon_{Xit} \tag{8.21}$$

$$I_{Xi} = I_{X0i} + \upsilon_{IXi} \tag{8.22}$$

$$S_{Xi} = S_{X10i} + \upsilon_{SXi} \tag{8.23}$$

Mediator Process:

$$M_{it} = I_{Mi} + S_{Mi}*t + \varepsilon_{Mit} \tag{8.24}$$

$$I_{Mi} = I_{M0i} + \gamma_1*I_{Xi} + \upsilon_{IMi} \tag{8.25}$$

$$S_{Mi} = S_{M10i} + \gamma_5*I_{Xi} + \gamma_2*I_{Yi} + a*S_{Xi} + \upsilon_{SMi} \tag{8.26}$$

Outcome Process:

$$Y_{it} = I_{Yi} + S_{Yi}*t + \varepsilon_{Yit} \tag{8.27}$$

$$I_{Yi} = I_{Y0i} + \gamma_3*I_{Xi} + \upsilon_{IYi} \tag{8.28}$$

$$S_{Yi} = S_{Y10i} + c′*S_{Xi} + \gamma_6*I_{Xi} + b*S_{Mi} + \gamma_4*I_{Mi} + \upsilon_{SYi} \tag{8.29}$$

Equation 8.21 specifies a model for individual i's data on X at time t that consists of an intercept, a slope factor, and error. Equations 8.22 and 8.23 represent models for the intercept (I_{Xi}) and slope (S_{Xi}) for the X variable, respectively. These two equations represent the intercepts and slopes that vary across persons. Equations 8.24 through 8.26 represent the growth model for the mediator where individual i's data on M is modeled by an intercept, a slope, and an error. Equation 8.25 specifies the predictors of the intercept of M, with an intercept (I_{M0i}) and γ_1 representing the relation of the intercept of X to the intercept of M. Equation 8.26 specifies the relation between the slope of M with an intercept (S_{M10i}), an a parameter reflecting the relation between the slope of X and the slope of M, γ_5 represents the relation between the intercept of X and the slope of M, and γ_2 represents the relation between the intercept of Y and the slope of M. Equations 8.27 through 8.29 are analogous to the mediator equations with the exception that there is an additional predictor of the slope in Y, c', which represents the direct relation between the slope of X and the slope of Y, b represents the relation between the slope of M and the slope of Y, γ_6 represents the relation between the intercept of X and the slope of Y, and γ_4 represents the relation between the intercept of M and the slope of Y.

The random intercepts (I_{Xi}, I_{Mi}, and I_{Yi}) in Equation 8.22, 8.25, and 8.28 represent the initial status of the independent variable, mediator and the dependent variable, respectively. The slope of the mediator (S_{Mi}) is influenced by the slope of the independent variable (S_{Xi}) and the initial status of the outcome process (I_{Yi}). The slope of the outcome (S_{Yi}) is influenced not only by the intercept (I_{Xi}) and slope (S_{Xi}) of the independent variable and the intercept of the mediator (I_{Mi}) but also by the slope of the mediator (S_{Mi}). In many cases it will be preferable to specify covariances among intercepts (and slopes) rather than directed paths in Equations 8.21 to 8.29.

Cheong, MacKinnon, and Khoo (2003) described a method to assess mediation of a prevention program in the LGC framework in which the growth curves of the mediator and the outcome were modeled as distinct parallel processes influenced by a binary independent variable. When the independent variable (X) is group membership under random assignment, the coefficients γ_1 and γ_3, denoting the relation between the independent variable and the random intercepts, are not different from zero. The mediated effect is estimated by the product of the coefficients $\hat{a}$ and $\hat{b}$. Figure 8.4 represents a parallel process growth curve model for mediation, for which the trajectories of the mediator and the outcome processes are modeled as linear.

One criticism of the parallel process model of mediation is that the mediation relation is correlational such that the slope in X is correlated with the slope in M and the slope in M is correlated with the slope in Y when X, M, and Y are assessed at the same occasions. The interpretation

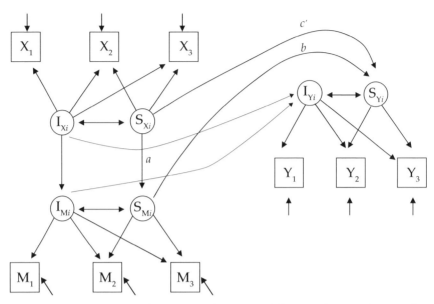

Figure 8.4. Latent growth curve mediation model. Note that $I_{Xi} \rightarrow S_{Mi}$, $I_{Yi} \rightarrow S_{Mi}$, $I_{Xi} \rightarrow S_{Yi}$, and $I_{Mi} \rightarrow S_{Yi}$ from Equations 8.21–8.29 not shown to simplify Figure 8.4.

of this correlation between the slopes is that the change in M is related to change in Y, not that prior change in M is related to later change in Y. An interesting alternative to this model is a two-stage piecewise parallel process model, which can be more sensitive than the single-stage parallel process model in estimating mediated effects in a situation in which the trajectory shape changes across time (Cheong et al., 2003). In a two-stage parallel process model, the growth of the mediator and the outcome process can be modeled separately for the earlier periods and for the later time periods. Thus, the mediated effects can be evaluated at different periods, that is, the mediated effect via the earlier growth of the mediator on the earlier growth of the outcome, the mediated effect via the earlier growth of the mediator on the later growth of the outcome, and the mediated effect via the later growth of the mediator on the later growth of the outcome.

Although specifying latent growth curve models addresses some limitations of autoregressive models, several criticisms of these models remain. Like autoregressive models, measurement is critical and may even be more important. The measure itself may change over time, which may yield a confusing representation of change over time. It is possible that what might be perceived as change over time is actually different measurement over time. As a result, investigation of measurement invariance is often conducted as part of LGC modeling. It is also helpful to test several different models of change over time for each variable separately before investing parallel process or two-stage LGC models. In this way, the change in each variable is established before the relation among the variables is assessed.

There are several steps in assessing mediation with latent growth curve modeling as described in Cheong et al. (2003). A first step requires detailed modeling of each individual variable over time, including assessment of different models for growth over time: linear, quadratic, exponential, logistic, cubic, and so on. This work includes plotting the data and studying the distribution of the dependent variable. The possibility of different growth rates among the variables, X, M, and Y, and the possibility of differential growth across levels of X can be investigated. If X codes assignment to conditions, this includes testing whether growth differs for treatment and control groups. The second step consists of combining the individual growth process models in a parallel process model and assessing mediation relations among the variables. Throughout this process standard methods for assessing model fit and χ^2 difference tests are applied. In the third step, estimates of the mediated effect and standard error are used to test mediated effects. If the coefficients in the mediated effect are random, that is, the relation of X to M and the relation of M to Y vary across participants, then a standard error that takes this into account is needed (Kenny, Bolger, & Korchmaros, 2003). The formula for the point estimate is shown in Equation 8.30 and the standard error is shown in Equation 8.31. Note that the formulas include the estimated covariance between the $\hat{a}$ and $\hat{b}$ paths (cov($\hat{a}\hat{b}$)) because these two coefficients represent random effects.

$$\hat{a}\hat{b}_{\text{random}} = \hat{a}\hat{b} + \text{cov}(\hat{a}\hat{b}) \tag{8.30}$$

$$s^2_{\hat{a}\hat{b}_{\text{random}}} = \hat{a}^2 s^2_{\hat{b}} + \hat{b}^2 s^2_{\hat{a}} + s^2_{\hat{b}} s^2_{\hat{a}} + 2\hat{a}\hat{b}\,\text{cov}(\hat{a}\hat{b}) + \text{cov}(\hat{a}\hat{b})^2 \tag{8.31}$$

An example using these formulas is shown in chapter 9 for the case of random effects in a multilevel model.

8.11 Mplus Code for the Three-Wave Latent Growth Curve Mediation Model

The program code for Mplus shown in Table 8.5 closely follows the Equations 8.21 and 8.29. In addition to the equations, covariances among measures are specified using the WITH command. The BY command specifies the variables that are related to intercept and slope for each variable. The @1 and @2 commands give the fixed values of the loadings relating each variable to the growth factors. Note that the loadings for intercepts are 1, 1, and 1, and the loadings for the linear growth are 0, 1, 2.

Table 8.5 Mplus Program for the Three-Wave Latent Growth Curve
Mediation Model

```
TITLE:
   LATENT GROWTH CURVE MODEL 3 WAVES 3 VARIABLES;
DATA:
   FILE IS c:\data;
VARIABLE:
   Names = X1 X2 X3 M1 M2 M3 Y1 Y2 Y3;
   Usevariables X1 X2 X3 M1 M2 M3 Y1 Y2 Y3;
ANALYSIS:
   TYPE IS meanstructure;
MODEL:
   i1 by Y1@1 Y2@1 Y3@1;
   s1 by Y1@0 Y2@1 Y3@2;
   i2 by M1@1 M2@1 M3@1;
   s2 by M1@0 M2@1 M3@2;
   i3 by X1@1 X2@1 X3@1;
   s3 by X1@0 X2@1 X3@2;
   s1 on i2 i3 s2 s3; s2 on i1 i3 s3;
   i2 on i3; i1 on i3;
   i1 with s1; i2 with s2; i3 with s3;
   [Y1@0 Y2@0 Y3@0
   M1@0 M2@0 M3@0
   X1@0 X2@0 X3@0
   i1-i3 s1-s3];
OUTPUT:
```

8.12 LISREL Code for the Three-Wave Latent Growth Curve Mediation Model

The specification of latent growth curve models in LISREL shown in Table 8.6 requires the addition of four new parameter matrices corresponding to the intercepts for the y variables, Tau-Y or τy, and for the x variables, Tau-X or τx, Alpha or α for the means of the endogenous latent variables η, and Kappa, κ, for the means of the exogenous latent variables ξ. Because an all-Y model is specified, the Kappa and Tau-X matrices are not specified in the LISREL program.

8.13 Latent Difference Score Models

The latent growth curve model estimates a slope based on several waves of data. Linear, quadratic, cubic, and higher way trends can be estimated to reflect the time effect across all waves of measurement. For the mediation

Table 8.6 LISREL Program for the Latent Growth Curve Mediation Model

```
LATENT GROWTH CURVE MODEL
DA NI=9 MA=CM ME=ML NO=100
RA FI=c:\data
LA
'X1' 'X2' 'X3' 'M1' 'M2' 'M3' 'Y1' 'Y2' 'Y3'
MO NY=9 NE=9 LY=FI BE=FU,FI PS=SY,FI TE=DI,FI TY=FU,FI AL=FR
FR PS(1,1) PS(2,2) PS (3,3) PS(4,4) PS(5,5) PS(6,6)
FR PS(2,1) PS(4,3) PS (6,5)
VA LY
1 0 0 0 0 0
1 1 0 0 0 0
1 2 0 0 0 0
0 0 1 0 0 0
0 0 1 1 0 0
0 0 1 2 0 0
0 0 0 0 1 0
0 0 0 0 1 1
0 0 0 0 1 2
PA BE
0 0 0 0 0 0
0 0 1 0 1 0
1 0 0 0 0 0
1 1 0 0 1 0
1 0 1 0 0 0
1 1 1 1 0 0
OU AL
```

model, the slope of X is related to the slope of M, which is related to the slope of Y. The two-stage piecewise parallel process latent growth model described earlier provides a way to evaluate the effect of earlier growth of mediator, for example, on later growth in the outcome variable Y. Similarly, it is often useful to examine the change between pairs of waves as described in a latent difference score model (Ferrer & McArdle, 2003; McArdle, 2001; McArdle & Hamagami, 2001; McArdle & Nesselroade, 2003). In this model, fixed parameters and hypothesized latent variables are used to specify latent difference (LD) scores. By specifying latent differences, the model represents dynamic change in terms of the difference between waves. A latent difference score mediation model is shown in figure 8.5. Looking at the model for X_1, X_2, and X_3, the latent difference is obtained by fixing two paths at 1, the path from the time 1 to the time 2 measure and the path from the latent difference to the time 2 measure. Because of these constraints, the latent difference between the two waves

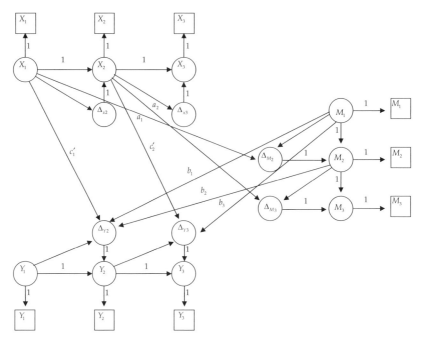

Figure 8.5.   Latent difference score mediation model.

is obtained. This model may be especially useful in situations in which it is expected that the predictors of change are different at different waves of measurement. One common example of these effects may occur in experimental research, in which the effects of a manipulation affect change early in a process, but these effects may not be present on the change at later waves. That is, the intervention affects change in a dependent variable at time 1 and time 2 but does not affect change between later waves. The latent difference score model is not necessarily constrained to represent change between two waves, and it is possible to devise models that represent the change in the change between waves (i.e., second derivatives; Malone, Lansford, Castellino, Berlin, Dodge, Bates & Pettit, 2004) and models representing moving averages are also possible.

Figure 8.5 shows a latent difference mediation model in which the relation of X_1 to the latent difference of Δ_{M2} represents the *a* path for relation of X_1 to the latent difference Δ_{M3}. The original formulation of the latent difference model was programmed in the reticular activation model (RAM) devised by McDonald and colleagues (McArdle & McDonald, 1984). The RAM model requires only three matrices to represent any covariance structure model, although the matrices do not directly represent substantive relations as with the EQS and LISREL formulation.

Another version of the latent difference score model includes paths relating the latent differences to each other. There are many different potential mediation effects in this type of model corresponding to mediation effects for contemporaneous change and mediation effects for longitudinal change. An example of contemporaneous change includes the relation between change in the same waves, for example, change in X_1 and X_2 being related to change in M_1 and M_2, the a coefficient, and change in M_1 and M_2 is related to change in Y_1 and Y_2, the b coefficient. Longitudinal mediation change corresponds to change in earlier waves that is related to change at later waves. An example of a mediation effect with contemporaneous and longitudinal change relations is the latent difference between X_1 and X_2 being related to the latent difference between M_1 and M_2, for the a coefficient, which is in turn related to the latent difference between Y_2 and Y_3, the b coefficient.

The original formulation of the latent difference score model (Ferrer & McArdle, 2003) is actually different from the models described earlier. In the classic latent difference score model, a latent factor is included in the same manner as described earlier with paths predicting each latent difference score. The paths from the latent factor to the latent difference scores are called α paths and are constrained to be equal to each other. That is, the latent factor predicts each difference score to the same magnitude and represents latent change across time. There would be separate latent factors for X, M, and Y for the multiple process mediation model. Similarly all paths from the earlier score of a wave to the subsequent latent difference score are constrained to be equal and these paths are called β paths. Different specifications of these α and β paths correspond to different models for change over time. If β is set to zero, then the model is a constant change score model quantified by the α coefficient. Specifying $\alpha = \beta = 0$ corresponds to a no change score model (McArdle & Hamagami, 2001).

8.14 Application of Autoregressive and Growth Curve Models to the Evaluation of a Prevention Program

To illustrate the longitudinal mediation models, the analyses of a study of the effects of an anabolic steroid prevention program are presented. Participants received either an anabolic steroid prevention program (X = 1) or a pamphlet (X = 0) designed to prevent steroid use. The participants in the study provided measures before the football season, immediately after the season, in the fall before next year's season, and in the fall at the end of the next season. There were a total of four waves of observation. The program was delivered to about half of the participants between the first and second measurement. Although there are many potential mediators to examine, the mediating effect of perceived severity of anabolic steroid use on intent to use anabolic steroids was selected for illustration here. A goal of the program was to increase the perceived severity of anabolic steroid use, which was hypothesized to reduce intentions to use anabolic steroids. The computer programs to estimate the parameters of this model and the output from the Mplus programs are shown in Tables 8.7 and 8.8.

The Mplus code, shown in Table 8.7, specifies the autoregressive model in Equations 8.3 through 8.8 extended to four waves. Note that this model includes autoregressive paths consistent with the mediation hypothesis. Only lag 1 relations are specified in this model. The "MODEL RESULTS" section contains the coefficients, standard errors, and critical ratios for the paths. For example, baseline intentions ($\hat{s} = 0.533$, $se = 0.037$), baseline perceptions of severity ($\hat{a} = -0.168$, $se = 0.036$), and group ($\hat{b} = -0.200$, $se = 0.084$) were significantly related to wave C intentions. At wave D, group is no longer statistically significant, but the mediator at wave C is significantly related to intentions at wave D, providing longitudinal evidence for the $\hat{b}$ path ($\hat{b} = -0.147$, $se = 0.046$). Group is significantly related to the mediator at wave C ($\hat{a} = 0.477$, $se = 0.106$), providing evidence for the $\hat{a}$ path. There are other statistically significant mediated effects from the mediator to the dependent variable at wave E, but there is only evidence for the $\hat{a}$ path at wave C for perceived severity. This significant $\hat{a}$ path is part of mediation effects at later waves.

The overall fit of the model is not very good with a root mean square error of approximation (RMSEA) = 0.116, suggesting that more analysis is necessary. In particular, the additional paths in the autoregressive II and III models provide better fit to the data as you are asked to do in exercise 8.4.

Table 8.8 shows the results for the latent growth curve model for a different mediator and different dependent variable than in the last example (Note that some relations in Equations 8.21 to 8.29 are not estimated in the model, e.g., $I_{Xi} \rightarrow I_{Mi}$). In the latent growth curve model, the mediated effect through belief that the media provides accurate information about health and nutrition on a nutrition behaviors measure was investigated. In the first model (not shown here), linear growth in the mediator and the dependent variable was specified as described earlier in this chapter. The problem with the initial growth curve model was that the main intervention was delivered before the second wave of measurement, and it was not increased at later measurements. To model both the slope over time in the mediator and the dependent variable and to model the effect of group, an additional slope variable was included with a zero for baseline and a one for all subsequent waves of measurement. The results from that analysis are shown in Table 8.8. The relation from group to the slope of the mediator was significant ($\hat{a} = -0.491$, $se = 0.069$), and there was evidence that the slope in the mediator was significantly associated with the slope in the

Table 8.7 Mplus Autoregressive Mediation Model and Selected Output

```
TITLE:
      AUTOREGRESSIVE MODEL FOUR WAVES;
DATA:
      FILE IS c:\Medbook h\New0204\c3medBtoG.csv;

VARIABLE:
      Names = ID GROUP SCHOOL INTENT NUTRIT STRTRN KNWAS
      CCHTL PERTL PERIN TEMIN NORMS RESIST SEVER SUSCEP
      MEDIA PROAS CONAS CINTENT CNUTRIT CSTRTRN CKNWAS
      CCCHTL CPERTL CPERIN CTEMIN CNORMS CRESIST CSEVER
      CSUSCEP CMEDIA CPROAS CCONAS DINTENT DNUTRIT
      DSTRTRN DKNWAS DCCHTL DPERTL DPERIN DTEMIN DNORMS
      DRESIST DSEVER DSUSCEP DMEDIA DPROAS DCONAS
      EINTENT ENUTRIT ESTRTRN EKNWAS ECCHTL EPERTL
      EPERIN ETEMIN ENORMS ERESIST ESEVER ESUSCEP EMEDIA
      EPROAS ECONAS FINTENT FNUTRIT FSTRTRN FKNWAS
      FCCHTL FPERTL FPERIN FTEMIN FNORMS FRESIST FSEVER
      FSUSCEP FMEDIA FPROAS FCONAS GINTENT GNUTRIT
      GSTRTRN GKNWAS GCCHTL GPERTL GPERIN GTEMIN GNORMS
      GRESIST GSEVER GSUSCEP GMEDIA GPROAS GCONAS
      cohort;
      Missing = all (-99);
      Usevariables= GROUP SEVER CSEVER DSEVER ESEVER
      INTENT CINTENT DINTENT EINTENT;
      useobservations = cohort<=1;
ANALYSIS:
      TYPE IS  meanstructure;
      iteration=50000;
      convergence=.000001;
      coverage=.05;
      h1convergence=.000001;
MODEL:
    CINTENT ON GROUP INTENT SEVER;
    DINTENT ON GROUP CINTENT CSEVER;
    EINTENT ON GROUP DINTENT DSEVER;
    CSEVER ON GROUP SEVER;
    DSEVER ON GROUP CSEVER;
    ESEVER ON GROUP DSEVER;
    GROUP WITH INTENT SEVER;
    INTENT WITH SEVER;
    CINTENT WITH CSEVER;
    DINTENT WITH DSEVER;
    EINTENT WITH ESEVER;
```

(continued)

Table 8.7 (Continued)

```
    OUTPUT:

Number of groups                                    1
Number of observations                            436

Number of y-variables                               6
Number of x-variables                               3
Number of continuous latent variables               0

Observed variables in the analysis
    GROUP     SEVER     CSEVER    DSEVER    ESEVER    INTENT
    CINTENT   DINTENT   EINTENT

Estimator                                          ML
Maximum number of iterations                    50000
Convergence criterion                      0.100D-05

Input data file(s)
  c:\Medbook h\New0204\c3medBtoG.csv

Input data format   FREE

TESTS OF MODEL FIT

Chi-Square Test of Model Fit

          Value                             103.257
          Degrees of Freedom                     15
          P-Value                            0.0000

Chi-Square Test of Model Fit for the Baseline Model

          Value                            1132.131
          Degrees of Freedom                     33
          P-Value                            0.0000

CFI/TLI

          CFI                                 0.920
          TLI                                 0.823
```

Table 8.7 (Continued)

Loglikelihood

H0 Value	-5405.114
H1 Value	-5353.486

Information Criteria

Number of Free Parameters	39
Akaike (AIC)	10888.228
Bayesian (BIC)	11047.256
Sample-Size Adjusted BIC	10923.490

Mplus VERSION 2.01
AUTOREGRESSIVE MODEL FOUR WAVES;

$$(n* = (n + 2) / 24)$$

RMSEA (Root Mean Square Error Of Approximation)

Estimate	0.116	
90 Percent C.I.	0.096	0.138
Probability RMSEA <= .05	0.000	

SRMR (Standardized Root Mean Square Residual)

Value	0.088

MODEL RESULTS

	Estimates	S.E.	Est./S.E.
CINTENT ON			
GROUP	-0.200	0.084	-2.384
INTENT	0.533	0.037	14.330
SEVER	-0.168	0.036	-4.677
DINTENT ON			
GROUP	0.003	0.109	0.029
CINTENT	0.351	0.045	7.732
CSEVER	-0.147	0.046	-3.169
EINTENT ON			
GROUP	0.042	0.092	0.456
DINTENT	0.424	0.040	10.587
DSEVER	-0.183	0.040	-4.584

(continued)

Table 8.7 (Continued)

CSEVER ON			
GROUP	0.477	0.106	4.479
SEVER	0.400	0.043	9.374
DSEVER ON			
GROUP	0.042	0.114	0.371
CSEVER	0.442	0.046	9.638
ESEVER ON			
GROUP	0.118	0.108	1.095
DSEVER	0.495	0.042	11.848
GROUP WITH			
INTENT	-0.014	0.027	-0.497
SEVER	0.014	0.030	0.470
INTENT WITH			
SEVER	-0.516	0.073	-7.115
CINTENT WITH			
CSEVER	-0.290	0.048	-6.028
DINTENT WITH			
DSEVER	-0.566	0.067	-8.436
EINTENT WITH			
ESEVER	-0.367	0.053	-6.863
Residual Variances			
CSEVER	1.220	0.083	14.765
DSEVER	1.342	0.091	14.765
ESEVER	1.240	0.084	14.765
CINTENT	0.759	0.051	14.765
DINTENT	1.224	0.083	14.765
EINTENT	0.897	0.061	14.765
Variances			
GROUP	0.247	0.017	14.765
SEVER	1.538	0.104	14.765
INTENT	1.320	0.089	14.765
Means			
GROUP	0.447	0.024	18.782
SEVER	5.865	0.059	98.743
INTENT	1.609	0.055	29.239

Table 8.7 (Continued)

Intercepts			
CSEVER	3.433	0.259	13.251
DSEVER	3.138	0.275	11.424
ESEVER	2.860	0.248	11.522
CINTENT	1.878	0.244	7.692
DINTENT	2.023	0.313	6.470
EINTENT	2.028	0.274	7.389

dependent variable ($\hat{b}$ = 0.823, *se* = 0.426) consistent with the mediation model. This model included both time trends and a code to test the program. The model also had an RMSEA = 0.026, which suggests good fit. It appears that the program altered change in the beliefs about media, and this was associated with better nutrition. Note that the estimation of the model was conducted using a missing data analysis strategy so that all data, even partial data, were used in the analysis. The "Missing = All *" indicates that missing data are indicated by a "*" and the "Type is missing h1 meanstructure" line selects full information maximum likelihood estimation.

8.15 Additional Longitudinal Models

There are other longitudinal models in addition to the autoregressive and latent growth models described here. Curran and Bollen (2001) and Bollen and Curran (2004) describe a model that combines features of the latent growth curve model with the autoregressive model (Curran & Hussong, 2003) called an autoregressive latent trajectory (ALT) model. The ALT model includes both latent growth along with paths between adjacent measures of the same variable. These models may be especially appropriate if the latent growth does not adequately reflect dependency across time. Another alternative model includes traits for measures over time along with dependence among adjacent waves (Jackson & Sher, 2003).

One other potential model for mediational relations is a differential equation model (Arminger, 1986; Boker & Nesselroade, 2002; Dwyer, 1992) for X, M, and Y. Differential equation models are generally considered the language of science because they represent relations among variables in continuous time. These models do not have the problem of different time intervals of measurement because the model parameters are in a continuous time metric. The models are dynamic and include negative and positive feedback loops, again in continuous time, which correspond most clearly to the notions of stability, feedback, and equilibrium. In this

Table 8.8   Mplus Latent Growth Curve Mediation Model and Selected Output

```
Mplus VERSION 4.1
MUTHEN & MUTHEN
08/30/2006  11:54 AM

INPUT INSTRUCTIONS

    TITLE:
        Chapter 8 Latent Growth Model with 4 Wave and 3
        Variables;
    DATA:
        FILE IS Chap8_ATLASBtoE.csv;

    VARIABLE:
        Names =  group nutrit media cnutrit cmedia
                 dnutrit dmedia enutrit emedia;
        Missing = ALL *;
        Usevariables= group media cmedia dmedia emedia
                      nutrit cnutrit dnutrit enutrit;
    ANALYSIS:
        TYPE IS missing h1 meanstructure;
        iteration=50000;
        convergence=.000001;
            coverage=.05;
        h1convergence=.000001;
    MODEL:
        i1 by media@1 Cmedia@1 Dmedia@1 Emedia@1;
        s1 by media@0 Cmedia@.3 Dmedia@1 Emedia@1.3;
        s3 by media@0 Cmedia@1 Dmedia@1 Emedia@1;

        i2 by nutrit@1 Cnutrit@1 Dnutrit@1 Enutrit@1;
        s2 by nutrit@0 Cnutrit@.3 Dnutrit@1 Enutrit@1.3;
        s4 by nutrit@0 Cnutrit@1 Dnutrit@1 Enutrit@1;

        s1 on i2;
        s2 on i1 s3 group;
        s3 on i2 group;
        s4 on s3 i1 group;

        [media@0 Cmedia@0 Dmedia@0 Emedia@0
        nutrit@0 Cnutrit@0 Dnutrit@0 Enutrit@0
        i1-s4];

    OUTPUT:
```

Table 8.8 (Continued)

Chapter 8 Latent Growth Model with 4 Wave and 3 Variables;

SUMMARY OF ANALYSIS

Number of groups	1
Number of observations	1506

Number of dependent variables	8
Number of independent variables	1
Number of continuous latent variables	6

Observed dependent variables

  Continuous
    MEDIA   CMEDIA   DMEDIA   EMEDIA   NUTRIT   CNUTRIT
    DNUTRIT   ENUTRIT

Observed independent variables
    GROUP

Continuous latent variables
    I1   S1   S3   I2   S2   S4

Estimator	ML
Information matrix	OBSERVED
Maximum number of iterations	50000
Convergence criterion	0.100D-05
Maximum number of steepest descent iterations	20
Maximum number of iterations for H1	2000
Convergence criterion for H1	0.100D-05

Input data file(s)
  Chap8_ATLASBtoE.csv

Input data format   FREE

SUMMARY OF DATA

     Number of patterns   21

COVARIANCE COVERAGE OF DATA

Minimum covariance coverage value   0.050

(*continued*)

Table 8.8 (Continued)

PROPORTION OF DATA PRESENT

Covariance Coverage

	MEDIA	CMEDIA	DMEDIA	EMEDIA	NUTRIT
MEDIA	0.973				
CMEDIA	0.778	0.801			
DMEDIA	0.555	0.497	0.569		
EMEDIA	0.321	0.295	0.325	0.331	
NUTRIT	0.973	0.779	0.556	0.322	0.974
CNUTRIT	0.780	0.801	0.499	0.297	0.782
DNUTRIT	0.559	0.501	0.569	0.327	0.560
ENUTRIT	0.323	0.297	0.326	0.331	0.323
GROUP	0.973	0.801	0.569	0.331	0.974

Covariance Coverage

	CNUTRIT	DNUTRIT	ENUTRIT	GROUP
CNUTRIT	0.804			
DNUTRIT	0.503	0.573		
ENUTRIT	0.298	0.328	0.332	
GROUP	0.804	0.573	0.332	1.000

THE MODEL ESTIMATION TERMINATED NORMALLY

TESTS OF MODEL FIT

Chi-Square Test of Model Fit

Value	33.908
Degrees of Freedom	17
P-Value	0.0086

Chi-Square Test of Model Fit for the Baseline Model

Value	2037.965
Degrees of Freedom	36
P-Value	0.0000

CFI/TLI

CFI	0.992
TLI	0.982

Table 8.8 (Continued)

```
Loglikelihood

          H0 Value                        -13124.173
          H1 Value                        -13107.219

Information Criteria

          Number of Free Parameters              35
          Akaike (AIC)                     26318.346
          Bayesian (BIC)                   26504.449
          Sample-Size Adjusted BIC         26393.263
            (n* = (n + 2) / 24)

RMSEA (Root Mean Square Error Of Approximation)

          Estimate                             0.026
          90 Percent C.I.                      0.013  0.038
          Probability RMSEA <= .05             1.000

SRMR (Standardized Root Mean Square Residual)

          Value                                0.029

MODEL RESULTS

                         Estimates     S.E.   Est./S.E.

  I1       BY
     MEDIA                 1.000      0.000      0.000
     CMEDIA                1.000      0.000      0.000
     DMEDIA                1.000      0.000      0.000
     EMEDIA                1.000      0.000      0.000

  S1       BY
     MEDIA                 0.000      0.000      0.000
     CMEDIA                0.300      0.000      0.000
     DMEDIA                1.000      0.000      0.000
     EMEDIA                1.300      0.000      0.000

  S3       BY
     MEDIA                 0.000      0.000      0.000
     CMEDIA                1.000      0.000      0.000
     DMEDIA                1.000      0.000      0.000
     EMEDIA                1.000      0.000      0.000
```

(continued)

Table 8.8 (Continued)

I2	BY			
	NUTRIT	1.000	0.000	0.000
	CNUTRIT	1.000	0.000	0.000
	DNUTRIT	1.000	0.000	0.000
	ENUTRIT	1.000	0.000	0.000
S2	BY			
	NUTRIT	0.000	0.000	0.000
	CNUTRIT	0.300	0.000	0.000
	DNUTRIT	1.000	0.000	0.000
	ENUTRIT	1.300	0.000	0.000
S4	BY			
	NUTRIT	0.000	0.000	0.000
	CNUTRIT	1.000	0.000	0.000
	DNUTRIT	1.000	0.000	0.000
	ENUTRIT	1.000	0.000	0.000
S1	ON			
	I2	-0.017	0.080	-0.210
S2	ON			
	I1	-0.159	0.065	-2.438
	S3	-0.236	0.373	-0.632
S3	ON			
	I2	-0.123	0.069	-1.769
S4	ON			
	S3	0.823	0.426	1.932
	I1	-0.060	0.062	-0.964
S2	ON			
	GROUP	-0.419	0.196	-2.143
S3	ON			
	GROUP	-0.491	0.069	-7.111
S4	ON			
	GROUP	0.951	0.223	4.259
I2	WITH			
	I1	0.208	0.038	5.510
S2	WITH			
	S1	0.132	0.057	2.304

Table 8.8 (Continued)

S4	WITH			
S1		-0.091	0.059	-1.543
S2		-0.208	0.191	-1.092
GROUP	WITH			
I1		-0.031	0.016	-1.910
I2		-0.036	0.015	-2.432
Means				
I1		2.766	0.033	84.950
I2		3.966	0.029	135.555
Intercepts				
MEDIA		0.000	0.000	0.000
CMEDIA		0.000	0.000	0.000
DMEDIA		0.000	0.000	0.000
EMEDIA		0.000	0.000	0.000
NUTRIT		0.000	0.000	0.000
CNUTRIT		0.000	0.000	0.000
DNUTRIT		0.000	0.000	0.000
ENUTRIT		0.000	0.000	0.000
S1		0.061	0.320	0.192
S3		0.531	0.282	1.882
S2		0.504	0.189	2.675
S4		0.112	0.187	0.598
Variances				
I1		0.709	0.046	15.359
I2		0.754	0.075	10.105
Residual Variances				
MEDIA		0.856	0.049	17.617
CMEDIA		0.811	0.055	14.822
DMEDIA		0.866	0.062	13.886
EMEDIA		0.867	0.091	9.532
NUTRIT		0.516	0.071	7.252
CNUTRIT		0.375	0.113	3.301
DNUTRIT		0.547	0.042	13.102
ENUTRIT		0.484	0.062	7.839
S1		0.152	0.067	2.264
S3		0.134	0.059	2.271
S2		0.333	0.178	1.869
S4		0.230	0.218	1.056

framework, the longitudinal model estimates are obtained using methods described earlier in this chapter, and these are treated as the integrated model. The task is to find the differential equation model that led to the integrated model. Arminger (1986) outlined this approach for stochastic differential equation models. Differential equation models seem especially promising, given the continuous time orientation of these models and the modeling of reciprocal relations and negative and positive feedback relations. These models have been used to model attitude changes over time (Arminger, 1986) and relative weight and blood pressure (Dwyer, 1992). Computer programs for these models have been written (e.g., DIFFLONG; MacKinnon, Dwyer, & Arminger, 1992) but not for mediation relations.

8.16 *Person-Centered Mediation Models*

The dominant view of mediation is a variable-centered approach with which relations among variables are investigated. In contrast, person-centered tests for mediation focus on patterns of responses for individuals that are consistent or inconsistent with mediation (Robins & Greenland, 1992; Witteman et al., 1998). The importance of developing person-oriented approaches to mediation is highlighted in an example in Collins, Graham, and Flaherty (1998) for a binary predictor (treatment/control), mediator (acquisition/failure to acquire refusal skills), and outcome (refused/failed to refuse drug offer). Collins et al. demonstrated that it is possible for traditional, variable-oriented approaches to detect mediated effects even when there are no differences between the treatment and control conditions in terms of the proportion of people with responses consistent with the mediational process. This may occur when the impact of the mediator on the outcome varies as a function of the treatment group or when the mediator has different construct validity between groups (i.e., moderated mediation).

Collins et al. (1998) specified three conditions for mediation, assuming three waves for binary X, M, and Y. Following Collins et al., let T represent being in the treatment condition and C represent being in the control condition, M denotes being in the mediator stage and nM denotes not being in the mediator stage, Y denotes being in the outcome stage, and nY denotes not being in the outcome stage. A later time is indicated by $t + x$, where x represents some elapsed time.

Condition 1: The probability of undergoing the mediator to outcome sequence, given starting in the no mediator stage and in the no outcome stage, is greater in the treatment group than in the control group, as shown in Equation 8.32.

$$P(M_{t+x} \text{ and } Y_{t+x+y} | T, nM_t, nY_t) > P(M_{t+x} \text{ and } Y_{t+x+y} | C, nM_t, nY_t) \quad (8.32)$$

Condition 2: The probability of a transition to the mediator stage, among those who are not already in the mediator stage, is greater in the treatment group than in the control group, as shown in Equation 8.33. This condition is analogous to the *a* parameter in the regression framework.

$$P(M_{t+x}|n_t, T) > P(M_{t+x}| nM_t, C) \qquad (8.33)$$

Condition 3: As shown in Equation 8.34, being in the mediator stage increases the probability of a transition to the outcome stage for those not already in the outcome stage in both the treatment and control groups.

$$P(Y_{t+x}|Mt, , nY, T) > P(Y_{t+x}|nMt, nYt, T) \text{ and}$$
$$P(Y_{t+x}|Mt, , nY, C) > P(Y_{t+x}|nMt, nYt, C) \qquad (8.34)$$

In the original description of the method, sampling variability is not taken into account when the probabilities are compared. It seems reasonable to conduct a *t* test of equal proportions for each condition using $p(1 - p)/N$ for the variance of each proportion to form the pooled standard rror of the difference of proportions.

Table 8.9 shows the data from Collins et al. (1998). The columns for Treatment, Mediator, and Outcome correspond to the different combinations of Treatment, (treatment = 1, control = 0), Mediator (has mediator = 1 and does not have mediator = 0), and Outcome (has the outcome = 1 and does not have the outcome = 0). For these data, Collins et al. assumed that all subjects start out without the mediator and without the outcome, so

Table 8.9 Frequencies from Collins et al. (1998) and One Actual Data Example

Treatment	Mediator	Outcome	Frequency			
			C1nC2	C1nC3	C2C3	MED
1	1	1	60	45	36	65
1	1	0	15	30	54	71
1	0	1	30	45	18	39
1	0	0	45	30	42	76
0	1	1	45	27	36	89
0	1	0	30	18	9	74
0	0	1	30	63	0	41
0	0	0	45	42	105	82
Total			300	300	300	537

it can be assumed that all frequencies are from subjects without these variables at baseline. The first column, C1nC2, of frequencies corresponds to the case where Condition 1 is met (0.3 – 0.4 = 0.1, $t = 1.8257$; marginally significant) and Condition 2 is not. The mediator has an effect on the outcome, but the treatment did not affect the mediator. Condition 2 is not met because the probability of acquiring the mediator is 0.5 whether or not an individual received the treatment. Condition 3 is met because the probability of acquiring the outcome is greater if the mediator was acquired in both the control ($t = 2.50$) and treatment groups ($t = 5.477$).

For the second column of numbers, C1nC3, Condition 1 is met because more persons acquired the mediator and the outcome in the treatment group compared with the control group (0.30 – 0.18 = 0.12, $t = 2.458$). Condition 2 is met because the probability of acquiring the mediator in the control group is lower than that for the treatment group (0.3 – 0.5 = 0.2, $t = -3.612$). However, Condition 3 is not satisfied as the probability that an individual acquires the outcome is the same for each group (0.6) and does not depend on whether they acquired the mediator or not.

Finally, the data in the third column, C2C3, illustrate some ambiguity for tests of Condition 3. Specifically, the probability of acquiring the mediator associated with acquiring the outcome is nonsignificant in the treatment group ($t = 1.27$) but statistically significant in the control group ($t = 13.42$). Condition 2 is satisfied because the probability of acquiring the mediator is higher in the treatment group than in the control group (0.6 – 0.3 = 0.3, $t = 5.477$). However, Condition 1 is not satisfied because the probability of acquiring the mediator (0.24) was the same in both treatment and control groups.

This method was applied to the data from the ATLAS example described earlier for longitudinal models with frequencies shown in the fourth column in Table 8.9. The median at baseline for nutrition behaviors and peer as an information source was used to dichotomize the third wave nutrition behaviors and second wave information source measure. These dichotomized measures were then classified by treatment condition and the resulting frequencies are shown in the last column of Table 8.9. The results of this analysis do not suggest evidence for either Condition 1 (0.3112 – 0.2590 = 0.0522, $t = 1.3422$) or Condition 2 (0.5699 – 0.5418 = 0.0281, $t = 0.6540$), but there was evidence for Condition 3 in the control ($t = 3.69$) and the treatment ($t = 2.35$) groups.

There are several limitations to this model (Fairchild & MacKinnon, 2005). First, the requirement of binary variables reduces the amount of information in the data and statistical power to detect effects. Second, the model as originally described requires that participants do not have the outcome or mediator at the beginning of the study, which may be unrealistic for most applications of mediation. Nevertheless, the notion of classifying individuals based on their scores on X, M, and Y is useful. For continuous data, it may be sensible to classify each individual according to whether they are consistent or inconsistent with an underlying mediational process. Fairchild and MacKinnon (2005) further investigated this method and found that Condition 2 is the same requirement as a statistically significant $\hat{a}$ path. There was no clear relation between Conditions 1 and 3 and values of the $\hat{c}'$, $\hat{c}$, or $\hat{b}$ coefficients.

Another development of person-oriented approaches is the mixture of person and variable relations, in which trajectories over time or other classes are identified in the data as well as modeling the change in the variables over time (Muthén & Muthén, 2004). These models allow for clustering of individuals on the basis of their change over time. Once these clusters of persons are identified, then variable-oriented methods are applied to each group. Here it may be possible to identify different mediators depending on the cluster of individuals.

8.17 Conclusions

The purpose of this chapter was to outline the strengths and limitations of several alternative approaches to investigating mediation in longitudinal data. Temporal precedence is a key idea in the identification of mediating processes, and longitudinal data shed more light on these mechanisms than cross-sectional data. In general, it is difficult to recommend one model in all research contexts, and in many cases it will be wise to estimate several of these longitudinal models for the same data set. The most convincing relations among variables will be those that are consistent across different models.

For designs with two waves of data, difference score, analysis of covariance, and residualized change scores are options for analysis. Each model provides a different approach to modeling change over time. Difference score models assume that differences at the first measurement will remain at the later measurement. Analysis of covariance and residualized change scores assume that scores will regress to the mean over time. Again the most convincing mediation relations are present for each model.

The strengths and weaknesses of each model suggest a general approach to longitudinal mediation analysis. First, the latent growth model provides a general way to investigate whether there is significant change over time and whether the change over time differs across participants. A first step in longitudinal growth modeling is to fit a growth model to each individual variable before estimating a model that includes all variables. If there is substantial growth in the variables over time, this suggests that a latent growth model may be ideal and subsequent analysis should be based on the latent growth model. Linear and nonlinear growth in each variable in the mediation model should be considered on the basis of theory and empirical work. Once satisfactory models for each variable are obtained, a combined model is tested in which the longitudinal relations between X, M, and Y are included. Estimates of the mediated effect and its confidence limits then provide some guidance regarding mediational processes.

In some cases, if changes between waves are expected or are observed, then the latent difference score or piecewise latent growth curve model may be ideal. These models allow for changes in mediators at different times to be related to changes in the dependent variable at different times. More convincing evidence for mediation is obtained when a change in a variable at earlier waves predicts change at later waves. Finally, the use of an X variable that represents random assignment to conditions also improves the interpretation of longitudinal relations because change in X must occur before a change in the mediator and the dependent variable.

If there is not significant growth over time, then the autoregressive model is often the ideal model because of the way that longitudinal and cross-sectional mediation relations can be investigated in cross-sectional models. More complicated patterns of mediation across waves, such as multiple path mediation, are also easily incorporated in this model along with standard errors used for creating confidence limits for the different mediated effects.

The importance of temporal precedence has led some researchers to recommend the sole use of longitudinal data to assess relations including mediation. There are situations in which cross-sectional models may provide information about mediation processes, but these relations must be interpreted in the context of the alternative models that may be operating when information on the timing of relations is not available. Many fields of science are based on cross-sectional data. The fields of geology and astronomy use cross-sectional data to examine longitudinal events. Aspects of cross-sectional data on geographic stratification, for example, are used to infer change over geologic time. Red shift information is used to incorporate time effects in astronomy. Furthermore, individuals in prestigious and effective jobs such as physicians and clinicians base diagnoses on cross-sectional measures of signs, symptoms, and tests. Physicians and clinicians study historical information based on forms completed at one time but also use longitudinal changes in response to treatments to diagnose and treat illness. Detectives complete entire investigations on the basis of cross-sectional analysis of crime scenes with inference regarding temporal precedence after the original event occurred. Timing of events is a critical component of cross-sectional interviews of suspects. In the social sciences, retrospective data regarding critical events in life history are used to map the temporal order of major events. The point is that longitudinal data provide both cross-sectional and longitudinal information that is likely to more accurately expose mediation relations.

As stated several times in this book, all studies can shed light on mediational processes including cross-sectional studies and case studies. The important point is the quality of the conclusions regarding mediational processes. Longitudinal data have the capacity to provide more detailed information about these processes. Several new approaches to mediation relations will probably receive more application. The person-oriented latent transition models proposed by Collins et al. (1998) also provide useful information regarding mediational processes. Current limitations to the model include the requirement of binary data. Differential equation models are also likely to receive additional development as they provide information on continuous time relations. To date, little is known about the correct models for longitudinal mediation. Advances in this area will probably require statistical development and theoretical development regarding the appropriate timing of mediation relations.

8.18 Exercises

8.1. The following code is the SAS code for the formula (Burr & Nesselroade, 1990, p. 9) for the reliability of the difference score, rdd, given the variance of the first measurement (s2x1), variance of the second measurement (s2x2), reliability of the first measurement (rx1x1), reliability of the second measurement (rx2x2), and correlation between the first and second measurements (rx1x2).

```
data diff;
input s2x1 s2x2 rx1x1 rx2x2 rx1x2;
sx1=sqrt(s2x1); sx2=sqrt(s2x2);
num=s2x1*rx1x1 - 2*sx1*sx2*rx1x2+s2x2*rx2x2;
den=s2x1-2*sx1*sx2*rx1x2 + s2x2;
rdd=num/den;
cards;
1 1 .8 .8 .5
```

   a. Verify the reliability of the difference score values in Table 8.1.
   b. If the true correlation between two waves is 0.6 and the reliability of the scale is 0.8, what is the ratio of difference score reliability to reliability of the individual score?

8.2. With your own four-wave data, estimate the mediated effect using an autoregressive, latent growth, and person-oriented approach. Compare the fit and interpret each model. Which model is most appropriate for your data? Why?

8.3. In what way can the estimate of the mediated effect from a parallel process growth curve model be considered correlational? How does the latent difference score model include time ordering in a way that may be more accurate than the latent growth curve model?

8.4. Estimate the second and third forms of the autoregressive model for the autrogressive example in the text.

8.5. How could the person-oriented methods of Collins et al. (1998) be extended to continuous data?

8.6. What are the equations for the autoregressive and LGM model for five waves of data?

9

Multilevel Mediation Models

> If there are effects of the social context on individu-
> als, these effects must be mediated by interven-
> ing processes that depend on characteristics of the
> social context, . . . The common core of these theo-
> ries is that they all postulate one or more psycho-
> logical processes that mediate between individual
> variables and group variables.
>
> **—Joop Hox, 2002, p. 7**

9.1 Overview

Chapter 9 extends the mediation model, described in chapters 3 and 5, to
data that are collected at more than one level, typically at the individual
and other levels such as schools, hospitals, or families. These multiple levels of data complicate mediation analysis but also increase the information available from mediation analysis. First, the statistical and conceptual
issues in multilevel analysis are described. Next the use of a multilevel
mediation model is described and illustrated with a hypothetical study
of the effects of two different types of group therapy on depression. SAS
and Mplus programs to conduct the analyses of the hypothetical data are
described. Finally, applications of the mediation model to more complicated patterns of mediation across and within different levels of analysis
are discussed.

9.2 Multilevel Data

Often studies are conducted in which the individuals measured are actually part of groups. Examples of these groups include schools, classrooms,
hospitals, businesses, school districts, communities, and families. Groups
may also correspond to geographical areas including census tracts, cities,
states, and countries. Because individuals from the same group are likely
to share characteristics, they are more likely to respond in the same way

on research measures compared with individuals in other groups. This dependency among individuals in the same group could be due to communication among members, similar backgrounds, or similar response biases. As a result, the data from each subject are not independent from those of other subjects, thereby violating the assumption of independent observations required for accurate analysis using the methods described earlier in this book. The violation of independence is important because it can compromise statistical tests (Barcikowski, 1981).

Perhaps the clearest example of dependency in groups occurs when multiple observations are obtained for the same individual as in the longitudinal studies discussed in chapter 8. In a longitudinal study, participants are measured at two or more waves and participants' scores tend to be more similar to each other than they are similar to scores for other participants. In this case, the repeated observations are obtained for individuals so that individuals are the groups and the repeated observations are the scores in each group. It is important to keep in mind that, although this chapter describes the multilevel model for individuals in groups such as schools or hospitals, the multilevel model also applies where the groups are individuals and the longitudinal measures are the scores in the groups defined by individual subjects.

9.3 Intraclass Correlation

A measure of the extent to which observations in the same group tend to respond in the same way is the intraclass correlation (ICC). The ICC has a long history. It was used by Fisher as a way to judge whether groups were significantly different from each other. Haggard (1958) provides a good overview of the early applications of the ICC, and McGraw and Wong (1996) give an overview of more recent applications. Equation 9.1 describes a classic equation for the ICC,

$$ICC = \frac{MS_B - MS_W}{MS_B + (k-1)MS_W} \tag{9.1}$$

where MS_B is the mean squared error between the groups, MS_W is the mean squared error within groups, and k is the number of subjects in each group. The value of the ICC ranges from 1 to $-1/(k-1)$. Examples of ICCs in the school-based drug use literature are 0.02 for weekly smoking and 0.01 for the number of cigarettes smoked (Murray et al., 1994). The average school level ICC for moderate physical activity for girls was .02 (Murray et al., 2004). The ICCs for mediating measures at the school level in Krull and MacKinnon (1999) ranged from 0.001 to 0.12. ICCs for the multilevel model for longitudinal data for which observations are the repeated measures from the same participants often have much higher ICCs.

If the subjects tend to respond in the same way, then there will be a positive ICC. When the ICC is nonzero, mediational analysis is subject to the violation of independence assumption as are other analytic techniques (Krull & MacKinnon, 1999; Palmer, Graham, White, & Hansen, 1998). Specifically, this analysis violates the independent observations assumption of ordinary least squares (OLS) estimation, and for a positive ICC the standard errors are too small and as a result, inflate Type I error rates (Barcikowski, 1981; Moulton, 1986; Scariano & Davenport, 1987; Scott & Holt, 1982; Walsh, 1947).

The significance of the ICC can be tested with Equation 9.2:

$$F_{g-1,g(k-1)} = \frac{1+(k-1)ICC}{1-ICC} \tag{9.2}$$

where g is the number of groups and k is the number of subjects in each group. Although testing the significance of the ICC is an important first step in determining the effect of the violation of independence in a sample of data, even very small ICCs can distort significance tests (Kreft, 1996; Muthén & Satorra, 1995). There are also various forms of the ICC that are a function of the design of a study and combinations of fixed and random effects (McGraw & Wong, 1996). Similarly, the size of the ICC may change substantially when covariates are included in the analysis. There are different views regarding when an ICC is so large that it must be included in the analysis. Kreft (1996) suggests that an ICC less than 0.1 may be safely ignored in some situations. Others, such as Barcikowski (1981), note that even small ICCs can have substantial effects on significance tests especially when the number of individuals in a cluster is large.

9.4 Traditional Analysis for a Nonzero ICC

Given the problem of a nonzero ICC on standard errors, researchers have typically used three options before multilevel models were introduced (Krull & MacKinnon, 1999). One option is to ignore the ICC and analyze the data as if there was no dependence among individuals, that is, ignore the groups altogether. More conservative significance values, such as 0.01 or .001, are then used to make some adjustment for the ICC effects on significance testing. This method is unlikely to precisely adjust for the violation of independence. Bias is also possible because the single regression relation is a mixture of individual and group levels of analysis.

Another option is to make an adjustment based on the value of the ICC. A measure called the variation inflation factor (VIF) or design effect

(DE) is a simple function of the ICC, DE = 1 + (ICC($k - 1$)), where k is the number of subjects in each group (Kish, 1965). If the number of subjects in each group is unequal, the harmonic mean of sample size for the groups is used for k. To correctly inflate standard errors, the standard error should be multiplied by the design effect (Hox, 2002, p. 5). A design effect of 1 is consistent with simple random sampling of units. However, this adjustment may not be optimal, and the multiple levels of the data may actually provide important additional information. The design effect is a good way to investigate the extent to which an ICC would affect results as it reflects the amount that standard errors are increased owing to the ICC.

A third option is to aggregate the data to the higher level of analysis and then analyze the data at the higher level. For example, if the data are from individuals in schools, then the data are aggregated to the school level, and the analysis is conducted on the school level means, ignoring the information from individuals (e.g., MacKinnon et al., 1991). This approach avoids the problem with the ICC, but it can reduce statistical power because the sample size is now the number of aggregated units, not the total number of individual subjects. It is also possible that most of the variability in the data is at the individual, not the aggregate, unit of analysis (de Leeuw, 1992). Furthermore, often the purpose of a study is to identify effects at the individual level of analysis, which is typically the theoretical level at which the analysis is based. Another related limitation, called the ecological fallacy (Robinson, 1950), is that the relation between two variables may differ and may even have a different sign across levels of analyses (Burstein, 1980; Robinson, 1950). Robinson (1950) found a 0.53 correlation between the percentage foreign born and the percentage illiterate for the 48 United States but a −0.11 correlation for the same variables measured from individuals. Relations between variables may also have different meanings at different levels of analysis.

9.5 The Multilevel Model

Multilevel analysis solves the statistical problems introduced by the violation of the independence assumption and allows for investigation of relations across and within levels of analysis such as the mediation effect at the group level on individual measures (Bryk & Raudenbush, 1992; Hedeker, Gibbons, & Flay, 1994; Murray, 1998; Palmer et al., 1998). Multilevel analysis provides correct standard errors for clustered data and consequently more accurate Type I error rates and appropriate statistical power. The model is considerably more complex than the single level mediation model and usually requires an iterative approach to estimate parameters and standard errors.

There are several published examples of multilevel mediation analysis. Krull and MacKinnon (1999) incorporated the clustering of football player respondents within teams in mediation analysis of an anabolic steroid prevention program. Komro et al. (2001) conducted a multilevel mediation analysis of the effects of an alcohol prevention program delivered to schools. For both studies, the multilevel nature of the data was treated as a nuisance, that is, adjusted for in the mediation analysis of individual-level data rather than examining effects at different levels of analysis. Krull and MacKinnon (2001) outlined models for investigating mediation at both individual and group levels and applied the models to a study of players from football teams. Sampson, Raudenbush, and Earls (1997) examined neighborhood effects on violent crime in neighborhoods in Chicago, Illinois. They tested a three-level model (where the first level was for measurement within each respondent) postulating that residential stability in a neighborhood reduces the collective efficacy of the neighborhood, which increases violence. The mediated effect of collective efficacy was tested by comparing the coefficient for the relation between residential instability and violence before and after adjustment for collective efficacy in a multilevel model. Raudenbush and Sampson (1999) later specified a three-level mediation model that included latent variables, missing data, and unbalanced multilevel designs. They found evidence that the relation between neighborhood poverty concentration and perceived violence was mediated by social control. Mensinger (2005) found that schools with higher levels of conflicting gender roles were associated with more idealization of a superwomen construct which was, in turn, associated with disordered eating.

9.6   Equations for Multilevel Mediation

There are many options for specifying multilevel mediation effects. One of the more common multilevel mediation models is discussed here as a start for describing additional models. For the case of individuals in groups and assignment of groups to one of two conditions, Equations 9.3 to 9.9 specify multilevel models based on individual (Level 1) and group (Level 2) levels. The independent variable is at the group level, and the mediator and the dependent variables are at the individual level. At Level 1, a model is specified for individuals within each group. Parameters in this model are assumed to be random and vary in part as a function of predictors at the group level. At Level 2, another linear model is specified, but the dependent variable is the intercept (and slopes although only random intercepts are shown in these equations) in the Level 1 model. As a result, there are individual- and group-level equations for each of the three mediation equations described in chapter 3 (Equations 3.1, 3.2, and 3.3) because there are both individual- and group-level coefficients as shown in Equations 9.3 to 9.9. In these equations, i subscripts refer to individuals and j subscripts refer to groups. Note that the value of the parameters β_{0j}, e_{ij}, γ_{00}, and u_{0j} differ across the three-mediation Equations 9.3 and 9.4, 9.6 and 9.7, and 9.8 and 9.9, even though the notation does not make this explicit.

9.6.1 Equations for Y Predicted by X

$$\text{Individual Level 1: } Y_{ij} = \beta_{0j} + e_{ij} \tag{9.3}$$

$$\text{Group Level 2: } \beta_{0j} = \gamma_{00} + cX_j + u_{0j} \tag{9.4}$$

In Equation 9.3, the individual-level score on the dependent variable is equal to a group-level intercept β_{0j}, plus an individual-level random error, e_{ij} associated with the ith individual in the jth group. The individual-level random error, e_{ij}, is assumed to have a normal distribution with $\text{Var}(e_{ij}) = \sigma^2$. In Equation 9.4, the dependent variable is the group-level intercept, β_{0j}, which is equal to the overall mean, γ_{00}, plus the slope, c, relating the independent variable, X, to the group-level intercepts and the random deviation of the predicted group-level mean from the observed group-level mean, u_{0j}. The deviations in the Level 2 group equation, u_{0j}, are assumed to have a normal distribution with variation between group means, $\text{Var}(u_{0j}) = \tau_{00}$. The c parameter is at the group level because assignment to condition is assumed to be at the group level for this example. The estimation of error terms at both levels of the model ($\hat{e}_{ij}$ at the individual level and $\hat{u}_{0j}$ at the school level) allows for a nonzero ICC to be incorporated in the analysis. As shown in Equation 9.5, random effect estimates of the variance between groups, $\hat{\tau}_{00}$, and the variance of the residuals at the individual level, $\hat{\sigma}^2$, provide an estimator of the residual ICC:

$$\widehat{\text{ICC}} = \hat{\tau}_{00} / (\hat{\tau}_{00} + \hat{\sigma}^2) \tag{9.5}$$

Using this equation, the ICC conditional on other effects in the model can be easily calculated. For Equations 9.3 and 9.4, the ICC is conditional on the relation between X and Y at the group level, which is why it is called a residual ICC (i.e., dependency in scores for two people who share the same treatment group membership).

9.6.2 Equations for Y Predicted by X and M

$$\text{Individual Level 1: } Y_{ij} = \beta_{0j} + bM_{ij} + e_{ij} \tag{9.6}$$

$$\text{Group Level 2: } \beta_{0j} = \gamma_{00} + c'X_j + u_{0j} \tag{9.7}$$

Equations 9.6 and 9.7 include two predictors, one at the individual level, M, and the other at the group level, X. The estimate of the b parameter is at the individual level, because the mediator is assumed to work through individual processes. The c' parameter, on the other hand, is in the group-level equation because the groups are assigned to conditions. There are several additional models that include the X and M predictors and that may be appropriate given the substantive context of the research. One such model investigates whether the slopes relating M to Y differ across the groups. This model would include two Level 2 regression equations, one for the random slope and one for the random intercept, so in principle b in Equation 9.6 could be random. Yet another model would include the group-level mean of M as an additional predictor to investigate both group-level and individual-level relations between M and Y. The random slope model and the school and group-level predictor multilevel model will be estimated for an example data set later in this chapter.

9.6.3 Equations for M Predicted by X

$$\text{Individual Level 1: } M_{ij} = \beta_{0j} + e_{ij} \tag{9.8}$$

$$\text{Group Level 2: } \beta_{0j} = \gamma_{00} + aX_j + u_{0j} \tag{9.9}$$

Equations 9.8 and 9.9 are analogous to Equations 9.3 and 9.4, but X predicts the dependent variable M rather than Y. The a parameter is estimated at the group level because the assignment to conditions is at the group level for this example. Definitions of the other parameters in the model are the same as those for Equations 9.3 and 9.4.

Because of the complex structure of the multilevel model, including the error terms at multiple levels, the parameters of the model are not estimated with exact formulas but are instead estimated using iterative methods such as restricted maximum likelihood (REML) techniques, rather than the OLS methods typically used to estimate the parameters of single-level models. The standard error estimates for the multilevel model are consequently more accurate than those for a single-level individual-as-unit-of-analysis model because they incorporate the dependence of subjects measured within groups (i.e., a nonzero ICC).

The $\hat{a}\hat{b}$ and $\hat{c} - \hat{c}'$ estimators of the mediated effect, algebraically equivalent in single-level models, are not exactly equivalent in the multilevel models (Krull & MacKinnon, 1999). This is because the weighting matrix used to estimate the model properly in the multilevel equations is typically not identical for each of the three equations. The non-equivalence between $\hat{a}\hat{b}$ and $\hat{c} - \hat{c}'$, however, is unlikely to be problematic because the discrepancy between the two estimates is typically small and unsystematic and tends to vanish at larger sample sizes (Krull & MacKinnon, 1999). The standard error of the mediated effect is calculated using the same formulas described in chapters 3 and 5, except that the estimates and standard errors of $\hat{a}$ and $\hat{b}$ may come from equations at different levels of analysis and may require the covariance between $\hat{a}$ and $\hat{b}$. As described later, there are situations in which $\hat{a}$ and $\hat{b}$ are random effects, and a different formula must be used to estimate the mediated effect (Kenny, Bolger, & Korchmaros, 2003).

Centering, which usually consists of removing the group mean from predictors, is important when both group and individual-level effects of the same predictor are analyzed. In general, it is important to center predictor variables before estimation of multilevel models because the value and meaning of the intercept depends on the coding of the X variable (Using X to represent a predictor variable and Y to represent the dependent variable). The intercept is the value of Y when all X variables are zero for any regression equation. If an X variable is not centered, then the intercept will be the value of Y when X is zero, even when a zero value of X is impossible or not sensible. After centering the X variables by subtracting the mean of the variable, the intercept is the value of Y at the average value of X. In the case of including both group and individual-level predictors, it is also important to create a new variable by subtracting the group-level mean for each observation in that group. This will simplify interpretation and reduce any correlation between the group and individual-level predictor (Kreft, de Leeuw, & Aiken, 1995). In summary, there are three major ways of scaling predictors in the Level 1 equation (Hofmann & Gavin, 1998): (a) raw metric—in which no centering occurs and Level 1 variables are left in their original metric; (b) grand-mean centering—in which the grand mean is subtracted from predictor variables; and (c) group mean centering—in which the mean of each group is subtracted from the score for each person in the group. These different options will be used in the multilevel analysis of an example later in this chapter.

9.7 Hypothetical Study of Exercise Therapy for Depression

The following data are from a hypothetical study of group therapy for depression. A total of 16 groups were randomly assigned to one of two conditions so there were 8 groups in each condition. In each of the 16 therapy groups, there were seven depressed persons. In one condition, the groups were assigned to receive a cognitive behavioral treatment program. The other eight groups had a cognitive behavioral program and a special exercise program. Because interaction within the groups is part of the group therapy, it was expected that there would be some dependence among subjects within each of the 16 groups. Indeed, the tasks required cooperation among group members, and in the exercise condition, all seven members of the group conducted the exercise program together. The independent variable was the assignment to the cognitive behavioral treatment or the cognitive behavioral treatment plus exercise program. The mediating variable was a measure of fitness taken at the end of six weekly sessions. The dependent variable was the measure on a happiness scale at the end of 12 weeks. The researchers were interested in whether the addition of the exercise program would enhance the effects of the cognitive behavioral therapy. Furthermore, they hypothesized that the exercise program would work by changing the fitness level of each person, which, in turn, would reduce depression and increase happiness. The researchers wanted to avoid a Type I error that could occur if they failed to include the clustering of subjects in groups in the data analysis. Furthermore, they did not want to reduce the power to detect a real effect by analyzing the group means.

Fabricated data for this hypothetical study of treatment for depression are shown in Table 9.1, where X is a binary independent variable (coded 0 for the standard program and 1 for the new exercise program), M is the mediating variable (mean = 35.3036 and variance = 136.8800), Y is the dependent variable (mean = 41.8571 and variance = 210.9344), j represents the groups, and i represents the individual subjects. Three other variables were used in the multilevel analysis based on how the fitness measure, M, was centered. First, the grand mean was subtracted from each value of the M variable to form the variable CM. Second, the average of the fitness-mediating variable in each group was used as a group-level measure of fitness. For this measure, the grand mean of the fitness measure was subtracted from the average fitness value for each group. The variable name for the group-level variable was MEANM. Third, the deviation of each participants' fitness score from the average fitness in their group was used as an individual-level measure; that is, fitness was centered within each group. The variable name for this variable was WITHINM.

There is evidence of clustering in the data for both the mediating and dependent variables. Applying Equation 9.2 for the dependent variable with $MS_B = 774.133$ and $MS_W = 122.935$, and $k = 7$, suggests a large ICC of .43 [$F(15, 96) = 6.30$, $p < .01$]. The ICC for the mediating variable was also large and equaled .38 [$F(15, 96) = 5.30$, $p < .01$]. These large ICCs suggest that participants in each group tend to respond in a more similar manner than participants in other groups.

Mediation analysis at the individual level ignoring the grouping using Equations 3.2 and 3.3, led to an estimate of the mediated effect of 9.0247 ($s_{\hat{a}\hat{b}} = 1.8410$) and zero was not in the interval formed by the lower confidence limit (LCL) of 5.4164 and upper confidence limit (UCL) of 12.6331. Ignoring

Table 9.1   Hypothetical Data for Exercise Group Therapy

Obs	X	M	Y	i	j	Obs	X	M	Y	i	j
1	1	23	31	1	1	57	0	23	2	1	9
2	1	32	41	2	1	58	0	28	24	2	9
3	1	32	41	3	1	59	0	28	24	3	9
4	1	35	50	4	1	60	0	14	20	4	9
5	1	42	41	5	1	61	0	28	24	5	9
6	1	38	44	6	1	62	0	18	20	6	9
7	1	38	44	7	1	63	0	23	10	7	9
8	0	54	61	1	2	64	1	41	38	1	10
9	0	32	42	2	2	65	1	41	38	2	10
10	0	54	61	3	2	66	1	54	50	3	10
11	0	15	33	4	2	67	1	44	25	4	10
12	0	32	14	5	2	68	1	54	50	5	10
13	0	22	26	6	2	69	1	44	42	6	10
14	0	38	44	7	2	70	1	61	53	7	10
15	0	24	44	1	3	71	0	28	19	1	11
16	0	27	45	2	3	72	0	21	36	2	11
17	0	24	44	3	3	73	0	28	19	3	11
18	0	27	35	4	3	74	0	25	22	4	11
19	0	31	35	5	3	75	0	25	22	5	11
20	0	27	35	6	3	76	0	34	43	6	11
21	0	4	25	7	3	77	0	16	31	7	11
22	1	40	31	1	4	78	1	44	39	1	12
23	1	33	47	2	4	79	1	44	45	2	12
24	1	33	47	3	4	80	1	22	36	3	12
25	1	33	50	4	4	81	1	44	45	4	12
26	1	53	59	5	4	82	1	40	50	5	12
27	1	53	59	6	4	83	1	44	45	6	12
28	1	42	73	7	4	84	1	25	38	7	12
29	1	47	74	1	5	85	1	42	47	1	13
30	1	38	43	2	5	86	1	42	47	2	13
31	1	18	45	3	5	87	1	47	45	3	13
32	1	47	74	4	5	88	1	39	40	4	13
33	1	38	43	5	5	89	1	39	45	5	13
34	1	38	56	6	5	90	1	39	53	6	13
35	1	26	57	7	5	91	1	39	45	7	13
36	0	20	26	1	6	92	0	28	29	1	14
37	0	32	43	2	6	93	0	24	24	2	14
38	0	20	26	3	6	94	0	28	29	3	14

Table 9.1 (Continued)

Obs	X	M	Y	i	j	Obs	X	M	Y	i	j
39	0	32	43	4	6	95	0	37	37	4	14
40	0	41	47	5	6	96	0	37	37	5	14
41	0	33	45	6	6	97	0	33	36	6	14
42	0	57	82	7	6	98	0	22	34	7	14
43	1	35	43	1	7	99	1	53	59	1	15
44	1	35	43	2	7	100	1	53	59	2	15
45	1	43	54	3	7	101	1	37	45	3	15
46	1	46	77	4	7	102	1	37	45	4	15
47	1	55	72	5	7	103	1	38	57	5	15
48	1	35	43	6	7	104	1	66	75	6	15
49	1	48	51	7	7	105	1	55	60	7	15
50	0	16	40	1	8	106	0	41	40	1	16
51	0	45	57	2	8	107	0	41	40	2	16
52	0	16	40	3	8	108	0	41	40	3	16
53	0	29	31	4	8	109	0	53	59	4	16
54	0	24	35	5	8	110	0	49	41	5	16
55	0	30	38	6	8	111	0	18	16	6	16
56	0	24	35	7	8	112	0	29	29	7	16

the individual-level data and analyzing the means for the 16 groups led to an $\hat{a}_1\hat{b}_2$ estimate of 6.9714, a larger standard error ($s_{\hat{a}\hat{b}} = 4.3324$), and a wider confidence interval (LCL = –1.5201 and UCL = 15.4630) than the individual-level analysis. Avoiding the problem with dependency within groups by conducting analysis of the 16 group means suggests that there is not statistically significant mediation because zero was included in the confidence limits in the analysis of the means from the 16 groups. The individual-level analysis led to the conclusion that the mediated effect was statistically significant, but the individual-level analysis does not adjust standard errors for the nonzero ICC and the estimates mix both group level and individual-level relations. A multilevel analysis is necessary to incorporate the dependency among subjects in the same group.

The presentation of the analysis of the example data is organized as follows. First, the results for a typical multilevel mediation analysis using Equations 9.3, 9.4, 9.6, 9.7, 9.8, and 9.9 are described along with a summary of the results of these analyses. Next three additional multilevel mediation models that correspond to models with both group and individual-level mediational processes are described. Related sets of analysis using the Mplus program are then described for the example.

9.8 MIXED Code and Output for Equations 9.3 and 9.4 (Y Predicted by X)

Table 9.2 shows the MIXED code to estimate the parameters of the multi-level model for Equations 9.3 and 9.4. The MIXED command actually inserts Equation 9.4 in Equation 9.3 to estimate the single equation $Y_{ij} = (\gamma_{00} + cX_j + u_{0j}) + e_{ij}$. Note that the group code j is in the class statement and also in the SUB option statement to indicate the groups in the analysis. The MODEL statement specifies fixed effects. Here the MODEL specifies that Y is predicted by X, and the /solution command requests that the regression coefficients and standard errors be printed in the output. The DDFM=BW command instructs SAS to use the between and within method for computing denominator degrees of freedom for the fixed effects. For unbalanced data DDFM=SATTERHWAITHE is often recommended. The RANDOM statement specifies random effects in the model. Here the intercept for Y is specified as random; that is, the group means are random, and the type=un statement indicates that covariance matrix among the error terms in the Level 2 random effect matrix is unstructured. The COVTEST command in the PROC MIXED line requests a hypothesis test of the significance of the random effects based on asymptotic methods, and these tests may not be highly reliable at smaller sample sizes (Singer & Willett, 2003).

The output shown in Table 9.3 consists of a summary describing the name of the data set WORK.BOTH, the dependent variable Y, the unstructured covariance structure for the error terms, the subject or group effect variable j, the type of estimation, REML or restricted maximum likelihood, the profile method of estimating residual variances, the model-based method to compute fixed effects standard errors, and the between-within method to compute degrees of freedom. Next, class level information is provided in the output identifying the class variable j, the fact that there are 16 levels, and the values for the 16 levels. The dimensions section is often useful for verifying the model and data specified for a multilevel analysis. The two covariance parameters are specified for the variance of the errors in the individual and the group-level equations. The columns in X represent the intercept and slope and the columns in Z represent the random slope for the intercept in the 16 groups. There are 16 groups and

Table 9.2   MIXED Program for Equations 9.3 and 9.4

```
proc mixed covtest;
class j;
model Y=X /solution ddfm=bw notest;
random intercept/type=un sub=j ;
```

Table 9.3 MIXED Output for Equations 9.3 and 9.4

```
                      The Mixed Procedure
                     Model Information
        Data Set                       WORK.BOTH
        Dependent Variable             y
        Covariance Structure           Unstructured
        Subject Effect                 j
        Estimation Method              REML
        Residual Variance Method       Profile
        Fixed Effects SE Method        Model-Based
        Degrees of Freedom Method      Between-Within
                   Class Level Information
Class      Levels                     Values
  J          16      1 2 3 4 5 6 7 8 9 10 11 12 13 14 15 16

                       Dimensions
        Covariance Parameters                2
        Columns in X                         2
        Columns in Z Per Subject             1
        Subjects                            16
        Max Obs Per Subject                  7
        Observations Used                  112
        Observations Not Used                0
        Total Observations                 112

                     Iteration History
Iteration Evaluations    -2 Res Log Like    Criterion
     0          1          878.20894206
     1          1          866.39597993     0.0000000
                  Convergence criteria met.
              Covariance Parameter Estimates
                             Standard       Z
Cov Parm    Subject   Estimate   Error    Value     Pr Z
UN(1,1)        j       41.1518  22.3361    1.84    0.0327
Residual              122.93    17.7441    6.93    <0.0001

                     Fit Statistics
        -2 Res Log Likelihood        866.4
        AIC(smaller is better)       870.4
        AICC(smaller is better)      870.5
        BIC (smaller is better)      871.9
```

(continued)

Table 9.3 (Continued)

		Null Model Likelihood Ratio Test			
	DF		Chi-Square	Pr > ChiSq	
	1		11.81	0.0006	

		Solution for Fixed Effects			
Effect	Estimate	Standard Error	DF	t Value	Pr > |t|
Intercept	34.6250	2.7091	14	12.78	<0.0001
x	14.4643	3.8313	14	3.78	0.0020

7 observations per group. The maximum number of observations for each group is 7. The number of possible observations used, observations not used, and total observations information is helpful to keep track of missing data. In this example, the number of observations per group is equal, and there are no missing data. A strength of multilevel data analysis is that it can appropriately analyze data with missing observations such as when some persons may be missing observations. The iteration history is then described; this model required one iteration to obtain maximum likelihood estimates that satisfied the convergence criteria.

The next sections of the output contain the estimates and standard errors of the multilevel equations in the "Covariance Parameter Estimates" section which contains the estimates for the random effects in the model with estimates for $\text{Var}(e_{ij}) = \hat{\sigma}^2 = 122.93$, which is the residual variation at the individual level, and $\text{Var}(u_{0j}) = \hat{\tau}_{00} = 41.1518$, which is the residual variation between groups after removing the effects of X. These values can be put in Equation 9.9 to estimate the residual ICC of .25 which is conditional on X as a group-level predictor.

After this section, several model fit statistics are included including –2 times the residual log likelihood, which represents a measure of the likelihood of observing the data given the model parameters, the Akaike Information Criterion (AIC), the Akaike Information Criterion Corrected (AICC) for degrees of freedom, and the Bayesian Information Criterion (BIC). Sometimes these measures of fit are used to compare across models.

Finally, the SOLUTION command presents the parameter estimates and standard errors for the intercept fixed effect, $\hat{\gamma}_{00} = 34.625$, which is the average group-level happiness score in the standard condition, its standard error, 2.7091, and the $\hat{c}$ coefficient, which is equal to 14.4643 with a standard error of 3.8313. There is a statistically significant effect of the fitness program of 14.4643 units on the happiness measure. The null model likelihood ratio test section presents a statistical test of whether the model estimated provides an improvement over a null model for the data. If this test was nonsignificant, it would suggest that the effects in the model do not provide an improvement in model fit more than a model without the effects. The Type 3 tests of fixed effect section is part of the default MIXED output and does not provide any information that was not in the solution for fixed effects section.

9.9 SAS Code and Output for Equations 9.6 and 9.7 (Y Predicted by Grand-Mean Centered M and X)

The MIXED code for the model in which X and M predict Y is given in Table 9.4 and output is shown in Table 9.5. Note that the program is very similar to the code for the aforementioned regression model except that there is an additional predictor, the grand-mean centered mediating variable, CM. The "Covariance Parameter Estimates" section again contains the estimates for the random effects in the model so $Var(e_{ij}) = \hat{\sigma}^2 = 62.8216$, which is the residual variation at the individual level, and for $Var(u_{0j}) = \hat{\tau}_{00} = 40.4209$, which is the residual variation between groups. The solution presents the parameter estimates and standard errors for the intercept fixed effect, $\hat{\gamma}_{00} = 39.4273$, which is the average group-level happiness score in the standard condition $(X = 0)$ and its standard error, 2.5330, and the $\hat{c}'$ coefficient equals 4.8598 with a standard error of 3.6489, and b equal to 0.8224, with a standard error of 0.0842. The mediator is significantly related to the dependent variable. The group-level coefficient for X changed 9.6045 units from 14.4643 to 4.8598 with the addition of the fitness mediator centered at the grand mean.

Output that is similar to the output for the first equation is not repeated here. The only difference with the previous MIXED output is that now there are three columns in X.

9.10 MIXED Code and Output for Equations 9.8 and 9.9 (Predicting M From X)

The MIXED code to estimate the independent variable effect on the mediator is analogous to the program effect on the dependent variable and

Table 9.4   Mixed Program for Equations 9.6 and 9.7

```
proc mixed covtest;
class j;
model y=X CM/solution ddfm=bw notest;
random intercept/type=un sub=j;
```

Table 9.5   Selected MIXED Output for Equations 9.6 and 9.7

The Mixed Procedure

Covariance Parameter Estimates

Cov Parm	Subject	Estimate	Standard Error	Z Value	Pr Z
UN(1,1)	j	40.4209	18.7552	2.16	0.0156
Residual		62.8216	9.1120	6.89	<0.0001

Fit Statistics

−2 Res Log Likelihood	801.6
AIC (smaller is better)	805.6
AICC (smaller is better)	805.7
BIC (smaller is better)	807.2

Null Model Likelihood Ratio Test

DF	Chi-Square	Pr > ChiSq
1	25.56	<0.0001

Solution for Fixed Effects

Effect	Estimate	Standard Error	DF	t Value	Pr > |t|
Intercept	39.4273	2.5330	14	15.57	<0.0001
X	4.8598	3.6489	14	1.33	0.2042
CM	0.8224	0.0842	95	9.77	<0.0001

is shown in Table 9.6. The output is shown in Table 9.7. The "Covariance Parameter Estimates" section again contains the estimates for the random effects in the model for $Var(e_{ij}) = \hat{\sigma}^2 = 86.6101$, which is the residual variation at the individual level, and for $Var(u_{0j}) = \hat{\tau}_{00} = 18.8538$, which is the residual variation between groups. Finally the solution presents the intercept of the fixed effect, $\hat{\gamma}_{00} = 29.4643$, its standard error, 1.9757, and the $\hat{a}$ coefficient relating X to M is equal to 11.6786 with a standard error of 2.7940. There is a significant effect of the program on the average fitness level.

9.11   Summary of the PROC MIXED Output

The SAS PROC MIXED provides the coefficients and standard errors for Equations 9.3, 9.4, 9.6, 9.7, 9.8, and 9.9 as shown:

$$\text{Individual Level 1: } Y_{ij} = \beta_{0j} + e_{ij} \tag{9.3}$$

Table 9.6 Mixed Program for Equations 9.8 and 9.9

```
proc mixed covtest;
class j;
model M=X /solution ddfm=bw notest;
random int/type=un sub=j ;
```

Table 9.7 Selected MIXED Output for Equations 9.8 and 9.9

Model Information

Data Set	WORK.BOTH
Dependent Variable	m
Covariance Structure	Unstructured
Subject Effect	j
Estimation Method	REML
Residual Variance Method	Profile
Fixed Effects SE Method	Model-Based
Degrees of Freedom Method	Between-Within

Class Level Information

Class	Levels	Values
J	6	1 2 3 4 5 6 7 8 9 10 11 12 13 14 15 16

Dimensions

Covariance Parameters	2
Columns in X	2
Columns in Z Per Subject	1
Subjects	16
Max Obs Per Subject	7
Observations Used	112
Observations Not Used	0
Total Observations	112

Iteration History

Iteration	Evaluations	−2 Res Log Like	Criterion
0	1	830.47132504	
1	1	823.93374022	0.00000000

(*continued*)

Table 9.7 (Continued)

Convergence criteria met.

Covariance Parameter Estimates

Cov Parm	Subject	Estimate	Standard Error	Z Value	Pr Z
UN(1,1)	j	18.8538	11.9369	1.58	0.0571
Residual		86.6101	12.5011	6.93	<0.0001

Fit Statistics

-2 Res Log Likelihood	823.9
AIC (smaller is better)	827.9
AICC (smaller is better)	828.0
BIC (smaller is better)	829.5

Null Model Likelihood Ratio Test

DF	Chi-Square	Pr > ChiSq
1	6.54	0.0106

Solution for Fixed Effects

Effect	Estimate	Standard Error	DF	t Value	Pr > |t|
Intercept	29.4643	1.9757	14	−2.96	0.0104
x	11.6786	2.7940	14	4.18	0.0009

$$\text{Group Level 2: } \beta_{0j} = 34.625 + 14.4643\ X_j + u_{0j} \qquad (9.4)$$
$$(2.7091)\quad(3.8313)$$

$$\text{Individual Level 1: } Y_{ij} = \beta_{0j} + .8224\ M_{ij} + e_{ij} \qquad (9.6)$$
$$(.0842)$$

$$\text{Group Level 2: } \beta_{0j} = 39.4273 + 4.8598 X_j + u_{0j} \qquad (9.7)$$
$$(2.5330)\quad(3.6489)$$

$$\text{Individual Level 1: } M_{ij} = \beta_{0j} + e_{ij} \qquad (9.8)$$

$$\text{Group Level 2: } \beta_{0j} = 29.463 + 11.6786 X_j + u_{0j} \qquad (9.9)$$
$$(1.9757)\quad(2.794)$$

The estimate of the total effect is 14.4693 (3.8313). In the multilevel model $\hat{c} - \hat{c}'$ is not exactly equal to $\hat{a}\hat{b}$ as for the ordinary regression model. In most situations, however, the two values are very close (Krull & MacKinnon, 1999). It is also not clear how to extend the formula for the standard error of $\hat{c} - \hat{c}'$ from the OLS regression model to the multilevel model. As a result, I focus on the $\hat{a}\hat{b}$ method of assessing mediation and its standard error. The estimate of the mediated effect at the individual level using the grand-mean centered mediator is equal to (11.6796)(.8224) = 9.6054, which is almost the same as $\hat{c} - \hat{c}' = 14.4643 - 4.8598 = 9.6045$. For the grand-mean centered mediator, $\hat{a}\hat{b}$ equals 9.6054 with a standard error of $s_{\hat{a}\hat{b}} = 2.4994$ and LCL = 4.7057 and UCL = 14.5032, consistent with a statistically significant multilevel mediated effect.

There are several additional multilevel mediation models that are possible because of the possibility of measures at multiple levels of analysis. Three of these different models are described in the following.

9.12 SAS Code and Output for Equations 9.6 and 9.7 (Y Predicted by Group-Mean Centered M and X)

For some models, it may be sensible to estimate the mediation effects of a group-mean centered mediating variable. The MIXED code for the model, in which X and M predict Y is given in Table 9.8 for group-mean centered M. The program is very similar to the code for the regression model for X and M predicting Y except that the predictor is WITHINM. In section 9.10, the grand-mean centered value of M was used as the additional predictor. The grand-mean centered predictor includes some aspects of the individual-level predictor, which is the relation between M and Y within each group and some aspects of the group-level relations among variables, that is, the relation between the group means of M and Y. If effects within each group are to be unambiguously examined and if both group and individual-level effects are simultaneously tested, group-mean centering is most appropriate. The group-mean centered variable represents how much an individual's score deviates from the average score of their group and the resulting coefficient is an estimate of the within-group association between M and Y.

Table 9.8 Mixed Program for Equations 9.6 and 9.7

```
proc mixed covtest;
class j;
model Y=X withinM/solution ddfm=bw notest;
random intercept/type=un sub=j ;
```

The "Covariance Parameter Estimates" section of Table 9.9 again contains the estimates for the random effects in the model with estimates for $Var(e_{ij}) = \hat{\sigma}^2 = 62.8432$, which is the residual variation at the individual level, $Var(u_{0j}) = \hat{\tau}_{00} = 49.7363$, which is the residual variation between groups. The solution presents the parameter estimates and standard errors for the intercept fixed effect, $\hat{\gamma}_{00} = 34.625$, which is the average group-level happiness score in the standard condition, and its standard error is 2.7091. The $\hat{c}'$ coefficient equals 14.4643 with a standard error of 3.8313, and $\hat{b}$ equals 0.8375 with a standard error of 0.0869. The mediator is significantly related to the dependent variable. The group-level coefficient for X is unchanged from the model without the fitness mediator because the WITHINM variable is centered within each group; that is, X and WITHINM are orthogonal predictors when centered at the group mean. The relation estimated is at the individual level and does not include group-level relations.

Table 9.9   Selected MIXED Output for Equations 9.6 and 9.7

Covariance Parameter Estimates

Cov Parm	Subject	Estimate	Standard Error	Z Value	Pr Z
UN(1,1)	j	49.7363	22.2300	2.24	0.0126
Residual		62.8432	9.1182	6.89	<0.0001

Fit Statistics

-2 Res Log Likelihood	804.0
AIC (smaller is better)	808.0
AICC (smaller is better)	808.1
BIC (smaller is better)	809.6

Null Model Likelihood Ratio Test

DF	Chi-Square	Pr > ChiSq
1	32.29	<0.0001

Solution for Fixed Effects

Effect	Estimate	Standard Error	DF	t Value	Pr > |t|
Intercept	34.6250	2.7091	14	12.78	<0.0001
X	14.4643	3.8313	14	3.78	0.0020
withinm	0.8375	0.08694	95	9.63	<0.0001

9.13 SAS Code and Output for Y Predicted by Group-Mean Centered M and X With Random Slopes Within Groups

This model is similar to the last model except that now both the intercepts and slopes relating M and Y are random effects as shown in Equations 9.10, 9.11, and 9.12. Note that there are now new coefficients. The term b_{1j} is the slope within each of the groups, c_{b0}' is the relation between the X variable and the intercepts in each group (depending on the coding of X and whether the data are balanced), c_{b1}' is the relation between the X variable and the slopes in each group, γ_{10} is the slope in the control condition, and u_{1j} is the residual in the equation predicting the slopes within each group.

$$\text{Individual Level 1: } Y_{ij} = \beta_{0j} + b_{1j} M + e_{ij} \tag{9.10}$$

$$\text{Group Level 2: } \beta_{0j} = \gamma_{00} + c_{b0}' X + u_{0j} \tag{9.11}$$

$$\text{Group Level 2: } b_{1j} = \gamma_{10} + c_{b1}' X + u_{1j} \tag{9.12}$$

With these equations, it is possible to test whether the relation between M and Y differs across groups by testing whether the $\hat{c}_{b1}'$ coefficient is statistically significant. The MIXED code for the model in which X and M predict Y is given in Table 9.10. Note that the program is very similar to the code for the aforementioned regression model except that there is an additional random effect in the RANDOM effect line so that the MIXED program estimates additional parameters. I have only included the "Covariance Parameter Estimates" section in Table 9.11 as this provides the information necessary to test whether the slopes differ across groups. The variation among individuals within groups, $\text{Var}(e_{ij}) = \hat{\sigma}^2 = 60.3643$, and the residual variation among group means, $\text{Var}(u_{0j}) = \hat{\tau}_{00} = 48.5354$, have the same meaning as described earlier except that the values are conditional on the additional parameters in the model. The UN(2,1) value of 1.9903 is the covariance between the intercepts and the slopes, with a standard error of 1.0326. The UN(2,2) coefficient provides the test of whether the slope varies across groups and is equal to 0.05166 with a standard error of 0.06075, which suggests that the variation in the slope relating Y to M does not significantly vary across groups. As a result, the parameter coding different slopes across groups is set to zero in further analysis. Note

Table 9.10   MIXED Program for Equations 9.10, 9.11, and 9.12

```
proc mixed covtest;
class j;
model Y=X withinm/solution ddfm=bw notest;
random int withinm/type=un sub=j;
```

Table 9.11 Selected MIXED Output for Equations 9.10, 9.11, and 9.12

Covariance Parameter Estimates

Cov Parm	Subject	Estimate	Standard Error	Z Value	Pr Z
UN(1,1)	j	48.5354	21.2022	2.29	0.0110
UN(2,1)	j	1.9903	1.0326	1.93	0.0539
UN(2,2)	j	0.05166	0.06075	0.85	0.1975
Residual		60.3643	9.3262	6.47	<0.0001

that a likelihood ratio test comparing the likelihood ratio for a model with UN(2,2) set to zero to the current model with UN(2,2) free is a more accurate test of the differential relation of Y to M. In addition, differential relations of M to Y can also be tested by including an XM interaction (and M main effect) in Equation 9.12.

9.14 SAS Code and Output for Y Predicted by X and Group-Mean Centered Individual M and Group-Mean M Predictors of Y

The next model estimates effects of both group and individual-level mediators as shown in Equations 9.13 and 9.14. There are now subscripts on the b parameters to indicate which b parameter is for the individual-level effect (b_i, where M_{ij} is the individual-level mediator) and which is for the group-level effect (b_j, where M_{+j} is the group level mean).

$$\text{Individual Level 1: } Y_{ij} = \beta_{0j} + b_i M_{ij} + e_{ij} \tag{9.13}$$

$$\text{Group Level 2: } \beta_{0j} = \gamma_{00} + c' X_j + b_j M_{+j} + u_{0j} \tag{9.14}$$

The SAS code for the model in which X, group-level M (M_{+j}), and individual-level M (M_{ij}) predict Y is given in Table 9.12. Note that the program is very similar to the code for the aforementioned regression model except that an additional predictor, the mediating variable, MEANM, is included as well as WITHINM. As shown in Table 9.13 the "Covariance Parameter Estimates" section contains the estimates for the random effects in the model. The estimates for $\text{Var}(e_{ij}) = \hat{\sigma}^2 = 62.8432$, which is the residual variation at the individual level, and for $\text{Var}(u_{0j}) = \hat{\tau}_{00} = 42.2698$, which is the residual variation between groups. The solution presents the parameter estimates and standard errors for the intercept of the fixed effect, $\hat{\gamma}_{00} = 17.0367$, which is the average group-level happiness score and its standard

Table 9.12 MIXED Program for Equations 9.13 and 9.14

```
proc mixed covtest;
class j;
model Y=X withinm meanm/solution ddfm=bw notest;
random int/type=un sub=j g;
```

error, 10.4007, and the $\hat{c}'$ coefficient equals 7.4929 with a standard error of 5.3666. The b_i coefficient equals 0.8375 with a standard error of 0.08694, and the group-level coefficient relating the average group fitness to happiness, b_j equals 0.5969 with a standard error of 0.3424.

The output for Equations 9.13 and 9.14 is shown in Table 9.13. Estimates and standard errors are

$$\text{Individual Level 1: } Y_{ij} = \beta_{0j} + \underset{(0.0870)}{0.8375} \, M_{ij} + e_{ij} \tag{9.15}$$

$$\text{Group Level 2: } \beta_{0j} = \underset{(10.4007)}{17.0367} + \underset{(5.3666)}{7.4929} \, X_j + \underset{(0.3424)}{0.5969} \, M_{+j} + u_{0j} \tag{9.16}$$

Two additional regression models are necessary to estimate the group-level and individual-level mediated effect. For the individual-level mediated effect, the $\hat{a}$ coefficient is obtained from a multilevel model with WITHINM as the dependent variable and is equal to 0.0000 with a standard error of 1.6430 so that the mediated effect $(0.0000)(0.8375) = 0$. For the group-level mediated effect the regression model relating X to the groups means (MEANM) is required, and $\hat{a}$ equals 11.6786 with a standard error of 2.7940. The difference between $\hat{c}$ and $\hat{c}'$, 14.4643 − 7.4929 equals 6.9714, which is very close to the sum of the individual-level mediated effect, $(0.0000)(0.8385) = 0.0000$ and the group-level mediated effect, $(11.6786)(.5969) = 6.9709$ for a total mediated effect of 6.9709. The individual-level mediated effect is nonsignificant. The group-level mediated effect equals 6.9714 ($s_{\hat{a}\hat{b}} = 4.3326$), and zero was contained in the confidence limit for the mediated effect, LCL = −1.5210 and UCL = 15.4628. These results suggest some evidence that the exercise program improved the fitness level, which increased happiness at the group level, but the effect was nonsignificant.

9.15 Multilevel Modeling in Mplus

The Mplus software has two ways to estimate multilevel models: one is to incorporate the clustering of observations within units for all variables (TYPE IS COMPLEX) and the other is to specify the relations at each level

Table 9.13 Selected MIXED Output for Equations 9.13 and 9.14

Class Level Information

Class	Levels	Values
j	16	1 2 3 4 5 6 7 8 9 10 11 12 13 14 15 16

Dimensions

Covariance Parameters	2
Columns in X	4
Columns in Z Per Subject	1
Subjects	16
Max Obs Per Subject	7
Observations Used	112
Observations Not Used	0
Total Observations	112

Iteration History

Iteration	Evaluations	-2 Res Log Like	Criterion
0	1	827.27501963	
1	1	801.42795022	0.00000000

Convergence criteria met.

Covariance Parameter Estimates

Cov Parm	Subject	Estimate	Standard Error	Z Value	Pr Z
UN(1,1)	j	42.2698	20.1430	2.10	0.0179
Residual		62.8432	9.1182	6.89	<0.0001

Fit Statistics

-2 Res Log Likelihood	801.4
AIC (smaller is better)	805.4
AICC (smaller is better)	805.5
BIC (smaller is better)	807.0

Null Model Likelihood Ratio Test

DF	Chi-Square	Pr > ChiSq
1	25.85	<0.0001

Solution for Fixed Effects

Effect	Estimate	Standard Error	DF	t Value	Pr > |t|
Intercept	17.0367	10.4007	13	1.64	0.1254
X	7.4929	5.3666	13	1.40	0.1860
meanm	0.5969	0.3424	13	1.74	0.1048
withinm	0.8375	0.08694	95	9.63	<0.0001

of the analysis (TYPE IS TWOLEVEL). The Mplus code (Table 9.14) and output (Table 9.15) identify the group-level cluster variable to estimate the multilevel model. The group variable is identified in the CLUSTER=j command in the program. The TYPE IS COMPLEX code specifies that the sampling is complex, meaning that the data are clustered in groups, here clustering in the *j* groups. The equations are specified in the MODEL statement where Y is regressed on M and X and M is regressed on X. Mplus first lists the characteristics of the data. Additional options are available, including listing of the observed data means, correlations, and covariances. Printed at the bottom are the regression estimates relevant for the multilevel model. These estimates are not identical to the results from PROC MIXED because a different estimation method is used, that is, a maximum likelihood estimator that corrects for nonindependence of observations within clusters. For Mplus multilevel analysis, the mediated effect $(11.679)(.773)$ was 9.0279 ($s_{\hat{a}\hat{b}} = 2.4591$) and LCL = 4.2081 and UCL = 13.8477, which are very similar to the results from PROC MIXED. The TYPE IS COMPLEX code is very useful as it provides a general adjustment for clustering in the data analysis for very complex mediation models.

9.16 Mplus Analysis Using the TWOLEVEL Option

The TYPE IS COMPLEX command is a very general way to adjust for clustering in data analysis. However, in some cases more detail regarding the

Table 9.14   Mplus Program Using TYPE IS COMPLEX

```
TITLE:    MULTLEVEL DATA COMPLEX
DATA:
FILE IS "E:\Chapter 9 Multilevel\exmult3.txt";
VARIABLE:
  NAMES ARE id x m y i j;
  USEVARIABLES ARE x m y i;
  CLUSTER IS j;
ANALYSIS:
  TYPE IS COMPLEX;
  ESTIMATOR IS MLR;
  ITERATIONS = 1000;
  CONVERGENCE = 0.00005;
MODEL:
Y ON X M;
M ON X;
OUTPUT:
```

Table 9.15 Mplus Output for TYPE IS COMPLEX

```
INPUT INSTRUCTIONS

  TITLE:  MULTLEVEL DATA COMPLEX
  DATA:
    FILE IS "E:\Chapter 9 Multilevel\exmult4.txt";
  VARIABLE:
    NAMES ARE id x m y i j;
    USEVARIABLES ARE x m y j;
    CLUSTER IS j;
  ANALYSIS:
    TYPE IS COMPLEX;
    ESTIMATOR IS MLM;
    ITERATIONS = 1000;
    CONVERGENCE = 0.00005;
  MODEL:
  Y ON X M;
  M ON X;
  OUTPUT;
MULTLEVEL DATA COMPLEX
SUMMARY OF ANALYSIS
Number of groups                                  1
Number of observations                          112
Number of dependent variables                     2
Number of independent variables                   1
Number of continuous latent variables             0

Observed dependent variables
  Continuous
  M       Y


Observed independent variables
  M

Variables with special functions
Cluster variable                                  J
Estimator                                         MLR
Maximum number of iterations                      1000
Convergence criterion                             0.500D-04
Maximum number of steepest descent iterations     20
Input data file(s)
  E:\Chapter 9 Multilevel\exmult4.txt
Input data format   FREE
```

Table 9.15 (Continued)

```
SUMMARY OF DATA
Number of clusters          16
Size (s)      Cluster ID with Size s
7             1  2  3  4  5  6  7  8
              9  10  11  12  13  14  15  16

Loglikelihood
H0 Value      -913.549

Information Criteria
  Number of Free Parameters      7
  Akaike (AIC)                   1841.097
  Bayesian (BIC)                 1860.127
  Sample-Size Adjusted BIC       1838.004
  (n* = (n + 2) / 24)

RMSEA (Root Mean Square Error Of Approximation)
  Estimate    0.000

SRMR (Standardized Root Mean Square Residual)
Value         0.000

MODEL RESULTS
             Estimates      S.E.    Est./S.E.    Std   StdYX
Y     ON
X            5.439         3.179     1.711      5.439 0.188
M            0.773         0.120     6.424      0.773 0.623

M     ON
X            11.679        2.614     4.468      11.679 0.501

Intercepts
M            29.464        1.949     15.118     29.464 2.530
Y            11.856        4.589     2.583      1.856 0.820

Residual Variances
M            101.560    14.727 6.896     101.560     0.749
Y            96.099     16.088 5.973     96.099      0.460

R-SQUARE
     Observed
     Variable      R-Square
     M             0.251
     Y             0.540
```

effects at different levels are important. To illustrate the multilevel option in Mplus, the parameters of Equation 9.6 and 9.7 are estimated. The program is shown in Table 9.16, and the output is shown in Table 9.17. For the ANALYSIS=TWOLEVEL keyword, Mplus requires additional information about variables measured within and between groups. For most applications, the between model represents relations among variables at the second level of analysis, which may consist of means in each of the groups. The within model represents relations among individual-level variables for the entire data set (Heck, 2001). The WITHIN keyword specifies the names of the variables measured only at the individual level and used only at the individual level of the analysis. In this case, the M variable is measured at the individual level and is used only at the individual level of analysis. The BETWEEN keyword lists the variables that are collected at the group level. In this case only the X variable is measured at the group level. The CENTERING=GRANDMEAN(M) centers the M variable at the grand mean. The MODEL keyword is used to specify the equations of the multilevel model. There are two sections, one keyword WITHIN to specify the individual-level analysis. For the mediation example, the effect of Y on M is the only individual-level relation. The BETWEEN section codes the equations for the between-group effects, which are the relation of Y on X.

Table 9.16   Mplus Program From Group Therapy Example

```
TITLE:   MULTILEVEL DATA TWOLEVEL
DATA:
  FILE IS "E:\Chapter 9 Multilevel\exmult4.txt";
VARIABLE:
  NAMES ARE id x m y I j ;
  USEVARIABLES ARE x m Y j;
  CLUSTER IS j;
  BETWEEN=X;
  WITHIN=M;
  CENTERING=GRANDMEAN(M);
ANALYSIS:
  TYPE IS TWOLEVEL random;
MODEL:
  %WITHIN%
  Y ON M;
  %BETWEEN%
  Y ON X ;

OUTPUT:
```

Table 9.17 Mplus Output for Multilevel Group Therapy Example

```
MULTLEVEL DATA TWOLEVEL

SUMMARY OF ANALYSIS

Number of groups                        1
Number of observations                  112

Number of y-variables                   1
Number of x-variables                   2
Number of continuous latent variables 0

Observed variables in the analysis

X    M    Y
Cluster variable           J
Within variables
M
Between variables
X
Centering (GRANDMEAN)
M
Optimization algorithm     EM

SUMMARY OF DATA

 Number of clusters    16
  Size (s) Cluster ID with Sizes
      7    1    2    3    4    5    6    7    8
           9   10   11   12   13   14   15   16

     Average cluster size       7.000

THE MODEL ESTIMATION TERMINATED NORMALLY

Loglikelihood
     H0 Value    -402.846
     H1 Value    -402.846

Information Criteria
Number of Free Parameters               5
Akaike (AIC)                            815.693
Bayesian (BIC)                          829.285
Sample-Size Adjusted BIC                813.483
(n* = (n + 2) / 24)
```

(*continued*)

Table 9.17 (Continued)

MODEL RESULTS

	Estimates	S.E.	Est./S.E.
Within Level			
Y ON			
M	0.820	0.093	8.780
Residual Variances			
Y	62.222	10.322	6.028
Between Level			
Y ON			
X	4.903	3.422	1.433
Intercepts			
Y	39.406	2.391	16.478
Residual Variances			
Y	34.078	12.632	2.698

The coefficients and standard errors are comparable to the results in MIXED but differ because a different estimation strategy is used. For the random effects in the model, the estimate for $Var(e_{ij}) = \hat{\sigma}^2 = 62.222$, which is the residual variation at the individual level, and for $Var(u_{0j}) = \hat{\tau}_{oo} = 34.078$, which is the residual variation between groups. The solution presents the parameter estimates and standard errors for the intercept fixed effect, $\hat{\gamma}_{00}$ =39.406, which is the average group-level happiness score in the standard condition and its standard error, 2.391, the $\hat{c}'$ coefficient equals 4.903 with a standard error of 3.422, and $\hat{b}$ is equal to 0.820 with a standard error of 0.093. Using programs analogous to TWOLEVEL for Equations 9.3 and 9.4 for X related to Y yielded estimates of $\hat{c}$ equal to 14.831 with a standard error of 3.570. Applying "Type is Twolevel" multilevel model Mplus estimates for Equations 9.8 and 9.9 yielded $\hat{a}$ equal to 11.668 with a standard error of 2.614. The resulting mediated effect (11.668)(.820) equals 9.568 with a standard error of 2.402 and UCL and LCL of 4.8589 and 14.2767. Analysis with the MPLUS TWOLEVEL option led to the conclusion that the mediated effect is statistically significant.

9.17 Random Coefficients in Multilevel Mediation Models

So far in this chapter, at least one of the coefficients in the mediation analysis has been fixed, that is, treated as constant across clusters (groups) such as schools, clinics, and therapy groups. If the coefficients instead vary across clusters, then the mediation analysis is more complicated as described by Kenny et al. (2003). For the group therapy example data analysis in this chapter, the a and the b parameters may vary across therapy groups. In other words, the *a* parameter may vary across the groups and the *b* parameter may vary across the groups so that no single *a* or *b* parameter applies for all groups. For this to occur, the X variable could not be treatment condition (unless conditions are assigned within groups) as it was in the example used in this chapter, which is generally a fixed effect, but would have to be a continuous measure (or a random X variable) for each group so that the *a* parameter could vary across groups. Kenny and colleagues refer to this type of mediation analysis as lower level mediation. They describe a daily diary example in which respondents indicate exposure to daily stressors, coping efforts, and mood states. The individual is the cluster for the multi-level analysis, and the parameters *a*, *b*, and *c'* in the mediation model may differ across individuals, so they may represent random effects.

The model for random effects for *a* and *b* is summarized in two individual-level Equations 9.15 and 9.16, representing the relation of X and M and the relation of X and M on Y at Level 1, respectively. There are three Level 2 equations corresponding to the average of each parameter *a*, *b*, and *c'* and the deviation in each of the groups.

$$\text{Individual Level 1: } M_{ij} = \beta_{1j} + a_j X_{ij} + e_{ij} \tag{9.15}$$

$$\text{Individual Level 1: } Y_{ij} = \beta_{2j} + c'_j X_{ij} + b_j M_{ij} + e_{ij} \tag{9.16}$$

$$\text{Group Level 2: } a_j = a + u_{1j} \tag{9.17}$$

$$\text{Group Level 2: } b_j = b + u_{2j} \tag{9.18}$$

$$\text{Group Level 2: } c'_j = c' + u_{3j} \tag{9.19}$$

In the case of random effects for *a* and *b*, Kenny et al. (2003) show that the mediated effect estimate equals $\hat{a}\hat{b}$ plus the covariance between $\hat{a}$ and $\hat{b}$ because the $\hat{a}$ and $\hat{b}$ coefficients vary across groups, and this variation must be included when $\hat{a}\hat{b}$ is calculated. The standard error of the product of random $\hat{a}$ and $\hat{b}$ coefficients adds $2\hat{a}\hat{b} \text{ cov}(\hat{a}\hat{b}) + \text{cov}(\hat{a}\hat{b})^2$ to Equation 3.9 for the standard error of $\hat{a}\hat{b}$ (see Equation 11 in Kenny et al., 2003). The formula for the mediated effect and its standard error for the case in which $\hat{a}$ and $\hat{b}$ are random effects is the same as the formula for the product of two correlated random variables. It is important to note also that the variance of $\hat{a}$ and $\hat{b}$ corresponds to the variance of the $\hat{u}_{1j}$ and $\hat{u}_{2j}$ terms in the equations, not the standard errors of $\hat{a}$ and $\hat{b}$ in Equations 9.15 and 9.16.

In this lower level mediation model, the independent, mediator, and dependent variables are continuous variables with random effects at the higher level of analysis. Kenny et al. (2003) described a model in which the genetic relatedness of a person leads to perceived similarity with that person, which leads to emotional closeness. Respondents named and reported several family members, and genetic relatedness was measured by the proportion of shared genes with the family member. The respondents then rated the emotional closeness and similarity of 10 persons from their list of family members. There were 72 participants (upper level units) and 10 family members (lower level units) for each participant. As expected, the $\hat{a}$ path relation between genetic relatedness and perceived similarity varied across persons and the $\hat{b}$ path relation between perceived similarity and emotional closeness varied across persons. The mediated effect required the addition of the covariance of $\hat{a}$ and $\hat{b}$, which was .348 and substantially increased the size of the standard error of the mediated effect.

To illustrate the random effects mediation model, simulated data provided by Kenny et al. are used. The data consist of 200 participants with 10 measures for each participant for each variable X, M, and Y. To add some context, assume a study similar to the group therapy study used in this chapter with X representing a continuous measure of how conducive the person's lifestyle and environment was to exercise. M is again fitness, and Y is feeling of happiness. A total of 200 participants had measures of X, M, and Y recorded on 10 different days. The Mplus program for this example is shown in Table 9.18. Note that 10 different environments allow for continuous measures of each variable rather than X representing exposure to one of two treatments. Here it is likely that the extent to which the environment on a particular day is conducive to exercise leads to physical activity that leads to feelings of happiness. The variables X, M, and Y are included along with the cluster variable subjid. It is noted that X is within subjects only. The model is specified in the type = twolevel random command and algorithmic integration is used. The %within% line specifies the estimation of the relation of Y on X, $\hat{c}'$, the relation of M on X, $\hat{a}$, and is the relation of Y on M, $\hat{b}$. The line after the %between% command tells Mplus to estimate the covariance between $\hat{a}$ and $\hat{b}$.

Selected output from the Mplus program in Table 9.18 is shown in Table 9.19. The output in Table 9.19 first shows means for each variable along with the covariances among the variables. The $\hat{a}$ coefficient equaled 0.589 with a standard error of 0.032. The $\hat{b}$ coefficient was equal to 0.633 with a standard error of 0.036. The variance of coefficient $\hat{a}$ equals 0.132 with a standard error of 0.020, suggesting significant variability of the $\hat{a}$ coefficient. The variance of coefficient $\hat{b}$ was 0.174 with a standard error of 0.024, suggesting significant variability. The covariance between $\hat{a}$ and $\hat{b}$ was equal to 0.126. These values were entered in Equation 8.31 for the variance of $\hat{a}\hat{b}$ equal to 0.2461 ($\hat{a}^2 s_b^2 + \hat{b}^2 s_a^2 + s_b^2 s_a^2 + 2\hat{a}\hat{b}\,\mathrm{cov}(\hat{a}\hat{b}) + \mathrm{cov}(\hat{a}\hat{b})^2 = 0.589^2(0.174)^2 + 0.633^2(0.132)^2 + (0.174)^2(0.132)^2 + 2(0.589)(0.633)(0.126) + (0.126)^2$), which differs only slightly from 0.2542 obtained in the Kenny et al. (2003) article using

Table 9.18 MPLUS Program for Random Effects Multilevel Mediation Model

```
title:
  kenny (2003)

  data:
  file=kenny.dat;
  variable:
  names=subjid meas X M Y constant;
  usevariables=x m y;
  cluster=subjid;
  within = x;
  analysis:
  type=twolevel random;
  algorithm = integration;
  ghfiml = on;
  model:
  %within%
  cprime | y on x;
  a | m on x;
  b | y on m;
  %between%
  a with b;
  output:
  sampstat tech1 tech3 tech8;
```

an ad hoc method rather than direct estimation with Mplus. The product of $\hat{a}$ and $\hat{b}$ equals 0.373 (0.589 × 0.633) but Kenny et al. show that cov($\hat{a}\hat{b}$) should be added to $\hat{a}\hat{b}$ to equal 0.373 + 0.126 = 0.5 as in Equation 8.30. The variance of the mediated effect across the 200 participants equals 0.2461. The estimated average mediated effect is statistically significant ($se = 0.041$, LCL = 0.420, UCL = 0.580). The variance of the estimated average mediated effect (Equation 9 in Bauer et al., 2006) adds the variance of the co-variance between $\hat{a}$ and $\hat{b}$ ($.017^2$) to Equation 8.11 and uses $s_{\hat{a}} = 0.032$, $s_{\hat{b}} = 0.036$, and Cov($\hat{a}\hat{b}$) = .0006 (Cov($\hat{a}\hat{b}$) not shown in Table 9.19).

A new method to estimate mediation for the case of random $\hat{a}$, $\hat{b}$, and $\hat{c}'$ coefficients has also been implemented in the SAS MIXED language (Bauer, Preacher, & Gil, 2006). The method used in Mplus, the SAS MIXED approach, and the ad hoc approach used in Kenny et al. have not yet been compared. However, the Mplus approach is integrated in the general statistical analysis of multilevel models, so it may be preferable.

Table 9.19 Selected MPLUS Output for the Random Effects Mediation Model

```
SAMPLE STATISTICS
Mean
```

	M	Y	X
1	0.004	−0.007	0.034

```
Covariances
```

	M	Y	X
M	2.131		
Y	1.767	2.929	
X	1.128	1.325	2.000

```
MODEL RESULTS
```

	Estimates	S.E.	Est./S.E.
Within Level			
Residual Variances			
M	0.645	0.023	28.647
Y	0.465	0.017	27.618
Between Level			
A WITH			
B	0.126	0.017	7.455
Means			
M	0.003	0.059	0.052
Y	0.001	0.050	0.016
CPRIME	0.176	0.027	6.446
A	0.589	0.032	18.402
B	0.633	0.036	17.601
Variances			
M	0.588	0.065	9.061
Y	0.398	0.048	8.328
CPRIME	0.056	0.013	4.320
A	0.132	0.020	6.711
B	0.174	0.024	7.300

9.18 Multilevel Mediation Models at Different Levels

Besides adjusting for a nonzero ICC, multilevel models can be used to investigate effects at the different levels of analysis, for example, the mediated effect when a group-level predictor changes an individual-level mediator. Kenny et al. (1998) briefly discussed two situations, termed lower level mediation, for mediation at the individual level, and upper level mediation at the group level, for example, for mediation in a multilevel framework. To date, these important cross-level effects have not been addressed in much detail (Palmer et al., 1998).

Krull and MacKinnon (2001) described three major types of multilevel models corresponding to the level of the independent variable, mediating variable, and dependent variable. They proposed a way to describe these models using arrows and numbers to indicate the level of analysis. For example, the $1 \rightarrow 1 \rightarrow 1$ model has an independent variable (X_{ij}), a mediator (M_{ij}), and a dependent variable (Y_{ij}) all measured at Level 1, or the lowest level of the data. As described earlier, the ij subscript on each variable indicates that the variable can take on a unique value for each individual i within each group j. In this simplest case, with all three variables measured at the individual level, it is only the clustered nature of the data that requires multilevel modeling to appropriately model the error structure. Examples of this model would be an experimental design in which assignment to conditions would be made within group so that some subjects in a group are in the control condition and other subjects are in the treatment condition. Another example of this type of analysis would be when all measures are taken at the individual level, but there is clustering in the data such as the primary sampling unit in a telephone survey.

A second type of model, which is the one described earlier in this chapter, has the independent variable at the group level but the mediator and dependent variable at the individual level. This $2 \rightarrow 1 \rightarrow 1$ model, has an independent Level 2 variable (X_j), representing a characteristic of the group, which affects an individual-level mediator (M_{ij}), which, in turn, affects an individual-level dependent variable (Y_{ij}). The single subscript j on the X variable indicates that this variable may take on a unique value for each group j. This type of multilevel mediation model is also common in the investigation of how group-level variables affect individual variables (Hofmann & Gavin, 1998). This model is very common in prevention research, in which assignment to conditions at the group level is the most practical level of assignment, but the mediating variable and the dependent variable are measured at the individual level. In management research, for example, mediators are hypothesized for how organizational climate affects individual performance, such as how level of centralization in a work unit affects the mediating variable of autonomy, which then affects job satisfaction. It is worth noting that the relation coded by a from X to M is at the group level whereas the relation b between M and Y is at the individual level, and the mediated effect combines relations at two levels.

In a large simulation study, Krull and MacKinnon (2001) found that group size, ICC of the mediator, and ICC of the dependent variable were identified as factors that increase the extent of underestimation of standard errors. As a result, multilevel mediation analysis may be most important in these situations. The simulation study also suggests that the Level 2 sample size (i.e., the number of groups in the analysis) plays at most a minimal role in determining the underestimation of single-level standard errors and the multilevel advantage in this regard. However, Level 2 sample size is known to play a key role in the statistical power of multilevel analysis (Kenny et al., 1998; Murray, 1998).

Another type of model is the $2 \to 2 \to 1$ model in which both the independent (X_j) and mediator (M_j) variables are measured at the group level, but the dependent variable (Y_{ij}) is measured at the individual level. Sampson et al. (1997) used a similar model (note that Sampson et al., 1977 actually had three levels with the first level within respondent) to study how neighborhood level measures of social composition (which reflect economic disadvantage and immigrant concentration) affect neighborhood level measures of collective efficacy (social cohesion and informal social control), which, in turn, influence individual-level measures of violence (such as perceived level of neighborhood violence and individual violent victimization). Sampson, Morenoff, and Gannon-Rowley (2002) described examples of this and other social process models in neighborhood research. An example of the $2 \to 2 \to 1$ model in management research occurs when individual psychological perceptions and meanings are shared in a group to the extent that individuals within the same group share the same perceptions and meanings (Griffin, Mathieu, & Jacobs, 2001). Because the individual-level measures of perceptions are so similar, the group-level perception measures are valid Level 2 predictors of individual variables (James, James, & Ashe, 1990).

These models can be extended to more than two levels such as individual, classroom, and school for educational data with correspondingly more complicated versions and types of multilevel models. In addition, many variables can be conceptualized at more than one level, making the clear interpretation of some multilevel models difficult. For example, any individual-level measure can be aggregated to the group level, by taking the mean for each group. Effects involving such a variable may operate at either or both levels, and individual and aggregate measures of the same variable may reflect different constructs at the different levels. One example of this type of mediator is social norms for which the individual measure of norm may reflect individual perceptions of social norms, whereas a norm measure at the school level may reflect general social attitudes. Burstein (1980, 1985) noted that individual student level responses about parental occupation and education may serve as indicators of home background and reflect parental commitment to the student's learning, whereas school level aggregates of the same responses more likely indicate the wealth and socioeconomic status of the community, which may determine the level of school resources. In general, true individual-level variables tend to be more psychological or specific in nature than group aggregates, which may be more indicative of social, organizational, or normative aspects of the environment. Aggregate measures may also represent contextual influences, which can operate in a different manner than the individual measure on which it was based as noted by Robinson (1950) in the well-known ecological fallacy that the effects of the same variable on the same outcome differ at different levels of analysis. For example, rebelliousness as an individual characteristic may encourage risk-taking and make an intervention less likely to be effective. Moreover, a group with a high average level of rebelliousness may create an environment in which discipline issues would make program delivery difficult, decreasing program effectiveness even for nonrebellious individuals (Palmer et al., 1998).

9.19 Summary

Many data sets are suitable for multilevel mediation modeling. The mediation model can be extended to multilevel analysis, but it is considerably more complicated and requires a new iterative estimation strategy. The multilevel model requires estimates of effects at more than one level. A hypothetical example was used to demonstrate the use of the model. Several additional models are described that differ on the level that is the focus of the analysis. As described in chapter 8, the multilevel model provides a general framework to incorporate longitudinal measures. In this regard, subject is a level of analysis, and the longitudinal measurements are clustered within each subject. This chapter presented Mplus and SAS MIXED programs for the estimation of multilevel models. There are other excellent programs for multilevel analysis including Mlwin and HLM as well as comprehensive covariance structure analysis programs with multilevel analysis capabilities such as LISREL and EQS.

9.20 Exercises

9.1.   What is the correlation between the same variable centered within each group and the group mean?

9.2.   Reparameterize the example used in this chapter so that there are random intercepts and slopes.

9.3.   In your own research describe examples of the following models: (a) $1 \rightarrow 1 \rightarrow 1$, (b) $2 \rightarrow 2 \rightarrow 2$, (c) $2 \rightarrow 1 \rightarrow 1$, (d), $3 \rightarrow 2 \rightarrow 1$, and (e) $3 \rightarrow 1 \rightarrow 1 \rightarrow 1$.

9.4. For the Sampson, Raudenbush, and Earls (1997) study described in section 9.5, describe each level of analysis. Suggest one additional level of analysis for these data, and discuss how you would model the data. The authors used a difference in coefficients test for the mediated effect. What coefficients would you use to obtain a product of coefficients mediated effect for each group?

10

Mediation and Moderation

> The value of a model is that it often suggests a simple summary of data in terms of the major systematic effects together with a summary of the nature and magnitude of the unexplained or random variation. Such a reduction is certainly helpful, for the human mind, while it may be able to encompass say 10 numbers easily enough, finds 100 much more difficult, and will be quite defeated by 1000 unless some reducing process takes place.
>
> **—Peter McCullagh & John Nelder, 1989, p. 3**

10.1 Overview

The strength and form of mediation effects may depend on other variables, called moderators. As described in chapter 1, moderators are variables that alter the relation between two variables. Many researchers advocate the evaluation of moderator variables and mediator variables in the same research study (Baron & Kenny, 1986; Kraemer, Wilson, Fairburn, & Agras, 2002; MacKinnon, Weber, & Pentz, 1989). This chapter describes how to incorporate moderators in mediation analysis. The moderator effect is more commonly known as an interaction effect (Baron & Kenny, 1986), and these two terms are used synonymously in this chapter. There are several different ways in which an interaction alters a mediation analysis and the different ways have different statistical and conceptual complexities. The chapter describes the most straightforward situation in which mediation differs across subgroups of a moderator. Next, moderators that are variables in the mediational process are described. An example is used to illustrate moderator and mediator effects. Finally, several other types of moderator and mediator models are described.

10.2 Moderators

A moderator is a variable that modifies the form or strength of the relation between an independent and a dependent variable. The examination of moderator effects has a long and important history in a variety of research areas. Moderator effects have been studied more extensively studied than mediator effects both in application and as a methodology, most notably in the context of analysis of variance. There are outstanding books on moderator effects (Aguinis, 2004; Aiken & West, 1991). Moderator effects are also called interactions to signify that the third variable interacts with the relation between two other variables. The third variable in this case is not part of a causal sequence but qualifies the relation between X and Y. The moderator variable can be continuous or categorical, although a categorical moderator variable will often be easiest to interpret. From a substantive perspective, interactions are especially interesting as they imply that an observed relation between an independent variable and a dependent variable can be strengthened, weakened, removed, or made opposite in sign when the third variable is considered. Although most moderator effects refer to the situation in which the relation between two variables differs across the levels of a third variable, higher order interactions involving more than one moderator are also possible.

A moderator may be a factor in an experimental manipulation, representing random assignment to levels of the factor. For example, participants may be randomly assigned to a moderator factor of treatment duration in addition to type of treatment received to test the moderator effect of duration of treatment across type of treatment. A moderator may also be a variable that is not manipulated, such as gender or age. For example, studies of racial or gender bias evaluate interactions corresponding to different relations between two variables across ethnic groups or gender. In treatment and prevention research, moderator variables may reflect subgroups of persons for whom the treatment or intervention is more or less effective than for other groups. In general, moderator variables are critical for understanding the generalizability of a research finding. Theory may be used to predict moderator effects and in other cases moderators may reflect a purely exploratory search for different relations across subgroups.

10.3 Moderator Effects

Sharma, Durand, and Gur-Arie (1981) described three types of moderator effects. The first type of moderator effect is called a homologizer for which the true relation between the independent variable and the dependent variable does not change across levels of the moderator, but the error variance does change across the levels of the moderator. If an effect is examined by subgroups, the strength of the standardized relation varies because the error variance varies across subgroups. The error variance may vary across subgroups because of different measurement properties such as response reliabilities across the subgroups. So a homologizer influences the strength of the link between the independent variable and dependent variable because of differences in error variance across groups.

The second and third forms of a moderator variable are consistent with most discussions of moderators. Here the moderator is a variable that changes the form of the relation between the independent variable and the dependent variable. If the moderator variable is also a significant predictor of the dependent variable, the moderator variable is called a quasi-moderator, the second type of moderator. If the moderator variable is not a significant predictor of the dependent variable it is called a pure moderator, the third form of a moderator. The pure moderator is also called a psychometric moderator because the form of the relation between the independent variable and the dependent variable changes as a function of the moderator.

The interaction effect model is shown in Equation 10.1.

$$Y = i_1 + c_1X + c_2Z + c_3XZ + e_1 \qquad (10.1)$$

where Y is the dependent variable, X is the independent variable, Z is the moderator variable, and XZ is the interaction of the moderator and the independent variable; e_1 is a residual, and c_1, c_2, and c_3 represent the relation between the dependent variable and the independent variable, the moderator variable and the dependent variable, and moderator by independent variable interaction, respectively. The interaction variable XZ is formed by the product of X and Z. Often X and Z are centered (i.e., the average is subtracted from each observed value of the variable, $Xc = X - \bar{X}$, $Zc = Z - \bar{Z}$) before the product is formed to improve interpretation of effects in the interaction model and to reduce collinearity among the measures, thereby improving the estimation of model parameters. In this model, centered X, centered Z, and the product of the centered X and Z variables are predictors.

If the XZ interaction is statistically significant, the source of the significant interaction is often explored by examining conditional effects with contrasts and plots. These contrasts, called tests of simple slopes, test the statistical significance of the relation between X and Y at different values of Z. There are several ways in which the XZ interaction may be statistically significant, which correspond to different simple slopes. For example, the size of the coefficient relating X and Y may be statistically significant at all observed values of Z and differ across levels of Z. Thus, in a two-group study with Z representing group membership, the effect in one group may be significantly different from the effect in the other group, and each effect may be individually statistically significant. To use the relation between stress and blood pressure as an example, the relation between these variables may be statistically significant for males and for females, but the relation may be significantly larger for males than for females. In another situation, the relation of the moderator to the dependent variable may be close to zero (i.e., $\hat{c}_2$ near 0) such that the relation between X and Y may have an opposite sign at different levels of Z. For example, for a two-group study, the coefficient relating X and Y may have a different sign in each group (a type of pure moderator). There are many other patterns of effects implied by a significant XZ interaction that are clarified by examining conditional effects with contrasts.

For a continuous moderator variable Z, tests of simple slopes are obtained by forming new variables so that the effect is computed at certain values of Z. For example, to obtain the simple effect of X at 1 standard deviation above the mean of Z, a new variable is made such that the zero value of Z is equal to 1 standard deviation above the mean of Z. The regression analysis is repeated, and the significance test for XZ is the significance test for the simple slope at the particular value of Z. More on interaction effects including procedures to plot interactions can be found in Aguinis (2004), Aiken and West (1991), and Keppel and Wickens (2004).

Plots of moderator effects are obtained by computing the predicted value of Y given the regression equation and values of X, Z, and XZ. Equation 10.2 shows a rearrangement of Equation 10.1 that makes plotting the data somewhat easier because the equation is recast in terms of the regression of Y on X at levels of Z.

$$Y = (c_1 + c_3 Z)X + (c_2 Z + i_1) \qquad (10.2)$$

The slope of Y on X, $c_1 + c_3 Z$, is called the simple slope and $c_2 Z + i_1$ is the simple (or conditional) intercept. In Equation 10.2, only the values of X and Z are necessary to compute predicted scores. The value of the interaction XZ is necessary for predicted means if Equation 10.1 is used. If X and Z are binary variables, then the predicted scores in each of the four groups defined by binary X and Z are plotted. If X is continuous and Z is binary, then the plots of the relation between X and Y at each level of Z represent the relation in each group. If X and Z are continuous, then the predicted scores are often plotted for the mean, 1 standard deviation above, and 1 standard deviation below the mean.

10.4 Moderation and Mediation

The definition and interpretation of mediation in the presence of moderation can be complex statistically and conceptually (Baron & Kenny, 1986; Hayduk & Wonnacott, 1980; James & Brett, 1984; Rogosa, 1988; Stolzenberg, 1980; Wegener & Fabrigar, 2000). In general, there are two types of effects that combine moderation and mediation (Baron & Kenny, 1986):

(a) moderation of a mediation effect in which the mediated effect is different at different values of a moderator and (b) mediation of a moderator effect in which the effect of an interaction on a dependent variable is mediated. Historically, the moderated mediation effect (Baron & Kenny, 1986) refers to different M to Y relations across levels of a moderator, different X to M relations across levels of the moderator or different M to Y and X to M relations across levels of the moderator.

An example of moderated mediation is a case in which a mediation process differs for males and females. A manipulation may affect social norms equally for both males and females, but social norms only significantly reduce subsequent tobacco use for females. A more complicated example of moderated mediation is a case in which social norms mediate the effect of a prevention program on drug use, but the size of the mediated effect differs as a function of risk-taking propensity. An example of mediated moderation is if the effect of a prevention program depends on risk-taking propensity, and this interaction changes a mediating variable of social norms, which then affects drug use. These types of effects are important because they help specify types of subgroups for whom mediational processes differ and help quantify more complicated hypotheses about mediation relations. Despite the potential benefits of testing for moderation of a mediated effect and mediation of a moderator effect, few research studies include both mediation and moderation, at least in part because of the difficulty of specifying and interpreting these models. An approach to models with both mediation and moderation is described in the next few sections.

10.5 Interaction Between the Mediator and the Independent Variable in the Single Mediator Model

The first type of moderator effect in a mediation model provides a test of one of the assumptions of the single mediator model. One of the assumptions of the mediation Equation 3.2 described in chapter 3 is that the relation from the mediator to the dependent variable is the same across levels of the independent variable; that is, the M to Y relation does not differ across levels of X. A nonzero XM interaction effect suggests that the independent variable alters the relation between the mediator and the dependent variable. The existence of this interaction also means that the relation of the independent variable to the dependent variable differs across levels of the mediator. To simplify the description, this chapter focuses on how the relation of M to Y differs across levels of X because X is often a variable representing an experimental manipulation. With X representing group random assignment, X is not a moderator. In situations in which the levels of X are not randomly assigned, then the researcher must decide whether X or M (or both X and M) is the moderator.

The test of the XM interaction has important substantive implications as well as providing a test of an assumption of the single mediator model. Substantive examples of a significant XM interaction are described in Judd and Kenny (1981a), in Merrill (1994), and more recently by the MacArthur group (Kraemer et al., 2002). As for any interaction effect, if the XM interaction is statistically significant, then the main effects of X or M do not necessarily provide a complete interpretation of the effects in the data. A statistically significant XM interaction means that the relation between M and Y differs for at least some values of X. Because the relation of M to Y differs across levels of X, the *b* path differs across groups. As described in Equation 10.3, the *h* coefficient codes the XM interaction.

$$Y = i_2 + c'X + bM + hXM + e_2 \qquad (10.3)$$

For the water consumption example in chapter 3, this interaction is not statistically significant ($\hat{h} = .0299$, $s_{\hat{h}} = .1198$, $t_{\hat{h}} = 0.25$, *ns*) suggesting that the assumption of no XM interaction is reasonable. That is, the significance test suggests that the relation of M to Y does not differ across levels of X for the water consumption study. If the XM interaction is statistically significant, it is important to explore the source of the significant interaction with contrasts including simple effects and plots following methods outlined in Aiken and West (1991) and Keppel and Wickens (2004). These contrasts test the significance of the $\hat{b}$ coefficient relating M to Y at different values of X. There are several ways in which the XM interaction may be statistically significant, which correspond to different simple slopes. For example, the size of the $\hat{b}$ coefficient may be statistically significant at all values of X but still differ across levels of X (i.e., for a two-group study, the $\hat{b}$ coefficient may be larger in one group than another). This pattern of effects may be predicted in treatment research in which the relation between M and Y is still substantial in each group, but the size of the relation is larger in one group, perhaps because the treatment increased (or decreased) the size of the relation. For example, assume that a drug prevention program reduces the relation between the number of offers of a drug and drug use. The relation between offers and drug use may be significantly lower in the treatment group than in the control group because the treatment reduced the strong influence of offers on drug use. Alternatively, the overall effect of M may be close to zero such that the $\hat{b}$ coefficient relating M and Y may have an opposite sign at different levels of X (i.e., for a two-group study the $\hat{b}$ coefficient may have a different sign in each group). In this case, the relation between M and Y is opposite in the two groups, which may lead to a nonsignificant $\hat{b}$ coefficient if the interaction is ignored, when in fact, the relation of M to Y may be statistically significant in both groups but opposite in sign. There are many other possible patterns of effects implied by a significant XM interaction that are clarified with simple slopes and other types of contrasts. Although the preceding discussion assumes slopes for linear relations, nonlinear relations may be tested in a similar manner.

Plots of effects are obtained by predicting scores for values of X and M. For example, the regression model equation for the XM interaction for the water consumption example in chapter 3 is shown in Equation 10.4. Note that the procedure for making plots described in the following is based on linear relations among variables, but nonlinear relations may be plotted using analogous procedures. The X variable (mean = 70.18, sd = 1.1373) and M variable (mean = 3.06, sd = 1.0382) were centered before forming their interaction and conducting the analysis.

$$\hat{Y} = 3.2272 + 0.2140\ X + 0.4542\ M + 0.0299\ XM \tag{10.4}$$

Putting values for X and M in the equation yields a predicted value for Y. These predicted values are used to make plots of the interaction. Predicted scores for this example at the mean, at 1 standard deviation above and 1 standard deviation below the mean for the variables in the interaction were (a) 1 sd below the mean for both X and M, 2.5476, (b) 1 sd below the mean for X and the mean of M, 2.9838, (3) 1 sd below the mean for X and 1 sd above the mean for M, 3.4200, (d) mean of X and 1 sd below the mean for M, 2.7557, (e) the mean of X and the mean of M, 3.4200, (f) the mean of X and 1 sd above the mean for M, 2.7557, (g) 1 sd above the mean for X and 1 sd below the mean for M, 3.6988, (h) 1 sd above the mean for X and the mean of M, 3.4706, and (i) 1 sd above the mean for X and 1 sd above the mean for M, 3.9774.

Equation 10.5 makes it easier to obtain predicted means because only the values for X and M are needed for the calculations:

$$\hat{Y} = (0.2140 + 0.0299\ M)X + 0.4542\ M + 3.2272 \tag{10.5}$$

To illustrate the calculation of the predicted scores, the predicted score for 1 standard deviation below the mean for both X and M is shown in Equation 10.6.

$$\hat{Y} = (0.2140 + 0.0299(-1.0382))(-1.1373) + 0.4542(-1.0382)$$
$$+ 3.2272 = 2.5476 \tag{10.6}$$

The predicted score for Y at 1 standard deviation below the mean of X and 1 standard deviation above the mean of M is shown in Equation 10.7.

$$\hat{Y} = (0.2140 + 0.0299(0))(-1.1373) + 0.4542(0) + 3.2272 = 2.9838 \tag{10.7}$$

It is clear from the predicted means that the two lines are nearly parallel, consistent with a nonsignificant interaction effect. If the interaction was statistically significant, then tests of simple slopes would be conducted. The test of simple slope is obtained by centering the data so that the slope is at certain values of X and M. For example, if the data are centered at 1 standard deviation above the mean, then the interaction tests the simple effect at 1 standard deviation above the mean for that variable. The aforementioned approach required computing six different means. An alternative approach to plotting the data would be to obtain the regression line relating M to Y at each of three values of X and plotting these regression lines.

Figure 10.1 shows a plot of the relation of M to Y for values of X equal to 1 standard deviation below the mean, the mean value, and 1 standard deviation above the mean. Note that the lines are almost, but not exactly, parallel, consistent with the nonsignificant and small XM interaction. The values of different effects can also be shown in the model extended from Merrill (1994), who presented graphs for these effects for the case of a binary X variable. The slopes represent different $\hat{b}$ coefficients for the three groups. Note that the slight distance between the lines differs at different values of M consistent with the different values of the $\hat{c}'$ coefficient at different values of M. The mediated effect $\hat{a}\hat{b}$, or the change in Y for a change in M of $\hat{a}$ units, is slightly different for the different groups.

Merrill (1994) described a substantive example in which there is an XM interaction, and X is a binary variable coding exposure to treatment or

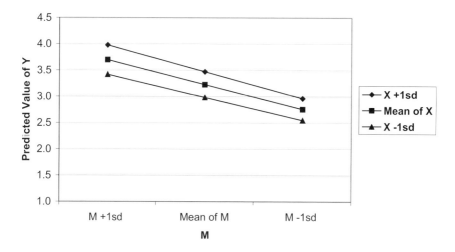

Figure 10.1. Relation of M to Y.

control. For treatment and prevention studies, a statistically significant XM interaction is sometimes expected with an effect of X on M. For example, a prevention program may increase achievement among school children that in turn reduces depression. However, the increase in this effect may depend on whether the persons had high or low achievement at the beginning of the study. So in this situation, the time 2 mediator is intermediate in the causal sequence relating the independent to the dependent variable, and the size of the mediated effect depends on the level of the mediator at baseline. For another example, imagine a program designed to increase social competence. The program increases social competence, which then subsequently increases achievement. Additionally, the size of the mediated effect depends on social competence such that more highly social competent participants do not improve as much as persons low in social competence.

Merrill (1994) described a set of procedures to test both the moderator effect and the mediator effect in this situation when the X variable is binary and the XM interaction is estimated. The estimator of the mediated effect is $\hat{a}\hat{b}$ and standard error is the same as described in chapter 3 of this book. The estimator of the moderator effect is $\hat{h}(\hat{i}_3 + \hat{a})$ with a standard error equal to $(\hat{i}_3^2 s_{\hat{h}}^2 + 2\hat{i}_3\hat{a}s_{\hat{h}}^2 + \hat{a}^2 s_{\hat{h}}^2 + \hat{h}^2 s_{\hat{i}_3}^2 + 2\hat{h}^2 s_{\hat{i}_3,\hat{a}} + \hat{h}^2 s_{\hat{a}}^2)^{1/2}$, where i_3 is the intercept in Equation 3.3 in which X predicts M, $\hat{a}$ is the coefficient relating X to M, and $s_{\hat{i}_3,\hat{a}}$ is the covariance between i_3 and $\hat{a}$. Estimates from Equations 3.3 and 10.3 are inserted in these equations to test statistical significance or to create confidence intervals for these effects. For the water consumption example, the moderator effect was equal to $0.0299(-20.7024 + 0.3386) = -0.6089$ with a standard error of 2.4527 and $t = 0.2482$ ($s_{\hat{i}_3,\hat{a}} = 8.5889$, *ns*). In a large simulation study, Merrill, MacKinnon, and Mayer (1994) demonstrated that the mediated effect is inflated in an analysis that ignores an XM interaction that is present in the population model generating the data.

10.6 Moderation and Mediation With Stacked Groups

A general approach to modeling mediation and moderation is described in the next few sections starting with a moderator with two different values. The approach is easily extended to moderators with more than two levels. The simplest way that an interaction is involved in a mediation effect is if the mediated effect differs between two different samples. For example, the mediated effect may differ for males versus females or for older versus younger persons. As described earlier, this would occur if mediation of a prevention program on drug use through social norms differed for males and females, for example. Such a model with a binary Z variable is shown in figure 10.2. In this situation, the estimation of the

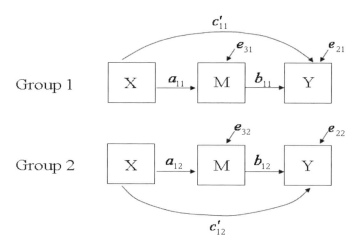

Figure 10.2. Moderation of a mediated relation.

mediated effect follows the procedures outlined in chapter 3 in each of the two groups. An example with two groups is shown in Equations 10.8, 10.9, and 10.10 for group 1 and Equations 10.11, 10.12, and 10.13 for group 2. Note that the second subscript for the parameters represents group membership and Z represents the moderator variable with groups as Z equals 1 or Z equals 2.

Group $Z = 1$

$$Y_1 = i_{11} + c_{11}X + e_{11} \tag{10.8}$$

$$Y_1 = i_{21} + c'_{11}X + b_{11}M + e_{21} \tag{10.9}$$

$$M_1 = i_{31} + a_{11}X + e_{31} \tag{10.10}$$

Group $Z = 2$

$$Y_2 = i_{12} + c_{12}X + e_{12} \tag{10.11}$$

$$Y_2 = i_{22} + c'_{12}X + b_{12}M + e_{22} \tag{10.12}$$

$$M_2 = i_{32} + a_{12}X + e_{32} \tag{10.13}$$

There are several interesting hypotheses that could be tested with these data, including a test of the equality of the a parameters ($H_0: a_{11} - a_{12} = 0$), a test of the equality of the b parameters (H$_o$: $b_{11} - b_{12} = 0$), or a test of the equality of the direct effect c', (H$_o$: $c'_{11} - c'_{12} = 0$). A test of the equality of the total effect c, (H$_o$: $c_{11} - c_{12} = 0$) is the test of the overall interaction effect of X on Y. Because the two groups are independent, the estimator of the standard error of the difference is the pooled standard error from each group. The tests of the equality of the a parameters is called a test of mediated moderation by Baron and Kenny (1986). The test of the equality of the b parameter is a test of moderated mediation in Baron and Kenny (1986). However these tests are not actually tests of mediation because they test the equality of only one link in the mediated effect. As a result, the test of equality of a parameters is a test of homogenous action theory (how X is related to M) and the tests of the equality of the b parameter across groups is a test for homogenous conceptual theory (how M is related to Y). These names clarify that the test is of either a or b separately and is not strictly a test of mediation. To test whether the mediated effect differs across levels of the moderator, a test of the equality of the mediated effect in each group is needed (H$_o$: $a_{11}b_{11} - a_{12}b_{12} = 0$). The standard error of this test is the pooled standard error of the mediated effect from each group. If there are more than two groups, then contrasts among the mediated effects are explored to find the source of the significant moderated mediation effect. With three groups for example, the main effect of any difference among mediated effects could be tested as well as contrasts between pairs of mediated effects.

10.7 Moderation and Mediation With a Continuous Moderator

There are many situations in which the moderator variable is continuous. In this case, one option would be to fit the mediation model treating each value of the continuous variable as a separate group (practical only if the moderator is an integer variable). A problem with this approach is that sample size may not be sufficient to estimate the model at all values of the continuous variable. There is an alternative setup of this moderator and mediator model that can be more easily generalized to moderator variables that are continuous. This model is described first for the two-group moderator variable.

The following models are used to test the same hypotheses described earlier for the two-group case for a binary or continuous moderator variable. Equation 10.14 represents the relation between the independent variable, the moderator, and the interaction of the moderator and the independent variable. Equation 10.14 combines Equations 10.8 and 10.11, which were separate equations for two groups when Z is binary. Equation 10.15 combines Equations 10.9 and 10.12. Equation 10.16 combines Equations 10.10

and 10.13. These are the equations implied by Baron and Kenny (1986, p. 1179). Equations 10.15 and 10.16 extend the single mediator model in several ways. First, the moderator variable, Z, is added along with its interaction with X, represented by XZ. The interaction of the moderator with M is represented by MZ. In this model, a test of homogeneous action theory is included in the test of the $\hat{a}_3$ coefficient because this coefficient tests whether the a parameter differs across the groups. A test of homogeneous conceptual theory is made with the $\hat{b}_2$ coefficient that tests whether the b parameter is different across values of Z. The test of whether the c' parameter is different across groups is obtained by testing the $\hat{c}'_3$ coefficient. The results from these tests are algebraically equivalent to the aforementioned model for which effects were estimated separately in each group. That is, H_o: $a_{11} - a_{12} = 0$ is the same as H_o: $a_3 = 0$, H_o: $b_{11} - b_{12} = 0$, is the same as H_o: $b_2 = 0$, and H_o: $c'_{11} - c'_{12} = 0$ is the same as Ho: $c'_3 = 0$.

$$Y = i_1 + c_1 X + c_2 Z + c_3 XZ + e_1 \tag{10.14}$$

$$Y = i_2 + c'_1 X + c'_2 Z + c'_3 XZ + b_1 M + b_2 MZ + e_2 \tag{10.15}$$

$$M = i_3 + a_1 X + a_2 Z + a_3 XZ + e_3 \tag{10.16}$$

In these equations with X and Z centered, Y is the dependent variable, X is the independent variable, M is the mediator, Z is the moderator, XZ is the interaction of the moderator Z and X, c_1, c_2, and c_3 represent the relation between the independent variable, moderator variable, moderator by independent variable interaction, and dependent variable, respectively; c'_1, c'_2, and c'_3 represent the relation between the independent variable, moderator variable, moderator by independent variable interaction, and dependent variable, adjusted for the other effects in Equation 10.15, b_1 is the coefficient relating the mediator to the dependent variable adjusted for the other effects in Equation 10.15, b_2 is the coefficient relating the mediator by moderator interaction to the dependent variable adjusted for the effects in Equation 10.16, a_1 is the coefficient relating X to the mediating variable, a_2 is the coefficient relating Z to the mediating variable, and a_3 is the coefficient relating XZ to the mediator, e_1, e_2, and e_3 represent error variability, and i_1, i_2, and i_3 are the intercepts in the Equations.

If a researcher assumes homogeneous conceptual theory but wishes to test for homogeneous action theory, then the coefficient b_2 would be zero and the interaction, MZ, would not be included as a predictor. If a researcher assumes homogeneous action theory but wishes to test for homogeneous conceptual theory then the a_3 parameter would be zero and XZ would not be included as a predictor in the model. Note that model tests with and without assuming an interaction is zero may lead to different research conclusions so it is often sensible to include the interactions in the analyses.

To investigate the value of the mediated effect as a function of Z it is useful to plot the value of the mediated effect as a function of the value of Z, where the X axis represents the value of Z and the Y axis represents the value of the mediated effect. If X codes random assignment to an experimental condition then X and Z should be uncorrelated. If Z codes a variable with one of two values, then the interaction codes the difference in the value of the coefficient between groups.

10.8 General Moderation and Mediation Model

The model can be made more general by adding two other interactions thereby allowing for testing more complicated forms of moderation and mediation. The XM and XMZ interactions can be added to the mediation and moderation equations to form a general model in Equation 10.17:

$$Y = i_2 + c_1'X + c_2'Z + c_3'XZ + b_1M + b_2MZ + hXM + jXMZ + e_2 \quad (10.17)$$

As described earlier (Equation 10.3) the h coefficient represents the test of whether the M to Y relation differs across levels of X. The j coefficient represents the three-way interaction effect where the relations between Z and M and Y differ across levels of X. If a statistically significant j coefficient is found, further simple interaction mediated effects and simple mediated effects are explored. In many situations the h and j parameters will be assumed to be zero. When time is included in this model, more general estimation strategies are needed such as the methods described in chapters 6, 7, and 8.

10.9 Mediated Baseline by Treatment Interaction Models

One example of a moderation and mediation model that explicitly includes a baseline score is the mediated baseline by treatment interaction model. These models are important because they may be the ideal model for the evaluation of treatment and prevention programs for which the effect of the program depends on baseline measures of the mediator or dependent variable. The XM interaction in the prediction of Y, described earlier in this chapter, was an example of a moderator variable in the mediational process. There are other more complicated forms of these models. I describe one of these models here, the mediation baseline by treatment interaction model.

Baron and Kenny (1986) and later Morgan-Lopez and MacKinnon (2006) specified the mediated baseline by treatment interaction model as shown in Equations 10.18 through 10.20:

$$Y = i_1 + c_1 X + c_2 Z + c_3 XZ + e_1 \tag{10.18}$$

$$Y = i_2 + c_1' X + c_2' Z + c_3' XZ + bM + e_2 \tag{10.19}$$

$$M = i_3 + a_1 X + a_2 Z + a_3 XZ + e_3 \tag{10.20}$$

where the variables and coefficients are the same as in the moderation and mediation model described in Equations 10.14 through 10.16, but here the Z variable corresponds to a baseline measure of M or Y (or X if it does not represent groups). Baseline values for M and Y are usually considered moderator variables, because X often codes an experimental manipulation occurring after the baseline measurement. And baseline values for M ($M_{Baseline}$) are somewhat more common moderators than baseline values of Y ($Y_{Baseline}$). In Equation 10.18, the XZ interaction tests whether the relation between X and Y differs as a function of baseline status. Using the baseline measure of Y as the moderator, Equation 10.19 would correspond to the prediction of Y with X, the baseline measure of Y, and the interaction of the baseline measure of Y with X. The XZ interaction in Equation 10.19 tests whether the relation between Y at baseline and follow-up differs across levels of X. The interaction has the same meaning in Equation 10.14, except that the effect is adjusted for M. In this model, there are three mediated effects corresponding to the effect of X to M to Y, Z to M to Y, and XZ to M to Y. The mediated $Y_{Baseline}$ by treatment interaction suggests that the size of the mediated effect depends on level of the outcome at baseline. This model is often appropriate when the mediated effect is different for persons at different levels on the outcome.

The interpretation of the mediated baseline by treatment interaction is similar if the baseline measure of the mediator is used as the moderator rather than the baseline measure of Y. The substantive interpretation of the mediated effect is that mediation depends on the baseline measure of the mediating variable. These types of effects are often observed in treatment research because the participants who benefit the most from a treatment are often the persons who start out at the lowest level on the mediator.

It is possible to include baseline measures of both M and Y in the mediated baseline by treatment equations. In this model, there would be additional interactions in each equation, and it may be appropriate to include the three-way interaction among baseline measures of M and Y and the

X variable. As described earlier, it is important to interpret these interactions with plots and contrasts. Morgan-Lopez and MacKinnon (2006) conducted a simulation study and found that mediated effect standard errors in a mediation of a moderator effect model generally underestimated true standard errors when there were smaller correlations among predictors, smaller sample sizes (N < 100), and nonzero direct effects.

10.10 More Complicated Moderation and Mediation Models

There are several more complicated models that include both moderation and mediation. One interesting method was developed recently for data that are entirely within subjects, for which the value of the independent variable is not assigned to individual participants (Judd, Kenny, & McClelland, 2001). For a single X variable, two measures of the mediator, M_1 and M_2, and two measures of the outcome, Y_1 and Y_2, test whether the change in Y depends on the level of the X variable. Mediator effects include a test of whether differences in the mediator between conditions is in the same direction as the difference in Y and a test that M predicts Y.

Other recent approaches include combining the identification of groups of persons with models for mediation, known as mixture models that identify subgroups of participants who serve as moderators of mediation effects. Participants are grouped in terms of their trajectory of change over time or grouped based on other variables. Mediation effects are then investigated within these groups. Recent advances in computing (Muthén & Muthén, 2004) should increase the application of these types of models. These models are likely to prove especially useful in the evaluation of prevention programs as they will allow for the examination of mediation models across unobserved groups. However, other research has demonstrated that violation of the normality assumption can have substantial effects on the accuracy of the subgroup trajectories (Bauer & Curran, 2003). The development and application of these models is an active area of research.

One common concern when interaction effects are examined is the effect of measurement error on the test of the interaction effect. Measurement error reduces the power to detect interaction effects and can distort parameter estimates. New approaches allow for the estimation of interactions among latent variables or latent interaction effects (Klein & Moosbrugger, 2000). Measurement error is modeled in these methods, thereby providing more accurate tests of interaction effects. These new methods should help further clarify mediator and moderator effects. Recent work, however, also suggests that these methods may be susceptible to violation of normality, and there has not been extensive research supporting the use of these methods for models with more than one interaction (Marsh, Wen, & Hau, 2004; Wall & Amemiya, in press).

Developments in generalized additive models (Brown, 1993) may allow for more accurate modeling of interaction effects and mediation effects. In these models, the relation between two variables is not restricted to linear relations and can model local relations among variables, where relations among variables are fit for different sized windows or ranges of values. The mediated effect is estimated within these windows defined by one or more of the variables in the mediation model. There is some question about whether these methods capitalize on chance relations and consequently whether the models replicate.

10.11 Example

The example used for the demonstration of moderation and mediation models assumes that the data described in chapter 3 for the influence of temperature on water consumed were actually for a sample of normal persons. Table 10.1 presents fabricated data from another sample consisting of 50 persons classified as fit. These data will be initially analyzed separately and then will be added to the data in Table 3.1 for the 50 normal persons. Assume that 1 year before the research study, half of the 100 total persons were randomly assigned to receive a specialized training program to improve fitness and the other 50 persons were not given any specialized training, called the normal group in the following analysis. After 1 year, both the persons in the fit group and the normal group participated in the water consumption study described in chapter 3. There are several ways in which mediation may differ for fit and normal persons. First, fit persons may be more sensitive to body functions and may more accurately judge their own thirst in relation to temperature. This type of moderator effect would be consistent with a statistically significant difference in the $\hat{a}$ path relating temperature to perceived thirst. Second, less fit persons may be less likely to translate their feelings of thirst to actual water consumption, which is consistent with a statistically significant difference in the $\hat{b}$ coefficient. Finally, both processes may be present.

SAS programs for the single mediator model were used to conduct the analysis yielding the following estimates for Equations 10.11 through 10.13 for 50 persons in the fit group:

Model 1: $Y = i_1 + cX + e_1$
$$\hat{Y} = -18.0323 + .3004X$$
$$(.1766)$$

Table 10.1 Hypothetical Data for a Study of Temperature (X) Self-Reported Thirst (M), and Water Consumption (Y) for Fit Participants

S#	X	M	Y	S#	X	M	Y
1	69	2	3	26	71	5	4
2	70	2	4	27	73	5	3
3	69	1	2	28	68	1	3
4	70	3	2	29	70	4	4
5	69	1	1	30	70	5	4
6	70	2	3	31	69	4	3
7	69	4	3	32	70	5	4
8	70	2	3	33	70	5	5
9	70	3	2	34	70	2	3
10	69	3	2	35	71	5	5
11	69	4	2	36	70	3	5
12	71	3	5	37	70	4	3
13	71	4	1	38	69	2	2
14	71	4	3	39	71	4	4
15	69	3	4	40	70	5	3
16	70	2	2	41	70	2	3
17	70	3	3	42	70	3	4
18	71	2	2	43	71	4	3
19	70	3	3	44	69	2	1
20	71	3	2	45	71	5	4
21	69	2	4	46	71	3	4
22	71	5	1	47	71	4	4
23	69	1	2	48	71	4	5
24	70	2	1	49	70	3	3
25	70	3	2	50	71	4	3

Model 2: $Y = i_2 + c' X + bM + e_2$
$$\hat{Y} = -0.6095 + 0.0359X + 0.3475M$$
$$\qquad\qquad\ (0.2035)\quad\ (0.1490)$$

Model 3: $M = i_3 + aX + e_3$
$$\hat{M} = -50.1371 + 0.7611X$$
$$\qquad\qquad (0.1637)$$

For the fit participants, temperature (X) was not significantly related to water consumption (Y) ($\hat{c} = 0.3004$, $s_{\hat{c}} = 0.1766$, $t_{\hat{c}} = 1.70$) although the size of the $\hat{c}$ coefficient was comparable to the value for the normal group (0.3604). There was a statistically significant effect of temperature on self-reported thirst for fit participants ($\hat{a} = 0.7611$, $s_{\hat{a}} = 0.1637$, $t_{\hat{a}} = 4.65$), which was almost twice the size as that for normal participants (0.3386). The relation of the self-reported thirst mediator on water consumption was also statistically significant ($\hat{b} = 0.3475$, $s_{\hat{b}} = 0.1490$, $t_{\hat{b}} = 2.33$) when controlling for temperature. The adjusted effect of temperature on water consumption was not statistically significant, ($\hat{c}' = 0.0359$, $s_{\hat{c}'} = 0.2035$, $t_{\hat{c}'} = 0.18$). The estimate of the mediated effect for the fit group was equal to $\hat{a}\hat{b} = 0.2645$ with asymmetric lower confidence limit (LCL) = 0.0430 and upper confidence limit (UCL) = 0.5395. The mediated effect of temperature through perceived thirst was equal to .2645 deciliters of water consumed. Using Equation 3.6 or 3.7, the standard error of the mediated effect was equal to 0.1269, and the mediated effect was statistically significant ($z_{\hat{a}\hat{b}} = 2.0846$). Note that all of the preceding standard errors are from the 50 persons in the fit group.

10.12 Tests of Moderator and Mediator Effects

Because the two samples of participants are independent, one way to test for moderator effects is to conduct a t-test comparing the regression coefficients in the two models divided by their pooled standard error. For example, the test of homogenous $\hat{a}$ coefficients could be conducted with a t-test as shown in Equation 10.21 where subscript 1 refers to the normal sample and subscript 2 refers to the fit sample. The difference between the two $\hat{a}$ regression coefficients is statistically significant ($t_{\hat{a}1-\hat{a}2} = -2.08$, p $<$ .05) as shown in the formula following Equation 10.21. Analogous tests of the equality of the $\hat{c}'$ coefficients ($t_{\hat{c}'1-\hat{c}'2} = 0.71$, ns), $\hat{b}$ coefficients ($t_{\hat{b}1-\hat{b}2} = 0.50$, ns), and $\hat{c}$ coefficients ($t_{\hat{c}1-\hat{c}2} = 0.27$, ns) were not statistically significant, suggesting that only the relation from the temperature to self-reported thirst significantly differed between the two groups. The test of equal mediated effects using Equation 6.18 was also not statistically significant ($t_{\hat{a}_1\hat{b}_1-\hat{a}_2\hat{b}_2} = .7608$).

$$t_{\hat{a}1-\hat{a}2} = (\hat{a}_1 - \hat{a}_2) / \sqrt{s_{\hat{a}_1}^2 + s_{\hat{a}_2}^2}$$

$$(0.3386 - 0.7611) / SQRT(0.1224^2 + 0.1637^2) = -2.08$$ (10.21)

A more general way to test moderated mediation effects is by combining the two data sets for a total of 100 participants and specifying interaction terms that correspond to the different tests as shown in Equations 10.14 through 10.16. A numeric value for group, X, is also needed, so here X = −1 for not fit and X = 1 for fit. The estimates and standard errors (in parentheses) for these equations are shown in the following:

$$\hat{Y} = -20.0414 + 0.3304X + 2.0091Z - 0.0300XZ$$
$$\qquad\qquad (0.1104) \qquad (7.7445) \qquad (0.1104)$$

$$\hat{Y} = -6.6612 + 0.1218X + 6.0517Z - 0.0859XZ + 0.3993M - 0.05178MZ$$
$$\phantom{\hat{Y} = -6.6612 + } (0.1201) \quad (8.2713) \quad (0.1201) \quad\quad (0.1045) \quad (0.1045)$$

$$\hat{M} = -35.4198 + 0.5498X - 14.7173Z + 0.2113XZ$$
$$\phantom{\hat{M} = -35.4198 + } (0.1015) \quad\quad (7.1189) \quad\quad (0.1015)$$

The test of homogeneous $\hat{a}$ paths corresponds to the test of the XZ interaction in the prediction of M ($\hat{a}_3 = 0.2113$, $s_{\hat{a}_3} = 0.1015$, $t_{\hat{a}_3} = 2.08$) and gives the identical test of significance to the two-sample independent t-test. The sign of the coefficient is reversed, and the value of the interaction effect, 0.2113, is half as large as the difference between the two coefficients because the groups were coded as 1 for fit and –1 for normal groups. Similarly the test of homogenous $\hat{b}$ paths is given in the MZ interaction coefficient for the prediction of Y, equivalent $\hat{c}'$ paths in the XZ interaction coefficient in the prediction of Y, and homogeneous $\hat{c}$ paths in the XZ interaction coefficient in Equation 10.14. The t-test for each effect is identical whether the variable is an independent group t-test or a test of an interaction effect. The test of equal mediated effects is a bit more complicated in these equations because the value of the mediated effect depends on the values of other predictors in the equations. To calculate the mediated effect at the average of the moderator, a method analogous to tests for simple effects is needed (Tein, Sandler, MacKinnon, & Wolchik, 2004). For the case of a moderator with two groups, the simple mediated effects are tested for each group. With a continuous moderator, it is necessary to select values to test the mediated effect. As for interaction effects, it is often sensible to test effects at 1 standard deviation above and below the mean.

The procedure for plotting simple regression lines for the XZ interaction is simpler than that described earlier for the continuous Z example, because for a binary Z variable there are separate plots for each level of Z. In this case, the plot consists of two lines or one line for each level of the moderator. The regression equation for the significant moderator by X interaction on M is shown, followed by the rearrangement of terms to make computation of predicted means easier.

$$\hat{M} = -35.4198 + 0.5498X - 14.7173Z + 0.2113XZ$$

$$\hat{M} = (0.5498 + 0.2113Z)X - 14.7173Z - 35.4198$$

For the fit group (Z = 1), the mean of M at 1 standard deviation below the mean of X equals

$$\hat{M} = (0.5498 + 0.2113(1))(69.1085) - 14.7173(1) - 35.4198 = 2.4614$$

For the fit group, the mean of M at the mean of X equals

$$\hat{M} = (0.5498 + 0.2113(1))(70.1300) - 14.7173(1) - 35.4198 = 3.2388$$

For the fit group, the mean of M at 1 standard deviation above the mean of X equals

$$\hat{M} = (0.5498 + 0.2113(1))(71.1515) - 14.7173(1) - 35.4198 = 4.0163$$

For the normal group (Z = –1), the mean of M at 1 standard deviation below the mean of X equals

$$\hat{M} = (0.5498 + 0.2113(-1))(69.1085) - 14.7173(-1) - 35.4198 = 2.6907$$

For the normal group, the mean of M at the mean of X equals

$$\hat{M} = (0.5498 + 0.2113(-1))(70.1300) - 14.7173(-1) - 35.4198 = 3.0365$$

For the normal group, the mean of M at 1 standard deviation above the mean of X equals

$$\hat{M} = (0.5498 + 0.2113(-1))(71.1515) - 14.7173(-1) - 35.4198 = 3.3823$$

As shown in the plot of these data in Figure 10.3, the two lines are not parallel, consistent with an interaction effect. The test of significant simple slopes indicates whether the $\hat{a}$ coefficient is different in each group. The

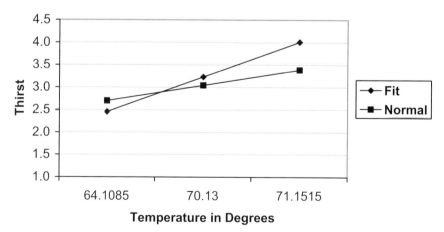

Figure 10.3. Simple effects of X to M for normal and fit groups.

test of simple slopes for the fit group is obtained by testing the regression coefficient relating X to M in that group. For this example, the simple slope is statistically significant in both the fit ($\hat{a}_1 = 0.7611$, $s_{\hat{a}_1} = 0.1637$, $t_{\hat{a}_1} = 4.65$) and normal ($\hat{a}_2 = 0.3386$, $s_{\hat{a}_2} = 0.1224$, $t_{\hat{a}_2} = 2.77$) groups. Setting the regression equation for fit group equal to the regression equation for the normal group and solving for X yields the point at which the two lines cross; for these data, the lines cross at X equal to 69.6679. It is possible to compute the regions of statistical significance for which the values of X correspond to significant differences on M using regions of significance procedures described in Huitema (1980). Regions of significance calculations are especially useful when lines do not cross, yet there is a statistically significant interaction (Preacher, Curran, & Bauer, 2006).

10.13 Summary

This chapter presents the basic statistical framework that can be used to estimate mediation models in the presence of moderator variables. There are several different types of potential moderator variables. For many situations, models with moderation and mediation require theoretical and empirical evidence for hypotheses. In the case of the XM interaction, the assumption that its value is zero should be routinely tested in mediation analysis. A statistically significant XM interaction will not negate findings of mediation but may in fact provide richer and more detailed information about an observed mediation effect. Hypotheses regarding moderation and mediation effects reflect a mature field of study that has progressed from initial work to detailed understanding of the mechanisms underlying relations that may differ across groups.

There are several limitations of models that combine moderation and mediation. All of the assumptions of the single mediator model outlined in chapter 3 apply. Several of these assumptions are more problematic for mediation models with moderators. First, as for the mediator case, it is assumed that measures have no, or negligible, error. Measurement error can seriously distort interaction effects. Results may not be as accurate with heterogeneous variances across levels of the moderator (Overton, 2001). Sufficient power to detect interaction effects often requires very large sample sizes or very large effect sizes (Aiken & West, 1991). The addition of moderators to mediator models also makes assumptions regarding true causal relations more complex, whereby some effects are only present at certain values of the moderator variable. Although richer understanding of the data is obtained with these models, the complexity of the model makes simple interpretations difficult. Nevertheless, models with mediators and moderators are important because they probably reflect the true complexity of relations among variables.

10.14 Exercises

10.1. Compare and contrast mediation, moderation, mediation of a moderator effect, and moderation of a mediated effect. Give examples of each type of effect.

10.2. A researcher wants to test whether the mediation effect differs for males and females. What methods would you recommend to her?

10.3. Do you think that moderation and mediation effects should be expected in your research area?

10.4. Assume that the data in this chapter and chapter 3 had an additional grouping variable. The first 25 observations in each data set were from participants who were told that their activities were all recorded and that their performance on the tasks they completed would be compared with that of all persons in the study. The last 25 observations were not given any instructions. Assume that participants were randomly assigned to conditions.

    a. Conduct a moderation and mediation analysis of these data.

    b. Does the mediation effect depend both on fitness and competition manipulation?

10.5. During the self-contained environment study, measures of work completed were obtained for the two groups. In general, the fit group participants completed twice as many tasks as the normal group participants. How would you interpret this effect in the context of the moderation and mediation effects?

11

Mediation in Categorical Data Analysis

> Above all else, we believe that the issue of when and how to use surrogate endpoints is probably the preeminent contemporary problem in clinical trials methodology, so it merits much extensive scrutiny.
>
> **—Colin Begg & Denis Leung, 2000, p. 27**

11.1 Overview

The purpose of this chapter is to describe methods to assess mediation when the dependent variable is categorical. First, logistic and probit regression, the appropriate regression methods for categorical dependent variables, are described. Second, the problems inherent in estimating mediation using logistic and probit regression are discussed. Two solutions for the problems involved in the estimation of mediation with categorical outcomes are proposed. A hypothetical example from the field of surrogate endpoints is used to illustrate the methods. Next, the multiple mediator model with categorical outcomes is presented.

11.2 Categorical Dependent Variables

Categorical outcome variables are common in many different types of studies. One of the outcomes in the Multiple Risk Factor Intervention Trial (MRFIT) was the presence or absence of coronary heart disease (Multiple Risk Factor Intervention Trial Research Group, 1990). Programs to prevent sexually transmitted diseases such as AIDS are designed to promote safer sex practices with binary outcome variables of reinfection or abstinence (Mays, Albee, & Schneider, 1989). Secondary prevention programs attempt to increase screening rates for serious illness with a binary outcome measure of whether the subject was screened for or not. Examples of binary outcome variables in psychology include clinical diagnosis, whether a subject littered or not, and whether a criminal was or was not recognized in a lineup.

An example of testing mediation with binary outcomes was described by Foshee et al. (1998). A program to prevent adolescent dating violence was hypothesized to prevent dating violence through the mediating variables of changing norms, decreasing gender stereotyping, improving conflict management, changing beliefs about the need for help, increasing awareness of services for victims and perpetrators, and increasing help-seeking behavior. The researchers compared the values of the logistic regression coefficient of treatment predicting outcome with and without controlling for the proposed mediators. The authors considered evidence of mediation to occur when the difference between the two values was attenuated by 20%. Given these criteria, results indicated that the treatment effect on sexual violence was mediated by changes in norms, gender stereotyping, and awareness of victim services. However, there are more accurate methods than proportion reduction to assess mediation, as described later.

Surrogate endpoint research is another area with categorical dependent variables. Surrogate endpoints are intervening or mediating variables that can be used instead of a dependent variable (Susser, 1973, 1991). In many areas of medical research, the length of time for a disease to occur and low incidence rates of the disease would require exorbitantly large sample sizes to study correlates of the disease. In this situation, researchers advocate the use of surrogate or intermediate endpoints (see special issue of *Statistics in Medicine*, Brookmeyer, 1989, and National Institutes of Health conference on surrogate endpoints, Henney, 1999). As described in chapter 2, surrogate endpoints are more frequent or more proximate to the prevention strategy and, as a result, are easier to study. Examples of surrogate endpoints are serum-cholesterol levels for the ultimate outcome of coronary heart disease and the presence of polyps for the ultimate outcome of colon cancer (Freedman & Schatzkin, 1992). The use of surrogate endpoints rests on the mediation assumption that the independent variable causes the surrogate endpoint that in turn causes the ultimate outcome. As a result, effects on the surrogate endpoints are important to the extent that the surrogate endpoint is causally related to the outcome.

Prentice (1989, p. 432) defined a surrogate endpoint as a "response variable for which a test of the null hypothesis of no relationship to the treatment groups under comparison is also a valid test of the corresponding null hypothesis based on the true endpoint." In an important article on identifying surrogate endpoints, Freedman, Graubard, and Schatzkin (1992) proposed the proportion mediated as a measure of a surrogate endpoint, where a value of 100% indicates that the surrogate endpoint explains all of the relation between the treatment and dependent variable. The proportion mediated measure includes the size of the surrogate endpoint effect as well as the amount of the treatment effect explained by the surrogate endpoint. The proportion mediated has been criticized, however, because proportion values are often very small and very large sample sizes are required for accurate confidence intervals.

In the situation in which the dependent variable is categorical, the estimation of the mediated effect is more complicated and requires logistic or probit regression because the categorical dependent variable violates several assumptions of ordinary regression analysis. The next section gives an overview of logistic and probit regression.

11.3 Introduction to Logistic and Probit Regression

Logistic regression is the most common method used to analyze data when the dependent variable is categorical (Hosmer & Lemeshow, 2000). Typically the dependent variable is binary or dichotomous, meaning it has two categories, although variables with ordinal categories can be easily incorporated in this analysis. The widespread application of logistic regression began after application for the analysis of binary dependent variables from the groundbreaking longitudinal study of cardiovascular disease conducted in Framingham, Massachusetts (Dawber, 1980).

To make regression work properly for a categorical dependent variable, the ordinary least squares regression model must be changed substantially. These changes are necessary because if ordinary regression procedures are used to analyze a binary categorical outcome variable, there are three major problems: (a) predicted values may be outside the possible range of possible values, for example, >1 or <0 for a variable coded as 0 or 1, (b) the residuals or errors from such a model will not be normally distributed, and (c) the standard errors of the estimates of the regression coefficients are inaccurate. Each of these problems with using ordinary least squares regression for binary outcome data is addressed in logistic regression. Once these changes have been made, logistic regression is similar to ordinary regression. These adjustments are made by the analysis of logits rather than the original binary dependent variable.

Logistic regression has become very popular in many fields for at least two reasons. First, logistic regression coefficients can be easily converted to odds ratios. Odds refers to the likelihood of one event relative to another event, for example, a horse has 2 to 1 odds of winning a horse race. The odds ratio is a ratio of odds; for example, horse A is two times more likely to win the race than horse B. The odds ratio is informative on a practical as well as a scientific level. Phrases such as "a person who smokes is two times more likely to die of coronary heart disease than a person who does not smoke" make intuitive sense. The logit is the natural logarithm of the odds ratio. The logit has several useful statistical properties that solve the problems with the analysis of a binary dependent variable. Second, logistic regression is more accurate than discriminant analysis, a method that is also used to analyze a binary dependent variable. The primary reason that logistic regression is preferable to discriminant analysis is a restrictive assumption of discriminant analysis. In discriminant analysis, it is assumed that for each level of the dependent variable, the independent variables have a multivariate normal distribution. But there are many predictor variables that are dichotomous or are not normally distributed, for example, gender and drug use, which will violate this assumption.

11.4 Logistic Regression Coefficients

Logistic regression coefficients are in the metric of the natural logarithm of the odds ratio, that is, the logit. To convert these coefficients to odds ratios compute $e^{\text{regression coefficient}}$ or the antilogarithm of the regression coefficient. For example, if the logistic regression estimate was equal to 0.34, then the odds ratio equals $e^{.34} = 1.4049$. If the logistic regression parameter was equal to 0.68, then the odds ratio equals 1.9739.

Table 11.1 presents the formulas for calculating the odds ratio and the variance of the logarithm of the odds ratio for data from a 2 × 2 table. Table 11.2 shows the data for a 2 × 2 table formed by a binary variable coding whether a subject was exposed to a smoking prevention program and a binary variable coding whether the subject smoked in the last month or not.

If group is coded 1 for program and 0 for control group, and cigarette use is coded 1 for use and 0 for no use, the logistic regression coefficient relating program exposure and smoking equals the logarithm of the odds ratio or –0.5057. If study participants received the program, they were 0.6 times less likely to smoke in the last month. The variance of the logarithm of the odds ratio equals 0.0316, so the standard error in logistic regression output is 0.1778. The coefficients of the logistic regression model can also be used to obtain predicted logits and predicted proportions as shown in Table 11.3.

Table 11.1   Frequencies and Formulas for the Odds Ratio and Its Standard Error

	Exposed		
	Yes	No	All
Cases	a	b	$a + b = N_1$
Controls	c	d	$c + d = N_0$
All	a + c	b + d	$a + b + c + d = N$

$$\frac{ad}{cb} = \frac{a/b}{c/d} = \text{odds ratio}; \quad \sigma^2_{\ln(\text{odds ratio})} = \frac{1}{a} + \frac{1}{b} + \frac{1}{c} + \frac{1}{d}$$

Table 11.2   Odds Ratio for the Relation Between Exposure to a Tobacco
Prevention Program and Smoking

	Smoked a Cigarette in the Last Month		
	Yes	No	All
Program	73	420	493
Control	83	288	371
All	156	708	864

$$\text{odds ratio} = \frac{73/420}{83/288} = 0.6031; \; \hat{\sigma}^2_{\ln(\text{odds ratio})} = \frac{1}{73} + \frac{1}{420} + \frac{1}{83} + \frac{1}{288} = 0.0316$$

$$e^{\ln(0.603) \pm 1.96\sqrt{.0316}} = e^{-0.8541, -0.1573} = 0.4257, 0.8544$$

The logistic regression equation is $\hat{Y} = -1.2441 - 0.5057\,X_1$. To get the predicted logit, insert values for X in the logistic regression equation. For the control group: $\hat{Y} = -1.2441 - 0.5057\,(X_1 = 0) = -1.2441$. For the program group: $\hat{Y} = -1.2441 - 0.5057\,(X_1 = 1) = -1.7498$. As shown in Table 11.3, these formulas are used to compute predicted proportions for each cell in the 2×2 table. These equations can be easily extended to the case of multiple independent variables.

11.5 Estimation

In Tables 11.1 and 11.2, logistic regression parameters were computed by hand using formulas for the regression coefficient, and standard error. These closed-form formulas are only available for the simplest

Table 11.3   Predicted Proportions and Predicted Logits

	Smoked	
	Yes	No
Program	0.1481	0.8519
Control	0.2237	0.7763

$$P = \frac{e^{Logit}}{1 + e^{Logit}} = \frac{e^{\beta_0 + \beta_1 X_1}}{1 + e^{\beta_0 + \beta_1 X_1}} = \frac{e^{-1.7498}}{1 + e^{-1.7498}} = \frac{0.1738}{1 + 0.1738} = 0.1481$$

$$P = \frac{e^{Logit}}{1 + e^{Logit}} = \frac{e^{-1.2441}}{1 + e^{-1.2441}} = \frac{0.2882}{1 + 0.2882} = 0.2237$$

logistic regression models. Often there are continuous predictors and more than one independent variable, making the estimation of parameters more complicated. In these more complicated situations, the parameters of the logistic regression model are estimated using an iterative procedure to determine the estimates that maximize the likelihood of observing the data. The purpose of the method is to find the value of the logistic regression estimates that maximizes the likelihood of observing the data that were actually observed.

The calculation of the odds ratio and standard error for the 2×2 table are shown here to explicitly show how the logistic regression model is a nonlinear model. In all of the logistic regression analyses described in this chapter, coefficients can be transformed in the same way from logit to odds to proportion. As described later the transformations to logits for statistical analysis and transformations to proportions and odds make standard approaches to mediation analysis inaccurate.

11.6 Probit Regression

Probit regression is very similar to logistic regression. In probit regression, the normal distribution rather than the logistic distribution is used. For example, rather than the logit of a proportion, the z-score corresponding to the cumulative proportion from the normal curve is the dependent variable. The predicted values in probit regression are the z-scores that correspond to the predicted proportion and are thus easily transformed to the proportion. The estimation of parameters follows an approach similar to that with logistic regression, and the conclusions from a probit regression analysis will be very similar, but not identical, to the conclusions from the logistic regression. In fact, the probit regression coefficients are approximately equal to 0.625 times the logistic regression coefficients (Amemiya, 1981). As will be seen later, there are several aspects of probit regression that make it preferable for mediation analysis. In particular, the mathematical tractability of the multivariate probit distribution makes it more widely used in advanced modeling of categorical variables using programs such as Mplus (Muthén & Muthén, 2004).

11.7 Mediation Analysis in Probit and Logistic Regression

As in the case of a continuous dependent variable, the mediated effect can be calculated in two ways when the dependent variable is categorical (MacKinnon, Warsi, & Dwyer, 1995). Both methods to calculate the mediated effect use information from the three equations described in chapter 3, but the notation has been changed in Equations 11.1, 11.2, and 11.3 to reflect the categorical dependent variable. Figure 11.1 displays the single mediator model with a categorical dependent variable.

$$Y^* = i_1 + cX + e_1 \tag{11.1}$$

$$Y^* = i_2 + c'X + bM + e_2 \tag{11.2}$$

$$M = i_3 + aX + e_3 \tag{11.3}$$

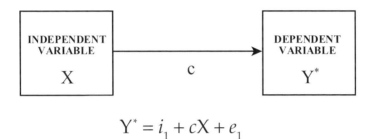

$$Y^* = i_1 + cX + e_1$$

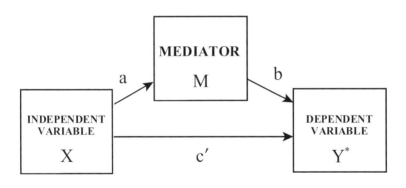

$$Y^* = i_2 + c'X + bM + e_2$$

$$M = i_3 + aX + e_3$$

Figure 11.1 Path diagram and equations for the mediation model.

The dependent variable, Y^*,

$$Y^* = \ln[P(Y_0 = 1)/(1 - P(Y_0 = 1))]$$

is the underlying latent continuous variable that is dichotomized into one of the categories of the outcome variable, where Y is the value of the outcome variable, either 0 or 1 for a binary dependent variable, X is the independent variable, and M is the mediator in the equations. The intercept and residual of each equation are i_i and e_i, respectively.

As described in chapter 3 for a continuous dependent variable, there are two methods to estimate the mediated effect in logistic or probit regression, the difference in the independent variable coefficients, $\hat{c} - \hat{c}'$, and the other based on the product of coefficients, $\hat{a}\hat{b}$. In logistic or probit regression, these values can be quite discrepant as will be shown later.

11.8 Standard Errors of the Mediated Effect in Logistic Regression

The standard error of $\hat{a}\hat{b}$ can be calculated using any of the standard error equations described in chapter 3 such as Equation 3.6. The standard error of $\hat{c} - \hat{c}'$ using formula 3.8 is more complicated because the covariance between $\hat{c}$ and $\hat{c}'$ for ordinary regression does not directly apply for logistic regression. Freedman et al. (1992) described a formula for the covariance between $\hat{c}$ and $\hat{c}'$, which is also described in Buyse and Molenberghs (1998). The steps required to compute the covariance between $\hat{c}$ and $\hat{c}'$ from logistic regression are presented in Table 11.4. The approach requires a matrix programming language such as SAS PROC IML.

When the dependent variable is continuous, and ordinary regression is used, the two methods for calculating the mediated effect are equivalent ($\hat{a}\hat{b} = \hat{c} - \hat{c}'$). This is not the case in logistic regression. The scale for the dependent variable, Y^*, in logistic regression equations is not directly observed. Unlike the error terms in ordinary linear regression with a continuous dependent variable, the residual variance in logistic regression is set to equal $\pi^2/3$ to fix the scale of the unobserved Y^* variable. In probit regression, the residual variance is fixed to 1. Because the residual variances are fixed in logistic and probit regression, the scale of the Y^* variable is not the same across models. Therefore, the $\hat{c} - \hat{c}'$ and $\hat{a}\hat{b}$ methods of estimating mediation are not equal and can be quite different.

A small simulation study conducted by MacKinnon and Dwyer (1993) compared the $\hat{c} - \hat{c}'$ and $\hat{a}\hat{b}$ estimates of the mediated effect in logistic and probit regression. The $\hat{c} - \hat{c}'$ estimates did not change even though the size of the mediated effect was increased and did not equal $\hat{a}\hat{b}$ for either logistic or probit regression for the effects studied. When the probit regression

Table 11.4   Steps to Compute Covariance of $\hat{c}$ and $\hat{c}'$

---

1. For each subject compute the predicted proportion, $\hat{p}$, using the model with just X. Remember that the predicted proportion is exp(equation)/(1 + exp(equation)).

2. For each subject compute the predicted proportion using the model with X and M.

3. Make a diagonal matrix from 1 with $\hat{p}(1 - \hat{p})$ along the diagonal. This is the V matrix.

4. Make a diagonal matrix from 2 with $\hat{p}(1 - \hat{p})$ along the diagonal. This is the Vs matrix.

5. Make X, which is the design matrix for the model with just X. It has a vector of 1s in the first column and the value of X in the second column. It is an $n \times 2$ matrix.

6. Make Xs, which is the design matrix for the model with X and M. It has a vector of 1s in the first column, the value of X in the second column, and the value of M in the third column. It is an $n \times 3$ matrix.

7. Compute the following matrix equation:

$$W = (X^{\mathrm{T}} V X)^{-1} X^{\mathrm{T}} V_s X_s (X^{\mathrm{T}} V X)^{-1}$$

where ^{T} indicates a transpose and $^{-1}$ is the inverse.

8. The element (2, 2) of the W matrix is the covariance between $\hat{c}$ and $\hat{c}'$ in logistic regression. The covariance is then included in formula 3.18 to compute the standard error of $\hat{c} - \hat{c}'$.

---

estimates were standardized using methods described later in this chapter, the $\hat{c} - \hat{c}'$ and $\hat{a}\hat{b}$ mediated effect estimates were approximately equal and increased as the population mediated effect increased. Standardization of logistic and probit regression coefficients is described in section 11.11.

Using true values based on a method described by Haggstrom (1983), MacKinnon, Lockwood, Brown, Wang, and Hoffman (in press) demonstrated the problems with the $c - c'$ method of testing mediation in probit and logistic regression. Figure 11.2 demonstrates how the ab method increases with increasing values of the mediated effect, but the $c - c'$ method flattens out and actually decreases, when, in fact, the mediated effect is increasing. The problem is present for probit regression for $c - c'$ versus ab as well. This occurs because the residual variance in logistic and probit regression is fixed so that the change in coefficients such as c and c' is due to fixing the residual variance across equations in addition to the change owing to adjusting for the mediator.

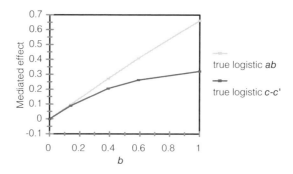

Figure 11.2

11.9 Solutions for the Problem with Mediation in Probit and Logistic Regression

One solution to different scales across logistic regression equations (Mac-Kinnon & Dwyer, 1993) is to make the scale equivalent across equations by standardizing regression coefficients before mediation is estimated (Winship & Mare, 1983). For example, in Equations 11.1 and 11.2, the variance of Y^* is equal to Equations 11.4 and 11.5, respectively, as described in Winship and Mare (1983):

$$\hat{\sigma}^2_{Y^*} = \hat{c}^2 \hat{\sigma}^2_X + \frac{\pi^2}{3} \tag{11.4}$$

$$\hat{\sigma}^2_{Y^*} = \hat{c}'^2 \hat{\sigma}^2_X + \hat{b}^2 \hat{\sigma}^2_M + 2\hat{c}'\hat{b}\hat{\sigma}_{XM} + \frac{\pi^2}{3} \tag{11.5}$$

Logistic regression estimates of $\hat{c}$ are divided by $\hat{\sigma}_{Y^*}$ from Equation 11.4, the estimates of $\hat{c}'$ and $\hat{b}$ are divided by $\hat{\sigma}_{Y^*}$ from Equation 11.5. Estimates of standard errors are similarly rescaled; that is, standard errors are divided by the square root of the variance of the equation. These standardized estimates are then used in the calculation of the mediated effect and its standard error. The mediated effect, $\hat{a}\hat{b}$, is then divided by its standard error and compared with a standard normal distribution to test for significance. Probit regression estimates are standardized in the same manner except that 1 replaces $\pi^2/3$ in Equations 11.4 and 11.5.

   As shown in Equation 11.6, another formula can be used to put the $\hat{c}$ coefficient in Equation 11.1 in the same metric as the $\hat{c}'$ coefficient in Equation 11.2. Coefficient $\hat{c}$ in Equation 11.1 is standardized by multiplying by the quantity in Equation 11.6, where $\hat{\sigma}^2_{\text{Equation 11.3}}$ is the residual variance in Equation 11.3, that is, the ordinary least squares regression of M predicted by X. This method of standardization preserves the original metric of the variables in Equation 11.2 and requires only standardizing coefficients from Equation 11.1.

$$\hat{c}_{corrected} = \hat{c}\sqrt{1 + \frac{\hat{b}^2 \hat{\sigma}^2_{Equation\ 11.3}}{\pi^2 / 3}} \tag{11.6}$$

Some researchers have assessed mediation by calculating the percentage drop between the unadjusted and adjusted coefficients, $(\hat{c} - \hat{c}')/\hat{c}$, and concluding that there is mediation if the drop is greater than a certain percentage. For example, Foshee et al. (1998) used a 20% reduction as evidence of mediation. In the continuous outcome case, however, the proportion mediated does not stabilize until a sample size of 500, making the use of this method to assess mediation questionable for small sample sizes (MacKinnon et al. 1995). Confidence limits for the proportion mediated, $1 - (c'/c)$, can be obtained using Fieller's theorem or the multivariate delta method. For Fieller's theorem the following equations are used to find the confidence limits (Herson, 1975);

$$A = \hat{c}\hat{c}' - z^2 s_{\hat{c}\hat{c}'} \tag{11.7}$$

$$B = \hat{c}^2 - z^2 s_{\hat{c}}^2 \tag{11.8}$$

$$C = \hat{c}'^2 - z^2 s_{\hat{c}'}^2 \tag{11.9}$$

$$\text{Upper confidence limit } (UCL) = 1 - \frac{A - \sqrt{A^2 - BC}}{B} \tag{11.10}$$

$$\text{Lower confidence limit } (LCL) = 1 - \frac{A + \sqrt{A^2 - BC}}{B} \tag{11.11}$$

The multivariate delta standard error for $1 - (\hat{c}'/\hat{c})$ is shown in Equation 11.12, which can be used to compute confidence limits using Equations 3.4 and 3.5. Other measures of the proportion mediated that are identical to $1 - (\hat{c}'/\hat{c})$ are $\hat{a}\hat{b}/\hat{c}$ and $\hat{a}\hat{b}/(\hat{c}' + \hat{a}\hat{b})$ in the ordinary least squares analysis but not logistic or probit analysis, in which these formulas may yield different values. The multivariate delta solution for the standard error of $\hat{a}\hat{b}/\hat{c}$ and $\hat{a}\hat{b}/(\hat{c}' + \hat{a}\hat{b})$ were shown in chapter 4:

$$\text{var}(1 - \hat{c}'/\hat{c}) = \frac{1}{\hat{c}^2} s_{\hat{c}'}^2 + (\frac{\hat{c}'}{\hat{c}^2})^2 s_{\hat{c}}^2 - 2\frac{\hat{c}'}{\hat{c}^3} s_{\hat{c}\hat{c}'} \tag{11.12}$$

11.10 Hypothetical Study of Pancreatic Cancer

To illustrate the mediation analysis of a binary dependent variable, a hypothetical data example is used. The data in Table 11.5 are from a hypothetical study of the relation between eating grilled meat and pancreatic cancer, which also included a mediating variable of blood fats. The data in Table 11.5 were simulated for an independent variable (X) that is the number of days eating grilled meat during a typical week, a mediator (M) that is the amount of fatty acids in the blood, and the binary dependent variable (Y) that is whether the person developed pancreatic cancer. The data, shown in Table 11.5, were simulated from a population with a very large mediated effect where $a = 0.2$, $b = 1.2$, and $c' = 0.6$.

SPSS and SAS Programs. The SAS statements and output, shown in Table 11.6, were used to obtain the logistic regression coefficient estimates used to compute the mediated effect and its standard error. For SPSS, the program and output are shown in Table 11.7. A new logistic regression statement is required for each regression equation. As a result, a researcher is more likely to have unequal numbers of subjects in the different regression models when SPSS is used. The researcher may want to remove cases that do not have measures of all three variables before estimating the regression models in SPSS. As shown in the output, all estimates are identical (within rounding) to those found in the SAS output.

Mediation Analysis for the Grilled Meat and Pancreatic Cancer Data. The regression estimates and standard errors (in parentheses) from the SAS or SPSS output for the three models are

Equation 11.1: $Y^* = i_1 + cX + e_1$

$$\hat{Y}^* = -3.9845 + 1.0065\, X$$

$$(0.1918)$$

Equation 11.2: $Y^* = i_2 + c'\, X + bM + e_2$

$$\hat{Y}^* = -11.0764 + 1.0499X + 1.7373M$$

$$(0.2287) \quad (0.2755)$$

Equation 11.3: $M = i_3 + aX + e_3$

$$\hat{M} = 3.1516 + 0.2149X$$

$$(0.0747)$$

Table 11.5 Hypothetical Data for a Study of Pancreatic Cancer
and Eating Grilled Meat

Obs	X	M	Y	Obs	X	M	Y
1	4	4	1	38	5	4	0
2	4	3	0	39	5	3	0
3	4	4	1	40	4	7	1
4	4	4	0	41	4	1	0
5	4	4	1	42	6	5	1
6	2	4	0	43	3	4	1
7	4	3	1	44	2	4	0
8	4	2	0	45	3	4	1
9	3	5	1	46	6	4	1
10	2	3	0	47	3	4	0
11	4	2	0	48	4	2	0
12	3	4	0	49	3	2	0
13	5	4	1	50	3	5	0
14	4	3	0	51	4	4	1
15	5	4	1	52	3	3	0
16	6	5	1	53	5	3	0
17	4	5	0	54	5	4	1
18	4	4	1	55	3	5	0
19	4	3	0	56	3	3	0
20	6	6	1	57	3	3	0
21	3	6	1	58	4	3	0
22	2	3	0	59	3	4	1
23	5	5	1	60	5	4	1
24	2	3	0	61	7	5	1
25	5	3	1	62	3	3	0
26	5	4	1	63	4	5	1
27	5	4	1	64	3	5	1
28	4	3	0	65	5	5	1
29	4	4	0	66	4	6	0
30	4	3	1	67	4	4	0
31	3	3	0	68	3	2	0
32	3	3	0	69	5	4	0
33	4	4	1	70	4	3	0
34	3	4	1	71	3	3	0
35	4	3	0	72	4	5	1
36	4	4	1	73	4	3	0
37	3	4	0	74	6	5	1

(continued)

Table 11.5 (Continued)

Obs	X	M	Y	Obs	X	M	Y
75	3	3	0	113	5	5	1
76	5	5	1	114	5	4	1
77	4	5	1	115	3	5	0
78	3	5	1	116	4	4	1
79	3	5	0	117	4	4	1
80	5	4	1	118	3	3	0
81	3	4	0	119	4	3	0
82	4	6	1	120	3	3	0
83	3	5	0	121	3	4	1
84	4	4	1	122	3	4	0
85	3	3	0	123	3	4	0
86	4	4	0	124	4	5	1
87	4	4	1	125	4	2	0
88	5	5	1	126	5	5	1
89	5	6	1	127	5	4	1
90	4	2	0	128	3	4	1
91	5	5	1	129	6	5	1
92	4	4	1	130	3	5	1
93	4	5	1	131	3	4	0
94	3	3	0	132	3	3	0
95	3	2	0	133	3	3	0
96	3	4	1	134	3	2	0
97	3	3	0	135	4	4	0
98	4	6	1	136	3	4	0
99	4	4	1	137	4	3	0
100	3	4	0	138	4	3	0
101	4	5	1	139	3	5	1
102	4	5	1	140	5	7	1
103	4	4	0	141	3	3	0
104	4	3	0	142	3	4	0
105	3	5	0	143	4	4	0
106	3	4	1	144	4	5	1
107	4	3	0	145	5	4	1
108	2	4	0	146	3	3	0
109	5	4	1	147	4	3	0
110	5	4	1	148	3	4	0
111	5	4	0	149	3	6	1
112	5	6	1	150	3	3	0

| | | | Table 11.5 (Continued) | | | |
Obs	X	M	Y	Obs	X	M	Y
151	4	5	1	176	4	5	1
152	5	4	0	177	4	5	1
153	4	3	0	178	3	3	0
154	3	4	1	179	5	4	0
155	4	5	1	180	3	4	0
156	3	4	0	181	4	4	1
157	5	6	1	182	4	4	0
158	3	3	0	183	3	5	0
159	4	4	1	184	4	4	0
160	5	4	0	185	4	5	0
161	3	3	0	186	5	5	1
162	3	4	0	187	4	2	0
163	5	3	0	188	5	4	1
164	4	4	1	189	1	5	1
165	3	3	0	190	4	4	1
166	3	4	1	191	4	5	1
167	5	3	0	192	4	3	0
168	3	5	0	193	2	4	0
169	3	4	0	194	6	3	1
170	5	4	1	195	5	4	1
171	4	6	1	196	3	4	0
172	3	3	0	197	4	5	1
173	5	3	0	198	4	3	1
174	5	3	0	199	4	5	1
175	4	5	1	200	3	5	1

Days eating grilled meat (X) was significantly related to pancreatic cancer (Y) ($\hat{c}$ = 1.0065, $s_{\hat{c}}$ = 0.1918, $t_{\hat{c}}$ = 5.2470, X^2 = 27.5314), providing evidence that there is a statistically significant relationship between the independent and the dependent variable. A 1-day increase in eating grilled meat is associated with an increase of 1.0065 in the logit of pancreatic cancer. There was a statistically significant effect of days eating grilled meat on levels of fatty acids ($\hat{a}$ = 0.2149, $s_{\hat{a}}$ = 0.0747, $t_{\hat{a}}$ = 2.8758). A 1-day increase in eating grilled meat was associated with change of 0.2149 in the blood measure of fat. The effect of the fat mediator on the logit of pancreatic cancer was statistically significant ($\hat{b}$ = 1.7373, $s_{\hat{b}}$ = 0.2755, $t_{\hat{b}}$ = 6.3053) even when controlling for days eating grilled meat. A 1 unit change in the blood measure of fat was associated with an increase of 1.7373 in the logit of pancreatic

Table 11.6   SAS Program and Output for Equations 11.1, 11.2, and 11.3

```
Proc logistic data=ex11.1 descending;
model Y=X ;
Proc logistic data=ex11.1 descending outest=covout;
model Y=X M ;
proc reg data=ex11.1;
model M=X;
```

Output for Equation 11.1

Analysis of Maximum Likelihood Estimate

Parameter	DF	Estimate	Std Error	Chi Square	Pr >ChiSq
Intercept	1	−3.9845	0.7549	27.8612	<0.0001
X	1	1.0065	0.1918	27.5314	<0.0001

Output for Equation 11.2

Analysis of Maximum Likelihood Estimate

Parameter	DF	Estimate	Std Error	Chi Square	Pr > ChiSq
Intercept	1	−11.0764	1.5653	50.0727	<0.0001
X	1	1.0499	0.2287	21.0674	<0.0001
M	1	1.7373	0.2755	39.7567	<0.0001

Output for Equation 11.3

Parameter Estimates

Variable	DF	Parameter Estimate	Std Error	t Value	Pr > |t|
Intercept	1	3.15163	0.29659	10.63	<0.0001
X	1	0.21488	0.07472	2.88	0.0045

cancer. The adjusted effect of days eating grilled meat on pancreatic cancer was statistically significant ($\hat{c}' = 1.0499$, $s_{\hat{c}'} = 0.2287$, $t_{\hat{c}'} = 4.5899$). Surprisingly, there was actually an increase in the value of $\hat{c}'$ ($\hat{c}' = 1.0499$) compared with $\hat{c}$ ($\hat{c} = 1.0065$), even though the data were generated from a population model with a very large mediation effect. This substantial discrepancy is the result of problems with estimating mediation using the $\hat{c} - \hat{c}'$ method.

The $\hat{a}\hat{b}$ estimate of the mediated effect, $(0.2149)(1.7373) = 0.3733$, is very different from $\hat{c} - \hat{c}' = 1.0065 - 1.0499 = -0.0434$. The reason for the large

Table 11.7 SPSS Program for Equations 11.1, 11.2, and 11.3

```
logistic regression variables = Y
  with X.
logistic regression variables = Y
  with X M.
regression
 /dependent=M
 /enter=X.
```

Output for Equation 11.1

Variables in the Equation

		B	S.E.	Wald	df	Sig.	Exp(B)
Step 1	X	1.007	0.192	27.531	1	0.000	2.736
	Constant	−3.985	0.755	27.861	1	0.000	0.019

a. Variable(s) entered on step 1: X.

Output for Equation 11.2

Variables in the Equation

		B	S.E.	Wald	df	Sig.	Exp(B)
Step 1	X	1.050	0.229	21.067	1	0.000	2.857
	M	1.737	0.276	39.757	1	0.000	5.682
	Constant	−11.076	1.565	50.073	1	0.000	0.000

a. Variable(s) entered on step 1: X, M.

Output for Equation 11.3

Coefficients

		Unstandardized Coefficients		Standardized Coefficients		
		B	Std. Error	Beta	t	Sig.
Model 1	(Constant)	3.152	0.297		10.626	0.000
	X	0.215	0.075	0.200	2.876	0.004

a. Dependent variable M

discrepancy is that the scaling of the $\hat{c}$ and $\hat{c}'$ coefficients differs across equations. To equate the scaling across equations, the standard errors and estimates must be scaled using formulas 11.4 and 11.5. Using Equation 3.6, the standard error of the mediated effect is equal to

$$0.1426 = \sqrt{(0.2149)^2(0.2755)^2 + (1.7373)^2(0.0747)^2}$$

As seen in the preceding example, when the regression coefficients and standard errors are small, it is very easy for rounding errors to affect the accuracy of the calculation of the standard error. Equation 3.7 gives the same answer, but it is less susceptible to computation errors because small numbers are not squared.

$$0.1426 = \frac{(0.2149)(1.7373)\sqrt{2.8758^2 + 6.3053^2}}{(2.8758)(6.3053)}$$

The 95% confidence limits for the mediated effect are equal to

$$\text{LCL} = 0.3733 - 1.96\,(0.1426) = 0.0938$$

$$\text{UCL} = 0.3733 + 1.96\,(0.1426) = 0.6529$$

The standard error of $\hat{c} - \hat{c}'$ in Equation 3.8 is equal to 0.1246 using the covariance between $\hat{c}$ and $\hat{c}'$ of 0.0368 based on the formulas described in Freedman et al. (1992):

$$0.1246 = \sqrt{0.1918^2 + 0.2287^2 - (2)(0.0368)}$$

The proportion mediated $1 - (\hat{c}'/\hat{c})$ equaled $1 - (1.0499/1.0065) = -0.0430$ with 95% confidence limits of -0.3122 and 0.2122 computed on the basis of Equations 11.7 through 11.11. The confidence limits based on the multivariate delta method were very similar and were equal to -0.2862 and 0.2001 for the lower and upper limits, respectively. The true percentage mediated for the population model was equal to $1 - (0.6/1.2) = 0.5$ which is not included in the confidence interval for $1 - (\hat{c}'/\hat{c})$. Again, the reason for the discrepancy is that the $\hat{c}$ and $\hat{c}'$ estimates are from models with a different scale. The proportion mediated measured by $\hat{a}\hat{b}/\hat{c}$ equaled 0.3709 and $\hat{a}\hat{b}/(\hat{c}' + \hat{a}\hat{b})$ equaled 0.2623 and are much closer to the true proportion mediated.

11.11 Standardizing Coefficients to Equate the Scale Across Logistic Regression Models

The first step in standardizing coefficients is to compute the variance of the dependent variable in logistic regression using Equations 11.4 and 11.5:

$$4.2001 = 1.0065^2 \, (0.8985) + \pi^2/3$$

$$8.1077 = 1.0499^2 \, (.8985) + 1.7373^2(1.0348) + 2(1.0499)(1.7373)(.1931) + \pi^2/3$$

The square roots of the variance for logistic regression Equations 11.1 and 11.2 were 2.0494 and 2.8474, respectively. As a result, the standardized logistic regression estimates were $\hat{c} = 0.4911$, $s_c = 0.0936$, $\hat{c}' = 0.3687$, $s_{\hat{c}'} = 0.0803$, $\hat{b} = 0.6101$, and $s_{\hat{b}} = 0.0968$. The estimates of the mediated effect are more similar for standardized logistic regression coefficients: $\hat{c} - \hat{c}' = 0.4911 - 0.3687 = 0.1224$ and $\hat{a}\hat{b} = 0.2149(0.6101) = 0.1311$. The standard error of the $\hat{a}\hat{b}$ estimate is 0.0506 with UCL = 0.1311 + 1.96(.0506) = 0.2303 and LCL = 0.1311 − 1.96(0.0506) = 0.0319. The proportion mediated measures were also very similar: $1 - \hat{c}'/\hat{c} = 0.2492$, $\hat{a}\hat{b}/\hat{c} = 0.2670$, and $\hat{a}\hat{b}/(\hat{c}' + \hat{a}\hat{b}) = 0.2623$. Note that the $\hat{a}\hat{b}/(\hat{c}' + \hat{a}\hat{b})$ measure is identical to the measure with unstandardized coefficients because the coefficients in the numerator, $\hat{b}$, are standardized by the same values as the coefficients in the denominator, $\hat{b}$ and $\hat{c}'$.

The second method is to put $\hat{c}$ and $\hat{c}'$ in the same metric using Equation 11.6:

$$\hat{c}_{corrected} = 1.0065\sqrt{1 + \frac{1.7373^2(0.998)}{\pi^2/3}} = 1.3931$$

Now the difference between $\hat{c}_{corrected}$ and $\hat{c}'$ equals 1.3931 − 1.0499 = 0.3442 for a difference in odds ratios of 4.03 and 2.86 and is now comparable to the $\hat{a}\hat{b}$ estimate of 0.3733.

11.12 Mediation Analysis in Probit Regression

As shown in Table 11.8, the conclusions from probit analysis are the same as those for logistic regression analysis. Nevertheless, the results for probit regression are presented because there is evidence that probit regression is more accurate for mediation with a categorical outcome. One limitation of probit regression is that the estimates do not have as clear an interpretation as the odds ratio from logistic regression. Another name for probit regression is normit regression, so the command to conduct probit regression requests the normit link function in PROC LOGISTIC. Probit regression is easily conducted in SAS with the following statements on the model line: Model Y=X/link=normit and Model Y=X M/ link=normit. Note that even though the output will say that the "LOGISTIC Procedure" is being used, the link function is included in the program to indicate that normit or probit regression is conducted in the program output, "Link Function Normit."

The probit regression estimates and standard errors (in parentheses) from the SAS output for the two probit regression models are shown in the following. The results for Equation 11.3 are not shown again as they are from ordinary least squares regression analysis.

Equation 11.1: $Y^* = i_1 + c\,X + e_1$
$$\hat{Y}^* = -2.3782 + 0.6012X$$
$$(0.1102)$$

Equation 11.2: $Y^* = i_2 + c'\,X + bM + e_2$
$$\hat{Y}^* = -6.5168 + 0.6252X + 1.0117M$$
$$(0.1296)\quad(0.1485)$$

Days eating grilled meat (X) was significantly related to pancreatic cancer (Y) ($\hat{c} = 0.6012$, $s_{\hat{c}} = 0.1102$, $z_{\hat{c}} = 5.4533$), providing evidence that there is

Table 11.8   SAS Probit Regression With Output for Equations 11.1 and 11.2

Output for Equation 11.1

The LOGISTIC Procedure

Analysis of Maximum Likelihood Estimate

Parameter	DF	Estimate	Standard Error	Chi Square	Pr > ChiSq
Intercept	1	−2.3782	0.4346	29.9492	<0.0001
X	1	0.6012	0.1102	29.7387	<0.0001

Output for Equation 11.2

Analysis of Maximum Likelihood Estimate

Parameter	DF	Estimate	Standard Error	Chi Square	Pr > ChiSq
Intercept	1	−6.5198	0.8346	60.9668	<0.0001
X	1	0.6252	0.1296	23.2887	<0.0001
M	1	1.0117	0.1485	46.3989	<0.0001

a statistically significant relationship between the independent and the dependent variable. A 1-day increase in eating grilled meat is associated with an increase of 0.6012 in the z-score relating eating grilled meat to pancreatic cancer. The effect of the fat mediator on the probit of pancreatic cancer was statistically significant ($\hat{b} = 1.0117$, $s_{\hat{b}} = 0.1485$, $z_{\hat{b}} = 6.8117$), when controlling for days eating grilled meat. A 1 unit change in the blood measure of fat was associated with an increase of 0.6252 in the z-score of pancreatic cancer. The adjusted effect of days eating grilled meat was statistically significant, ($\hat{c} = 0.6252$, $s_{\hat{c}} = 0.1296$, $z_{\hat{c}} = 4.8258$). As in logistic regression, there was an increase in the value of $\hat{c}'$ ($\hat{c}' = 0.6252$) compared with $\hat{c}$ ($\hat{c} = 0.6012$), even though the data were generated from a population model with a very large mediation effect.

The $\hat{a}\hat{b}$ estimate of the mediated effect is equal to $(0.2149)(1.0117) = 0.2174$ which is very different from $\hat{c} - \hat{c}' = 0.6012 - 0.6252 = -0.0240$. The reason for the large discrepancy is that the scaling of the c and c' coefficients differs across equations, and if the scale is not made consistent across the equations, then the two methods to assess mediation will not be equal. The standard error of the $\hat{a}\hat{b}$ mediated effect was equal to 0.0828. The proportion mediated measure, $1 - (\hat{c}'/\hat{c}) = -0.0400$, differed from the other proportion measures, $\hat{a}\hat{b}/\hat{c} = 0.3616$ and $\hat{a}\hat{b}/(\hat{c}' + \hat{a}\hat{b}) = 0.2580$.

The 95% confidence limits for the mediated effect are equal to:

$$LCL = 0.2149 - 1.96 \, (0.0828) = 0.0526$$

$$UCL = 0.2149 + 1.96 \, (0.0828) = 0.3772$$

The first step in standardizing coefficients is to compute the variance of the dependent variable in probit regression. The probit estimates for the standard deviation using Equations 11.4 and 11.5 are equal to 1.1510 and 1.6293, respectively, with the following standardized estimates for probit regression, $\hat{c} = 0.5223$, $s_{\hat{c}} = 0.0958$, $\hat{c}' = 0.3837$, $s_{\hat{c}'} = 0.0795$, $\hat{b} = 0.6210$, $s_{\hat{b}} = 0.0912$. The difference and product estimates of the mediated effect are now very close, $\hat{c} - \hat{c}' = 0.1386$ and $\hat{a}\hat{b} = 0.1334$. The standard error of $\hat{a}\hat{b}$ equals 0.0508. The three measures of the proportion mediated are now also quite similar as well, $1 - (\hat{c}'/\hat{c}) = 0.2653$, $\hat{a}\hat{b}/\hat{c} = 0.2555$, and $\hat{a}\hat{b}/(\hat{c}' + \hat{a}\hat{b}) = 0.2580$.

11.13 Multiple Mediator Models

Models for continuous variables outlined in earlier chapters can also be evaluated when the dependent variable is categorical. As shown in the following, for the case of multiple mediators, Equations 11.2 and 11.3 may be modified to include more mediators as was done for the continuous

Table 11.9   Mplus Program and Output for Data in Table 11.5

TITLE: Example 11.10 Binary Dependent Variable
DATA:
FILE IS "e:\chapter 11 Cat. med\ex111";
 VARIABLE:
  NAMES ARE id x m y ;
  USEVARIABLES ARE x m y;
  CATEGORICAL Y;
 ANALYSIS:
  TYPE IS general;
  ESTIMATOR IS WLSMV ;
  ITERATIONS = 1000;
  CONVERGENCE = 0.00005;
 MODEL:
 Y ON X M;
 M ON X;
 OUTPUT: STANDARDIZED;

MPLUS Output
Example 11.1 Binary Dependent Variable
MODEL RESULTS

Example 11.1 Binary Dependent Variable

		Estimates	S.E.	Est./S.E.	Std	StdYX
Y	ON					
X		0.448	0.083	5.385	0.448	0.369
M		0.713	0.070	10.140	0.713	0.629
M	ON					
X		0.215	0.082	2.615	0.215	0.201

Residual Variances

	Estimates	S.E.	Est./S.E.	Std	StdYX
M	0.988	0.096	10.291	0.988	0.960

R-SQUARE

Observed Variable	Residual Variance	R-Square
M	0.040	
Y	0.497	0.624

dependent variable case in chapter 4. The equations for the four mediator model are

$$Y^* = i_1 + cX + e_1 \tag{11.13}$$

$$Y^* = i_2 + c'X + b_1M_1 + b_2M_2 + b_3M_3 + b_4M_4 + e_2 \tag{11.14}$$

$$M_1 = i_3 + a_1X + e_3 \tag{11.15}$$

$$M_2 = i_4 + a_2X + e_4 \tag{11.16}$$

$$M_3 = i_5 + a_3X + e_5 \tag{11.17}$$

$$M_4 = i_6 + a_4X + e_6 \tag{11.18}$$

The same mediation analysis steps for the single categorical dependent variable are followed for multiple mediators. As described in chapter 6, there are now four mediated effects, one transmitted through each of the four mediators. The total mediated effect can be calculated in the same way as that described in chapter 6, that is, $\hat{a}_1\hat{b}_1 + \hat{a}_2\hat{b}_2 + \hat{a}_3\hat{b}_3 + \hat{a}_4\hat{b}_4$, which is not equal to $\hat{c} - \hat{c}'$ for the same reasons that the two total mediated effect measures are not equal using logistic regression for the single mediator model. Standardizing coefficients and standard errors can be used to appropriately model the different scales across the two logistic regression Equations 11.4 and 11.5 (or Equation 11.6). The matrix routine to calculate the covariance between $\hat{c}$ and $\hat{c}'$ is accurate for this situation as well.

Mplus, SAS, and SPSS programs are easily expanded for the multiple mediator case by adding additional predictors in the equation relating X and the mediators to the binary dependent variable, and additional regression statements are needed to estimate the parameters for each mediator.

11.14 Mediator Models With Combinations of Categorical and Continuous Variables

With more than two categorical dependent variables, the parameters of the model must be estimated with more complicated iterative approaches such as the Mplus covariance structure analysis. These models are based on the multivariate probit distribution. Because the models are standardized as part of the analysis, these models solve the scaling problem for the different types of mediated effects. This approach uses probit regression to estimate thresholds for categorical variables. These thresholds are then included in the estimation of a model that can be used for a large number of models. The Mplus program in Table 11.9 is used to analyze the data in

Table 11.5. The Y variable is specified as categorical. Even though Mplus uses probit regression, the results are not the same as described earlier because a weighted least squares estimation procedure is used to estimate parameters. However if Mplus uses the ESTIMATOR IS ML, then the same results as with SAS and SPSS are obtained.

Days eating grilled meat (X) was associated with fatty acids ($\hat{a} = 0.215$, $s_{\hat{a}} = 0.082$, $t_{\hat{a}} = 2.615$). A 1 day a week increase in eating grilled meat was associated with a change of 0.21 in the blood measure of fat. The effect of the fat mediator on the probit of pancreatic cancer was statistically significant ($\hat{b} = 0.713$, $s_{\hat{b}} = 0.070$, $t_{\hat{b}} = 10.140$) even when controlling for days eating grilled meat, providing evidence for Step 3. A 1 unit change in the blood measure of fat was associated with an increase of 0.713 in the probit of pancreatic cancer. The adjusted effect of days eating grilled meat on pancreatic cancer was statistically significant, ($\hat{c}' = 0.448$, $s_{\hat{c}'} = 0.083$, $t_{\hat{c}'} = 5.385$). The estimate of the mediated effect is $\hat{a}\hat{b} = (0.215)(0.713) = 0.1533$ with a standard error of 0.0604 and UCL = 0.2717 and LCL = 0.0349.

Mplus has two types of standardized variables, one based on standardizing the dependent variable, Std and the other based on standardizing both the X and the Y variable, StdYX. Using the coefficients standardized on the basis of the X and Y variable, $\hat{a} = 0.201$, $s_{\hat{a}} = 0.0717$, $t_{\hat{a}} = 2.615$, and $\hat{b} = 0.629$, $s_{\hat{b}} = 0.0618$, $t_{\hat{b}} = 10.140$. The estimate of the mediated effect is then 0.1264 with a standard error of 0.0468, which gives UCL = 0.2181 and LCL = 0.0347. As described in the next section, the INDIRECT command can be used to compute the indirect effects and standard errors using Mplus.

Even though Mplus conducts probit regression, the estimation procedure leads to different results. In fact, the Mplus program does not estimate the univariate probit regression model. The probit is used to model the relationship between the observed categorical variable and the latent normally distributed variable. The entire model is then estimated using the probit as the threshold value. Mplus applies this same approach to estimate more complicated models for any number of latent variables as well as measured variables.

11.15 Mediator Models for Other Categorical Variables

There are other possible combinations of categorical variables in mediation analysis. For example, the mediator may be a categorical variable. For instance, assume that marital quality predicts a binary variable of whether the couple divorces or not, which is then related to a continuous measure of children's symptomatology. In this case, Equation 11.3 is estimated using logistic or probit regression, and the other equations are estimated using ordinary regression. Thus, the $\hat{c} - \hat{c}'$ and $\hat{a}\hat{b}$ methods of estimating mediation will not be equal, but both methods should provide similar conclusions about the significance of the mediated effect.

Another prominent model with a categorical outcome is survival analysis. For example, in the evaluation of a smoking cessation program, researchers may be interested in the mediators of time until relapse in addition to whether a client relapses or not. These types of models share the same type of problems outlined in this chapter for logistic regression. More on mediation in survival analysis is described in Tein and MacKinnon (2003).

11.16 Summary

The purpose of this chapter was to describe important issues in the estimation of mediated effects for categorical data dependent variables. Methods to assess mediation based on the difference in coefficients $\hat{c} - \hat{c}'$ method or the $1 - (\hat{c}'/\hat{c})$ measure of the proportion mediated are incorrect unless model parameters are standardized. Methods based on the product measure of mediation, $\hat{a}\hat{b}$, are more accurate and are not susceptible to the scaling problem as only the $\hat{b}$ coefficient is from a logistic regression analysis.

11.17 Exercises

11.1. Why is the estimate $\hat{c} - \hat{c}'$ not equal to $\hat{a}\hat{b}$ in logistic and probit regression? Use Example 11.10 to illustrate how these two quantities are not equal.

11.2. In the pancreatic cancer example, what are the odds ratios and confidence limits for each of the logistic regression coefficients? Interpret these values.

11.3. Imagine a study like the one described in the chapter in which the amount of grilled meat a person eats in a typical week is the independent variable on a scale of 0, 1, 2, and 3, a mediator is the amount of fatty acids in the blood coded 1, 2, 3, or 4, and the dependent variable is whether the person developed pancreatic cancer. The frequency of subjects in each of the possible categories is given by the FREQ variable. Using the steps in section 11.4, the covariance between $\hat{c}$ and $\hat{c}'$ was found to be 0.0125.

Hypothetical data for a replication study of pancreatic cancer and eating grilled meat.

```
data pancreas;
input X M Y freq;
cards;
0 1 1 26
1 1 1 1
```

```
  2 1 1 1
  3 1 1 2
  0 2 1 12
  1 2 1 1
  2 2 1 3
  3 2 1 3
  0 3 1 4
  1 3 1 2
  2 3 1 5
  3 3 1 5
  0 4 1 1
  1 4 1 8
  2 4 1 10
  3 4 1 12
  0 1 0 42
  1 1 0 8
  2 1 0 12
  3 1 0 9
  0 2 0 25
  1 2 0 3
  2 2 0 4
  3 2 0 4
  0 3 0 8
  1 3 0 2
  2 3 0 2
  3 3 0 1
  0 4 0 10
  1 4 0 1
  2 4 0 1
  3 4 0 6
  ;
  Proc logistic data=pancreas descending
  outest=covout; weight freq;
  model Y=X ;
  Proc logistic data=pancreas descending
  outest=covout; weight freq;
  model Y=X M ;
  proc reg data=pancreas; weight freq;
  model M=X;
```

The output from SAS is shown. These are the numbers that can be used in the calculation of the mediated effect and its standard error.

Output for Equation 11.1

Analysis of Maximum Likelihood Estimate

Parameter	DF	Estimate	Std Error	Chi Square	Pr > ChiSq
Intercept	1	-0.6409	0.1768	13.1317	0.0003
X	1	0.2771	0.1118	6.1435	0.0132

SAS Output for Equation 11.2

Analysis of Maximum Likelihood Estimate

Parameter	DF	Estimate	Std Error	Chi Square	Pr > ChiSq
Intercept	1	-1.4507	0.2955	24.1005	<0.0001
X	1	0.1390	0.1213	1.3127	0.2519
M	1	0.4406	0.1244	12.5376	0.0004

SAS Output for Equation 11.3

Root MSE	1.10853	R-Square	0.1177
Dependent Mean	2.11111	Adj R-Sq	0.1139
Coeff Var	52.50910		

Parameter Estimates

Variable	DF	Parameter Estimate	Std Error	t Value	Pr > |t|	Corr Type I
Intercept	1	1.78228	0.09352	19.06	<0.0001	
X	1	0.33748	0.06067	5.56	<0.0001	0.11768

a. Write the three equations with coefficients and standard errors based on the SAS output.
b. Compute the two estimates of the mediated effect.
c. Compute the standard errors and confidence limits for the two estimates of the mediated effect. Do the mediated effect estimates differ?
d. Compute the proportion mediated and its confidence limits.
e. Compute the two mediated effect estimates with one of the two methods to standardized coefficients.

11.4. Write an Mplus program to analyze the data in 11.3. How does the estimate of the mediated effect and its confidence interval compare to the values in your answer to 11.3?

12

Computer Intensive Methods for Mediation Analysis

In recent years tests using the physical act of randomisation to supply (on the Null Hypothesis) a frequency distribution, have been largely advocated under the name of "Non-parametric" tests. Somewhat extravagant claims have often been made on their behalf. The example of this Section, published in 1935, was by many years the first of its class. The reader will realise that it was in no sense put forward to supersede the common and expeditious tests based on the Gaussian theory of errors. The utility of such nonparametric tests consists in their being able to supply confirmation whenever, rightly or, more often, wrongly, it is suspected that the simpler tests have been appreciably injured by departures from normality.

They assume less knowledge, or more ignorance, of the experimental material than do the standard tests, and this has been an attraction to some mathematicians who often discuss experimentation without personal knowledge of the material. In inductive logic, however, an erroneous assumption of ignorance is not innocuous: it often leads to manifest absurdities. Experimenters should remember that they and their colleagues usually know more about the kind of material they are dealing with than do the authors of text-books written without such personal experience, and that a more complex, or less intelligible, test is not likely to serve their purpose better, in any sense, than those of proved value in their own subject

—Ronald Aylmer Fisher, 1960, pp. 48–49

12.1 Overview

The purpose of this chapter is to describe computer-intensive methods to estimate mediated effects, construct confidence limits, and conduct significance tests. In general, these computer-intensive methods use the observed data to determine the significance of an effect and do not make as many assumptions about underlying distributions as methods described earlier in this book (Manly, 1997; Mooney & Duval, 1993; Noreen, 1989). There has been enormous growth in the application of computer-intensive methods during the last 30 years, primarily because of improvements in computing power. Computer-intensive methods are often the method of choice when exact formulas for statistical quantities are not available or are too complicated, when unknown distributions or outlier observations may bias results, or when sample size is small. First, different computer-intensive methods are described and applied to the case of mediation analysis. Second, each method is illustrated with data from chapter 3 and software to conduct these tests is described. Strengths and limitations of the methods are discussed.

12.2 Single Sample and Resampling Methods

Each of the methods described so far in this book is based on a single sample. Formulas for the point estimator of the mediated effect and its standard error were described that can be used to test the significance of a mediated effect and construct confidence intervals for the effect in the population based on data from the single sample. One assumption of this approach is that the population distribution underlying both the point and standard error estimates of the mediated effect is normal. As discussed in chapter 4, there is reason to believe that the mediated effect is not distributed normally. Similarly, outliers and other types of non-normal data may make tests based on normal theory assumptions invalid.

Several computer-intensive statistical methods have been developed that are more accurate than traditional methods in many situations including situations in which the data are not normally distributed. These methods use repeated samples from the original sample to conduct analyses. The repeated samples from the original data are used to form an empirical version of a sampling distribution of a statistic (Efron & Tibshirani, 1993; Manly, 1997; Mooney & Duval, 1993; Noreen, 1989). The empirical distribution of the statistic formed by repeated sampling from the original data is used to determine the significance of the effect and to construct confidence intervals. The bootstrap (Efron & Tibshirani, 1993), permutation (Edgington, 1995), randomization (Edgington, 1995), and jackknife (Mosteller &

Tukey, 1977) are examples of computer-intensive tests. Because most computer-intensive tests entail repeated sampling from the observed data, they are also called resampling methods. The methods differ in how the resampling is accomplished, but each method consists of taking repeated samples from the original sample to create a new sampling distribution to which the results from the observed sample are compared.

Resampling methods show considerable promise for the estimation of mediated effects. Bollen and Stine (1990) and Lockwood and MacKinnon (1998) applied the bootstrap method to examine the confidence intervals of mediated effects. In general, confidence limits constructed using the bootstrap were asymmetric, consistent with the asymmetric distribution of the mediated effect. Shrout and Bolger (2002) recently suggested that the bootstrap methods should be used instead of the single sample methods because the distribution of the mediated effect is unknown. MacKinnon, Lockwood, and Williams (2004) compared a large number of single sample and resampling methods to assess the mediated effect and found several bootstrap methods had more accurate confidence limits than the single sample methods. Several other resampling methods did not differ substantially from the single sample methods. The material in this chapter provides an overview of current applications of computer intensive methods for mediation analysis.

12.3 Permutation Test for Mean Differences

Although computer-intensive tests appear to be a modern method, these methods were originally discussed much earlier by R. A. Fisher, one of the most well-known developers of statistical methods. Fisher outlined a resampling method known as the permutation test, which is now also called the exact randomization test. When the F (named the F-test by Snedecor to honor R. A. Fisher) and t-tests were first proposed, one of the criticisms was the rather stringent assumptions required for the methods. For example, normally distributed data and independent observations were assumptions of the t-test for the difference between two groups. Critics argued that these assumptions were rarely met, and data that departed from the normal distribution would make the methods inaccurate. To address this criticism, Fisher and others (Eden & Yates, 1933; Pitman, 1937) used a permutation test to evaluate the accuracy of the t-test.

The data for Fisher's permutation test example were from a study of the effects of self- versus cross-fertilization on the height of plants (Darwin, 1876). For each of 15 matched pairs of plants, one plant was self-fertilized and the other plant was cross-fertilized. Fisher used a permutation test to determine the accuracy of the t-test comparing the height of self- versus cross-fertilized plants. The permutation test compares the difference in mean height for the observed data to all data sets that could have occurred. "All data sets" refers to all of the unique data sets that can be made by rearranging the observed data; for example, one permuted data set would consist of switching the height of the self-fertilized plant in the first pair with that of the cross-fertilized plant in the second pair. For 15 pairs of plants, there were a total of $2^{15} = 32{,}768$ possible data sets. Fisher found that 863 of these 32,768 permuted data sets had a group difference equal to or larger than the observed difference for an exact one-tailed probability of 0.02634 (863/32,768) compared with 0.02485 from the ordinary t-test (and 0.02529 with a slight correction to the t-statistic, see, Fisher, 1960, Table 5, p. 48). His conclusion was that the use of the t-test was justified because the significance level was so close to the results of the permutation test. The permutation test was used as the true test to verify the traditional test.

In general, Fisher did not promote the use of these exact randomization tests because traditional methods were expeditious (see quote at the beginning of this chapter) and presumably because of the large number of computations necessary to conduct such an analysis in the pre-computer era (Ludbrook & Dudley, 1998). He used the permutation test as a way to demonstrate the accuracy of parametric methods. Interestingly, the t-test, F-test, and related methods are sometimes called classic methods and the resampling approaches are called modern methods, yet it appears that the two approaches appeared at similar times. Here I refer to the classic tests as traditional tests to avoid the ambiguity of when these tests were developed. I call them traditional tests because these statistical tests reflect the most widely used statistical methods.

For a two-group matched pair design, the permutation test proceeds as follows: (a) Compute the difference between means in the two groups for the original data. (b) Make all possible data sets by rearranging observed data and compute the difference between the means in each group for each of the possible data sets. The number of these data sets can be very large if there are a lot of subjects. For example, for the two-group matched-pairs design with 15 plants in each group, there are a total of 32,768 different data sets. (c) Tabulate all the possible values of the mean difference between groups for all the data sets. (d) Compare the observed difference between groups with the entire distribution of possible differences. The proportion of differences as big as or bigger than the observed difference is the exact probability or significance level. The exact probability is then compared with a specified significance level such as 0.05. If the probability from the empirical distribution is smaller than the significance level, then the difference would be considered statistically significant. Note that if it is a two-tailed test, then the test uses the distribution of the absolute value of the differences in means to determine the significance level.

12.4 Permutation Test for the Correlation Coefficient

The permutation test for a correlation follows the same logic as for the difference between the mean in two groups. The observed value of the correlation between two variables is compared with the entire distribution of possible correlations in the N! (factorial) possible data sets. With N = 2 there are 2! = 2 data sets. For N = 3, there are 6, and for N = 4, there are 24 data sets. The number of possible data sets gets very large very quickly; for example, for N = 10 there are 3,628,800 different possible data sets and, as a result, 3,628,800 correlations must be computed for the permutation test.

The data in Table 12.1 are the number of cases of malaria per 1,000 persons during the building of the Panama Canal during 1906, 1909, and 1912 (Gorgas, 1915, p. 275). These data are used to illustrate a permutation test for N = 3 and 3! = 6 different data sets as in Noreen (1989, p. 198).

The correlation in the observed sample was −0.926. The correlations in the other five data sets were −0.789, −0.137, 0.789, 0.137, and 0.926. Two of the six data sets had an absolute value of 0.926, so the two-tailed probability is 2/6 = 0.333 based on the permutation test.

12.5 Approximate Randomization Tests

Permutation tests require the analysis of a large number of data sets for even modest sample sizes. Because the number of possible data set gets

Table 12.1 Data for Correlation Permutation Example

Permutation 1 Observed Data		Permutation 4	
X	Y	X	Y
1906	821	1906	110
1909	215	1909	215
1912	110	1912	821
Permutation 2		Permutation 5	
X	Y	X	Y
1906	821	1906	215
1909	110	1909	110
1912	215	1912	821
Permutation 3		Permutation 6	
X	Y	X	Y
1906	215	1906	110
1909	821	1909	821
1912	110	1912	215

very large even with small sample sizes, researchers (Edgington, 1995) have advocated taking a random sample of all of the possible data sets rather than using all possible data sets. Tests based on a random sample of permuted data sets are called approximate randomization tests, and the permutation test is sometimes called an exact randomization test because it is based on all possible data sets and is therefore exact (Noreen, 1989). For example, for the test of a correlation in a sample of size 10, a random sample of 999 of the 3,628,800 data sets are taken, and the correlation is computed for these 999 samples. The distribution of the correlation is based on these 999 correlations plus the one observed correlation (the fact that the total is 1,000 makes it easier to calculate significance level), and the significance test is based on the number of cases for which the correlation is as large as or larger than the observed correlation in the sample of 1,000 correlations. Typically, the steps in this analysis are (a) randomly shuffle the Y variable, (b) compute the statistic, (c) repeat steps (a) and (b) for a certain number of replications (e.g., 999), and (d) find the proportion of shuffled data sets in which the statistic is equal to or greater than the statistic in the original data and that is the exact probability. This exact probability is compared with a specified significance level such as 0.05 to determine whether the observed correlation is statistically significant for the approximate permutation test.

12.6 Randomization Tests for the Mediated Effect

Randomization tests for the mediated effect are complicated because two separate equations are involved in the analysis of three variables. As a result, the number of potential data sets is even larger than that for the correlation coefficient. The first step in the development of an exact randomization test is the creation of all possible data sets. There are three variables in each of the data sets for the single mediator model. The total number of unique data sets is equal to $N!^2$, so for a sample size of 4, there are 576 different data sets. For N = 5, 6, 7, or 8, there are 14,400, 518,400, 25,401,600, and 1,625,702,400 different data sets, respectively.

The exact randomization test or permutation test for the mediated effect proceeds as follows: (a) estimate the mediated effect from the original sample of data, (b) create each possible permuted data set and estimate the mediated effect, (c) construct the distribution of these mediated effects in each possible data set along with the mediated effect in the original data to form a distribution of the mediated effect, and (d) locate the percentile of the observed mediated effect in the distribution of mediated effects. The corresponding percentile is the probability level and does not make many of the assumptions of the usual tests of mediation (MacKinnon & Lockwood, 2001).

The data in Table 12.2 are provided only to illustrate the $N!^2 = 2!^2 = 4$ possible sets of data for two observations and three variables. It is not possible to estimate the mediated effect with $N = 2$ because there are not sufficient degrees of freedom. If there are $N = 3$ observations, then the model (Equation 3.2) with two predictors has 0 degrees of freedom. With $N = 4$ there is 1 degree of freedom for the regression model with two predictors, making $N = 4$ the lowest possible sample size for mediation analysis that includes the direct effect.

The small data set presented in Table 12.3 is provided to demonstrate an exact randomization (permutation) test of the mediated effect with four observations. Imagine that these data are per capita values from four cities (of equal miles driven) in which the independent variable, X, is the change in per capita money spent yearly on the prevention of driving while under the influence of alcohol, the mediator, M, is the yearly change in the average from a survey of individuals' perception of being caught if a person drives under the influence of alcohol in each city, and Y is the yearly change in per capita number of alcohol-related accidents in each city. Each variable was the change from the previous year for each city so that some numbers are negative. There are a total of $N!^2 = 4!^2 = 576$ unique permuted data sets, including the observed data in Table 12.3. Each of these data sets generates a mediated effect, which results in a distribution of the mediated effect. Using methods described in chapter 3, the mediated effect in the original sample of 4 was equal to 76.3799 with a standard error of 4.09638, t value of 18.6457 ($p < 0.0001$) and lower confidence limit (LCL) = 68.3510 and upper confidence limit (UCL) = 84.4088. The mediated effect value of 76.3799 was at the 93.9th (554/576) percentile of the permutation distribution as plotted

Table 12.2   Permuted Data Sets for $N = 2$

Original Data		
X	M	Y
1	2	3
4	5	6
Permutation 1		
4	2	3
1	5	6
Permutation 2		
1	5	3
4	2	6
Permutation 3		
4	5	3
1	2	6

Table 12.3   Data for N = 4 Permutation Test Example

Obs	I	X	M	Y
1	1	−0.42761	−3.9026	−33.365
2	2	0.44967	4.2594	34.484
3	3	2.24475	18.7894	154.468
4	4	0.63210	6.3242	52.358

in figure 12.1. The data were generated from a population model with an extremely large mediated effect, $a = 8$, $b = 8$, and $c' = 2$, so the mediated effect was present in the population model. The exact randomization test was not as highly significant as the normal theory test, that is, $p = .061$ versus $p < .0001$. The confidence limits for the randomization test are complicated and require iteratively searching for the upper and lower limit and are thus not presented here. Confidence limits based on the permutation methods are described in Taylor and MacKinnon (2006).

Because of the large number of possible data sets for even small sample sizes, the exact randomization test is unrealistic for many situations. To conduct an exact randomization test for the example with N = 50 in chapter 3 would require making the $N!^2 = 50!^2 = 9.2502 \times 10^{128}$ different data sets. An alternative is to conduct an approximate randomization test, in

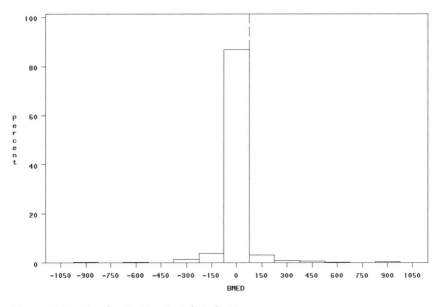

Figure 12.1.   Randomization test distribution.

which the values of variables are shuffled to select a random sample of all possible data sets. As described earlier, because only a sample of all possible data sets are selected, this type of test is called an approximate randomization test (Noreen, 1989). There are several options for selecting data sets for this test, including shuffling the mediator, randomly shuffling the dependent variable, or randomly shuffling both variables. An approximate randomization test would proceed as follows: (a) estimate the mediated effect from the whole sample of data, (b) randomly shuffle the mediating variable and the dependent variable, (c) estimate the mediated effect, (d) repeat Steps 2 and 3 a large number times (e.g., 999 times) to form a distribution of the mediated effect, and (e) locate the percentile of the value of the mediated effect from the original data set in the distribution of 1,000 (999 permuted and 1 observed data sets) mediated effects. Later in this chapter, an approximate randomization test is applied to the data in chapter 3.

12.7 Bootstrap Sampling

The bootstrap is now a widely used resampling method (Efron, 2000; Efron & Tibshirani, 1993; Yung & Bentler, 1996). Assume that you have a sample of size N. The bootstrap method consists of randomly sampling with replacement from the original N observations so that a new sample of N observations is obtained, which is the first resample (or the first bootstrap sample). Because there is sampling with replacement, one case in the original data set may be included 0, 1, 2, 3, 4, or more times in the bootstrap sample. For example, using the four cases in Table 12.3 for a pedagogical illustration, the first bootstrap sample may select the 4th, 3rd, 4th, and 3rd observations, the second bootstrap sample may consist of the 3rd, 1st, 2nd, and 1st observations, a third bootstrap sample may consist of the 2nd, 3rd, 2nd, and 1st observations, and so on for a large number of bootstrap samples. Typically, at least 1,000 of these bootstrap samples are selected to compute confidence limits (Efron & Tibshirani, 1993), although ways to determine the optimal number of bootstrap samples have been discussed (Fay & Follmann, 2002). A statistic, such as the correlation, is calculated for each of these 1,000 samples. The average of the correlations across the 1,000 samples is the bootstrap estimate of the correlation and the bootstrap standard error of the correlation is the standard deviation of the estimate of the correlation across the 1,000 samples. In the simplest form of bootstrapping, called the percentile bootstrap, upper and lower confidence limits are obtained by finding the values of the correlation in the 1,000 samples that correspond to the 2.5% and 97.5% percentiles. There are several variations of the bootstrap method that are useful in some situations.

Another bootstrap method, called the bias-corrected bootstrap, is important for mediation analysis because of its accuracy for computing confidence intervals for the mediated effect when the mediated effect is nonzero (Efron, 1987). The method consists of adjusting each bootstrap sample for potential bias in the estimate of the statistic. The bias-corrected bootstrap method removes bias that arises because the true parameter value is not the median of the distribution of the bootstrap estimates. The bias correction is used to obtain a new upper and lower percentile used to adjust the confidence limits in the bootstrap distribution. The steps in the bias-corrected bootstrap are as follows: (a) Find the observed value of the statistic in the bootstrap distribution and determine the proportion of bootstrapped values that are as large as or larger than the observed statistic. (b) Find the value from the normal distribution that corresponds to the proportion of bootstrap samples that are as large as or larger than the statistic from the observed sample found in (a). The z value from the standard normal distribution corresponding to the proportion, called z_0, is the bias correction. (c) For the lower confidence limit subtract the t value for the upper confidence limit; that is, $2z_0 - 1.96$. Determine the proportion on the normal distribution that corresponds to this new z value for the lower confidence limit. Find the percentage in the bootstrap distribution that corresponds to the percentage for the new z value. (d) For the upper confidence limit add $2z_0$ to the t value for the upper confidence limit ($2z_0 + 1.96$). Determine the percentage on the normal distribution that corresponds to this new z value for the upper confidence limit. Find the percentage in the bootstrap distribution that corresponds to the percentage for the new z value for the bias-corrected bootstrap. This percentage is then the probability of observing a mediated effect as large as or larger than the observed value. The probability level can be used to test the significance of the mediated effect.

Another resampling method, the jackknife (Mosteller & Tukey, 1977), preceded the development of the bootstrap. For a sample size N, there are N jackknife samples, each corresponding to removing one observation at a time from the original sample, so that each jackknife sample has N – 1 observations. The jackknife estimate is the average estimate across the N jackknife samples. The standard error of the jackknife estimate is a function of (N – 1)/N times the squared deviations of the mediated effect in each jackknife sample from the jackknife estimate of the mediated effect. The number of possible data sets is N because each jackknife data set consists of the original data set with one observation removed.

There are other forms of the bootstrap method, including the accelerated bias-corrected bootstrap, bootstrap t, bootstrap Q, resampling residuals and iterated bootstrap methods, which are not discussed here. More on these methods can be found in several sources: Chernick (1999), Edgington (1995), Efron and Tibshirani (1993), Good (2000), Manly (1997), and Noreen (1989). Cross-validation was also not discussed here but it is a computer intensive method that entails dividing an observed sample and evaluating the correspondence between the mediated effects between the two samples.

12.8 Bootstrap Estimates of the Mediated Effect

Bootstrap estimates of the mediated effect and its confidence limits are straightforward to obtain. First, the mediated effect estimate is obtained from the sample of data. In a bootstrap analysis of a sample of N = 100, for example, a new sample of 100 is taken with replacement from the original sample of 100, and the mediated effect is estimated. Then a second sample of 100 is taken from the original sample, and the mediated effect is estimated. The process is repeated a large number of times, usually at least 1,000. The mediated effect estimated in each bootstrap sample is used to form a distribution of the bootstrap mediated effect estimates, and confidence limits are obtained from the bootstrap distribution. Using the distribution of mediated effect estimates, the 95% confidence limits of the mediated effect are then the values of the mediated effect at the 2.5th and 97.5th percentiles in the distribution of bootstrapped mediated effects. The bias-corrected bootstrap is more complicated in that the difference between the observed sample mediated effect and the average mediated effect in the bootstrap distribution are used to correct the percentiles in the bootstrapped distribution. Other types of bootstrap methods such as the bootstrap *t* differ only in which value is evaluated in the bootstrap distribution.

12.9 Software for Computer Intensive Methods

A bootstrap procedure suitable for mediation analysis is included in the AMOS (Arbuckle & Wothke, 1999), Mplus (Muthén & Muthén, 2004), and EQS (Bentler, 1997) covariance structure analysis programs. The jackknife method is also included as part of the EQS program. A SAS program to compute the bootstrapped confidence limits of the mediated effect is described in Lockwood and MacKinnon (1998). This program has been expanded to include several versions of the bootstrap, randomization, and jackknife tests for the mediated effect. Preacher and Hayes (2004) provide SPSS and SAS programs for resampling. There are other statistical packages that conduct resampling tests such as StatXact (StatXact, 1999), Resampling Stats (Blank, Seiter, & Bruce, 1999), and SPSS Exact (SPSS Inc., 1999, at an extra cost), but few programs include options specific for the mediated effect. The bootstrap approaches for models larger than the single mediator model are straightforward extensions of the single mediator methods described in this chapter. A bootstrap sample is taken from the observed data and the larger model is estimated in the bootstrap sample, a second bootstrap sample is taken, and the larger model is estimated again and so on to construct bootstrap distributions for the coefficients in these larger models. The randomization test, on the other hand, is more complicated for larger models and would entail shuffling each mediator separately, increasing the time to conduct the analysis. The randomization test developed here may prove useful for covariance structure analysis of mediation. No software now exists to conduct the randomization test for covariance structure analysis for larger models. The AMOS program does include a randomization test in which the variables in a model are randomly rearranged, but this is a different test from the randomization test described here, in which the position of variables themselves are rearranged in the model.

12.10 Resampling Methods Applied to the Data in Chapter 3

In chapter 3, mediation analysis was conducted using data from a hypothetical study of the effect of temperature on water consumption through the mediator self-reported thirst. The data for the 50 subjects were shown in Table 3.1, where X is the temperature in degrees Fahrenheit, M is a self-report of thirst at the end of a 2-hour period, and Y is the number of deciliters of water consumed during the last 2 hours of the study. In this section, computer intensive methods are applied to these data. The estimates and standard errors for the regression analysis are given in chapter 3.

The estimate of the mediated effect is equal to $\hat{a}\hat{b} = (0.3386)(0.4510) = \hat{c} - \hat{c}' = 0.3604 - 0.2076 = 0.1527$. Using Equation 3.6, the standard error of the mediated effect is equal to 0.0741. The 95% confidence limits for the mediated effect based on normal theory are LCL = 0.0033 and UCL = 0.2979. The 95% confidence limits for the mediated effect based on the distribution of the product are LCL = 0.0329 and UCL = 0.3197.

12.11 SAS Program to Conduct Resampling Analyses

The data in chapter 3 were analyzed with the two-shuffle randomization (i.e., shuffled the mediator and shuffled the dependent variable), percentile bootstrap, bias-corrected bootstrap, bootstrap *t*, bootstrap Q, and jackknife methods using a SAS program (MacKinnon et al., 2004). Computer-intensive methods for the single mediator model can be easily tested with this program. The program requires that the original data set be identified as part of a SAS LIBNAME statement and that the independent, mediator, and dependent variables are labeled, X, M, and Y in this data set (i.e., upper case letters). The data containing the results of the computer intensive tests are written to another directory defined by the user.

For the present analysis, none of the 999 mediated effects from any of the permuted data sets from the approximate randomization test had a mediated effect as large as or larger than the observed mediated effect, so the significance level value was $1/1000 = 0.001$. The same program was run with 10,000 data sets, and there were seven data sets for which the mediated effect was as large as or larger than the observed mediated effect, so the resulting significance level was 0.0008. The confidence limits using the SAS program are shown in Table 12.4. The EQS and AMOS programs to conduct resampling analysis are described in the next section. Note that there are some minor differences among the confidence limits, but, overall, the confidence limits for all tests are very close for this data set. The original data were simulated to have a multivariate normal distribution, so the assumptions of each of the procedures are met, and different approaches are not expected to yield very different results. The resampling tests were based on 1,000 resamples, with the exception of the jackknife and the normal theory test.

12.12 EQS Program for Resampling Tests

The EQS (Bentler, 1997) computer program has several resampling options under the /SIMULATION command. The bootstrap and the jackknife method are conducted using the BOOTSTRAP (and JACKKNIFE) commands as shown in Table 12.5. The EQS program below was used to generate the data for a bootstrap analysis.

The SIMULATION command is used to conduct resampling analysis. Here a total of 1,000 bootstrapped data sets are requested. A separate data file called "boot" is written and saved separately. In the OUTPUT section, a file called boot.rst contains the results of the analysis of each bootstrap

Table 12.4 Confidence Limits for Single Sample and Resampling Tests of the Mediated Effect

	LCL	UCL
Normal	0.0033	0.2979
Percentile SAS	0.0395	0.2876
Percentile EQS	0.0405	0.2756
Percentile AMOS	0.0275	0.3130
Bias-corrected SAS	0.0604	0.3322
Bias-corrected EQS	0.0567	0.3237
Bias-corrected AMOS	0.0465	0.3700
Jackknife EQS SAS	0.0239	0.2813

Table 12.5 EQS Program for Bootstrap Estimation of Chapter 3
Water Consumption Data

```
/TITLE
   CHAPTER 3 EXAMPLE EQS MEDIATION ANALYSIS
/SPECIFICATIONS
   CAS=50; VAR=4; ME=ML; DA='a:cpt3.txt';MA=RAW;
/LABEL
  V1=s; V2=X; V3=M; V4=Y;
/EQUATIONS
   V4 = 1*V2 + 1*V3 + E2;
   V3 = 1*V2 + E3;
/VARIANCES
   V2  = 1*;
   E2 TO E3 =  2*;
/SIMULATION
  replications=1000;
  BOOT=50;
  DA='boot';
  save = separate;
/OUTPUT
  DA='BOOT.RST'; STANDARD ERRORS; PARAMETER ESTIMATES;
/END
```

sample. The first line of this data set contains information about the model estimation. The second line contains the six parameter estimates of this model. The third line contains the six estimates of the standard error of each parameter estimate in the model. EQS does not provide a summary of these results. A separate program must be written to analyze the data. Although the lack of summary analysis in the EQS output makes computer-intensive analysis more difficult than the AMOS program, which summarizes these results, the availability of an output file with the information for each bootstrap sample makes it possible to bootstrap many additional mediation measures such as the proportion mediated or the ratio of the mediated to the direct effect.

The SAS program in Table 12.6 was used to read the data file and compute resampling tests. This program is necessary to compute the mediated effect in each of these samples and to construct confidence limits from the results and relevant bootstrap results.

For the data from chapter 3, the percentile bootstrap confidence limits were 0.0405 and 0.2756 with an average bootstrap estimate of 0.1473 and an average standard error of 0.0745. The bias-corrected confidence limits are adjusted by the proportion of bootstrap estimates to the right of the sample estimate of the mediated effect. The mediated effect estimate of

Table 12.6 SAS Program to Read EQS Bootstrap File

```
data a;
infile 'c:\btstrap\boot.rst';
input
#1
#2 e1 e2 e3 a b cp
#3 see1 see2 see3 sea seb secp;
ab=a*b;
seab=sqrt(a*a*seb*seb+b*b*sea*sea);
t=ab/seab;
;
proc means;
proc univariate normal freq; var ab;
run;
```

0.1527 was at the 57.8th percentile in the bootstrap distribution, which corresponds to a z value of 0.1968. The corrected upper and lower z values equaled 2.3536 (2(.1968) + 1.96) and −1.5664 (2(0.1968) − 1.96), respectively, which correspond to the 99.07th and 5.86th percentiles, respectively. These values are 0.3237 and 0.0567, which are the bias-corrected bootstrap upper and lower 95% confidence intervals.

The EQS program in Table 12.7 was used to conduct the jackknife analysis of the chapter 3 data using EQS. The results of each separate jackknife sample

Table 12.7 EQS Code to Conduct Jackknife Analysis of the Chapter 3 Water Consumption Data

```
/TITLE
   CHAPTER 3 EXAMPLE EQS MEDIATION ANALYSIS
/SPECIFICATIONS
   CAS=50; VAR=4; ME=ML; DA='a:cpt3.txt';MA=RAW;
/LABEL
  V1=s; V2=X; V3=M; V4=Y;
/EQUATIONS
   V4 = 1*V2 + 1*V3 + E2;
   V3 = 1*V2 + E3;
/VARIANCES
   V2  = 1*;
   E2 TO E3 =  2*;
/SIMULATION
  REP=50;JACKNIFE;
/OUTPUT
  DA='JACK.RST'; STANDARD ERRORS; PARAMETER ESTIMATES;
/END
```

are not saved by EQS because it simply deletes the data from one subject to create each new data set. The data, with estimates and standard errors, are saved in a file called Jack.rst. The average jackknife mediated effect estimate was 0.1526. The standard error from the jackknife was equal to 0.0656, which led to lower and upper confidence limits of 0.0239 and 0.2813 respectively.

Another important use of EQS is the bootstrap estimation of other mediation statistics, such as the proportion mediated and the ratio of the mediated to the direct effect. Figure 12.2 shows the bootstrap distribution of the proportion mediated. The observed proportion mediated was 0.1527/(0.1527 + 0.2061) = 0.4344, which was at the 97.5th percentile in the bootstrap distribution of the proportion as shown in Figure 12.2. The ratio was equal to 0.1527/0.2061 = 0.7333, which was located at the 98.4th percentile of the bootstrap distribution of the ratio.

12.13 AMOS Program for Resampling Tests

AMOS has options for the percentile and bias-corrected bootstrap and unlike EQS, the AMOS output includes the upper and lower confidence limits for the mediated effect. To date, no computer program conducts the randomization test for the mediated effect with the exception of the SAS program described above. Models can be entered either by drawing a figure in the AMOS graphics input option or by writing code in the AMOS basic input option. The graphics method is an easy way to set up the program because it is based on a detailed figure for the model to be tested.

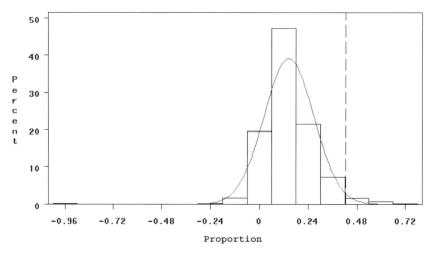

Figure 12.2. Bootstrap distribution for proportion.

Options to conduct the bootstrap analysis are obtained with options from a window in the program. It is important to request estimates of indirect effects so that they are included in the resampling routine.

The percentile bootstrap confidence limits for the mediated effect were 0.0275 and 0.3130 and for the bias-corrected percentile bootstrap 0.0465 and 0.3700, as shown in Table 12.8. The mediated effect is significant with both of these methods. AMOS prints out the upper and lower bounds of the estimates as shown below for the bias-corrected bootstrap. Note that the (BC) refers to the bias-corrected confidence limits. The corresponding values for the percentile method have the code (PC).

12.14 Mplus Resampling for the Two Mediator Model

The Mplus program for bootstrap analysis of the two mediator model, described in chapter 5, is shown in Table 12.9. In the analysis section, 500 bootstrap samples are selected by the command BOOTSTRAP=500 (for 1,000 bootstrap samples use BOOTSTRAP=1000). The MODEL INDIRECT command, Y IND X, requests that all specific indirect effects of X on Y are estimated: the specific effect X to M1 to Y and the specific indirect effect X to M2 to Y. The asymmetric percentile bootstrap confidence intervals are selected by the CINTERVAL(BOOTSTRAP) command. The bias-corrected bootstrap would be selected by CINTERVAL(BCBOOTSTRAP).

Selected output from the Mplus program is shown in Table 12.10. First the total indirect and specific indirect effects obtained from the bootstrap analysis are presented. The values for the total indirect and specific indirect effects are very similar to those for the single sample analysis described in chapter 5. In the next section, the 99% and 95% confidence limits are shown. For example, the 95% confidence interval for X to M1 to Y was 0.207 to 0.791, compared with normal (0.1842 to 0.7719) and distribution of product (0.1654 to 0.7906) confidence limits described in chapter 5. The 95%

Table 12.8 AMOS Output for Bias-Corrected Bootstrap of the Water Consumption Data

	X	M
Indirect effects lower bounds (BC)		
M	0.0000	0.0000
Y	0.0465	0.0000
Indirect effects upper bounds (BC)		
M	0.0000	0.0000
Y	0.3700	0.0000

Table 12.9   Mplus Program for the Two-Mediator Model

```
TITLE:   TWO MEDIATOR MODEL;
DATA:    FILE IS c:\twomed.dat;
VARIABLE:
    NAMES= S X M1 M2 Y;
    USEVARIABLES=X M1 M2 Y;
ANALYSIS:
    BOOTSTRAP=500;
MODEL:
    M1 ON X; M2 ON X;Y ON M1 M2 X;M1 WITH M2;
MODEL INDIRECT:
    Y IND X;
OUTPUT:
    CINTERVAL(BCBOOTSTRAP);
```

confidence interval for the X to M2 to Y specific indirect effect was −0.029 to 0.306 which is also similar to the normal (−0.0467 to 0.2817) and distribution of product (−0.0261 to 0.3106) confidence intervals from chapter 5. Mplus can be easily used to conduct resampling analysis of complicated models including the models described in chapters 6, 7, and 8.

12.15 Pros and Cons of Resampling Versus Single Sample Methods

First, consider the arguments in favor of resampling methods. Often a resampling method is the only way to find a standard error to test significance or create confidence intervals because the analytical derivations for these quantities are not available. This may be useful in mediation analysis because of the non-normal distribution of the product in some cases and also for tests based on functions of mediated effects. Traditional procedures require generalizing sample results to a theoretical population, which in turn, requires assumptions about distributions. In many situations, the characteristics of the population are not clear and invalid assumptions about the population may render traditional methods inaccurate. Resampling methods apply to nonrandom (but with restricted generalization) as well as random samples, and most traditional methods assume random sampling. Resampling methods, especially randomization tests, may handle small samples better than alternative tests and may provide more accurate results than traditional tests in this situation. Similarly, resampling methods handle outliers and other violations of assumptions. Replication is an important aspect of scientific research, and the repeated samples in resampling approaches are like replications, but, of

Table 12.10 Mplus Resampling Output

TOTAL, TOTAL INDIRECT, SPECIFIC INDIRECT, AND DIRECT EFFECTS

	Estimates	S.E.	Est./S.E.
Effects from X to Y			
Total	0.708	0.174	4.075
Total indirect	0.596	0.174	3.429
Specific indirect			
Y			
M1			
X	0.478	0.154	3.096
Y			
M2			
X	0.118	0.084	1.405

TOTAL, TOTAL INDIRECT, SPECIFIC INDIRECT, AND DIRECT EFFECTS

	Lower .5%	Lower 2.5%	Estimates	Upper 2.5%	Upper .5%
Effects from X to Y					
Total	0.324	0.368	0.708	1.056	1.189
Total indirect	0.221	0.286	0.596	0.991	1.113
Specific indirect					
Y					
M1					
X	0.125	0.207	0.478	0.791	0.961
Y					
M2					
X	-0.050	-0.029	0.118	0.306	0.374

course, these replications are different from independent research studies. Resampling methods such as the permutation test are also intuitively appealing given that they consider all, or a sample of all, possible data sets. Finally, R. A. Fisher and others used it to determine the accuracy of their traditional tests, at least suggesting that that test may be used as a gold standard for significance testing.

Now consider arguments against resampling methods. The researcher may get more from the data than what actually exists. Resampling may just magnify the bias in biased samples. Generalizing beyond the particular sample may be problematic. There is evidence that resampling methods do not work well if the sampling of bootstrap samples differs from the sampling that generated the data such as for goodness-of-fit indices as described by Bollen and Stine (1993), but this limitation is not problematic for mediation effect estimation. The computing power is adequate for most computer-intensive methods, but the software to make these routines simple is only beginning to be widely available. For example, a SAS macro had to be specifically written to conduct bootstrap analysis and randomization tests of the mediated effect for this chapter. Furthermore, the difference between resampling and traditional tests is often minuscule, so why bother with resampling methods that can be complicated and time-consuming? Another criticism is based on Gleser's first law of applied statistics, "Two individuals using the same statistical method on the same data should arrive at the same conclusion" (Gleser, 1996, p. 210). Because resampling methods, with the exception of the jackknife and the exact randomization test, entail repeated random samples of observations, it is possible that different individuals would come to different conclusions in a resampling analysis of the same data set. Finally, as Fisher's quote at the beginning of this chapter describes, resampling approaches may reflect a certain lack of knowledge about important aspects of substantive problems such as the correct underlying distribution.

12.16 Summary

Resampling approaches for testing mediation effects hold considerable promise for mediation analysis. There is evidence that the resampling methods generally have more accurate Type I error rates and more statistical power than single sample methods that assume a normal distribution for the mediated effect (MacKinnon et al., 2004). There is also some evidence that the percentile bootstrap is preferred over the bias-corrected bootstrap because in some rare cases the bias-corrected bootstrap has excess Type I error rates. Resampling methods are also a good general option for more complicated models with mediated effects. The availability of bootstrap resampling methods in the AMOS, EQS, and Mplus computer programs should make the application of these methods more common. Resampling methods are often useful for any mediation model to obtain accurate confidence limits, especially for models with complex mediated effects such as three-path mediated effects. It is likely that computer-intensive methods will continue to be an active area of research for mediation analysis.

12.17 Exercises

12.1. How many unique data sets of three variables can be made with eight subjects?

12.2. Why are approximate rather than exact randomization tests conducted?

12.3. Why does the bootstrap yield more accurate confidence limits for the mediated effect than normal theory methods?

12.4. Why is it not possible to conduct a resampling analysis for the achievement model in chapter 6?

12.5. Describe how the words *jackknife* and *bootstrap* are appropriate names for resampling tests. (Hint: think of the typical definitions of jackknife and bootstrap.)

12.6. Read R. A. Fisher's quote at the beginning of this chapter again. Do you think he is correct about resampling tests? Do you think that resampling methods just display ignorance or blind analysis? Discuss the arguments for and against resampling tests.

13

Causal Inference for Mediation Models

> Two roads diverged in a yellow wood, / And sorry
> I could not travel both, / And be one traveler long I
> stood, / And looked down one as far as I could
>
> **—Robert Lee Frost, 1920**

13.1 Overview

The purpose of this chapter is to describe modern causal inference approaches to evaluating mediating variables. These approaches specify the criteria for causal relations that clarify the limitations of mediation models and suggest additional methods to identify mediating processes. Several approaches to demonstrating causal relations are briefly described, followed by a description of the Rubin causal model (RCM), one of the most widely used models to interpret causal relations. Compliance with a treatment regimen as a mediator is then described along with instrumental variable approaches to investigating mediating variables. Holland's extension of the RCM to mediation is presented, followed by more recent extensions based on principal stratifications of participants in a study.

13.2 Causal Inference

Causal interpretation is the motivation for many research studies even though researchers may not claim that their results provide causal conclusions (Pearl, 2000). The identification of causes has been a primary focus of knowledge since the time of Aristotle (Wheelwright, 1951). General methods to identify causes based on research are relatively recent. Robert Koch, the famous 19th century biologist, outlined a set of rules for determining whether an agent is a cause of disease (cited in Last & Wallace, 1992). First, the agent must be present in organisms with the disease. Second, the agent must be isolated from diseased organisms. Third, introduction of the agent into a new organism must create disease in the new organism. These rules were developed when the bacterial causes of many diseases were being discovered. Koch used these rules to prove the bacterial causes of anthrax and tuberculosis.

Primarily in response to the question of whether smoking was a cause of lung cancer, criteria for causal relations were described by Hill (1965) and the U.S. Surgeon General's report on Smoking and Health (U.S. Department of Health, Education, and Welfare, 1964). Hill (1971) outlined these criteria for statistical evidence of causal relations: (a) strength of association, that the size of the relation between two variables provides evidence for a causal relation, (b) consistency, that the same effect is observed by different researchers, on different subjects (animal or human) in different circumstances and times, (c) specificity, that there is a clear link from exposure to a certain disease and other exposures do not lead to the disease, (d) temporal precedence, that a relation in time such that exposure to the risk factor occurs before the disease, (e) biological gradient, that the likelihood of the disease increases as the exposure increases, that is, there is a dose-response curve, (f) biological plausibility, that the relation makes sense from biological theory, (g) coherence of the evidence, that the cause and effect hypothesis should not conflict with what is known about the natural history and biology of the disease, (h) experimental results, that an experimental intervention designed to reduce the risk factor has expected effects on the outcome, (i) reasoning by analogy, that the action of the disease under study is similar to the action of other exposures and diseases, and (j) common sense and figures, that the observed effects should be evident in statistical analysis as well as make common sense. Hill (1971) provides these criteria as guidelines, not as set rules for causation. Several of these criteria are especially relevant for mediation studies. Specificity of an effect through one mediator and not other mediators adds credence to a mediator. Temporal precedence provides evidence such that a change in the mediator leads to a later change in the dependent variable. Perhaps most important is the consistency criteria for which mediated effects should be observed by other researchers using other experimental designs. Similarly, as in the biological gradient criterion, larger effects on the mediator should be associated with larger changes on the outcome.

During the last 30 years, new methods for making causal interpretations of research results have been developed. The purpose of these models is to provide a framework to carefully consider the different information and assumptions necessary for causal interpretation of research results and to add to the previous criteria required for causal statements, such as the temporal precedence and specificity criteria outlined in the Surgeon General's 1964 Report on Smoking (Hill, 1965; U.S. Department of Health, Education, and Welfare, 1964). Unlike the biological transmission of disease and smoking and lung cancer motivations of earlier criteria, these new methods were designed for the interpretation of medical and social policy research, which often used observational as well as experimental designs. These new developments in causal interpretation of research results incorporate the causal criteria of Koch and Hill to form a broader interpretation of causal evidence. An important benefit of these methods is that they elucidate the difficulty of establishing causal relations and often suggest that mediation methods provide only descriptive information about relations, rather than identifying causal relations. In many cases, the methods suggest alternative information or designs that bolster the evidence for a mediational relation among variables. Overall, these methods provide a sound theoretical basis for conclusions drawn from mediation studies.

13.3 The RCM

The RCM (Rubin, 1974, 1977) provides a basis for causal inference in research designs including the mediation model. One common theme of the RCM is the distinction between the effects of a cause versus the cause of effects (Holland, 1986, 1988b). It is often easier to define the effects of a cause than it is to infer the cause of an effect. As described by Holland, the statement that A is a cause of B is usually false because it represents a summary of current knowledge, and what is considered a cause now may be incorrect when more information becomes available. It is more sensible to focus on statements from experimental results such as, "An effect of A is B" because the effect of A will be B in future studies as well as in the current study.

A second and most important theme of the RCM and related approaches is the notion of a counterfactual. The counterfactual is central to causal inference. The counterfactual is common in everyday thinking such as when one is considering possible actions other than the action the person actually took, for example, if I had left for work at 6 this morning rather than 8, then I would not have been in so much traffic. The Robert Frost quote at the beginning of the chapter also refers to the counterfactual case in which only one road was actually taken, but the author is considering what would have happened if the other road had been taken. In the RCM, the counterfactual is more specific. It refers to conditions in which a participant could serve, not just the condition they did serve in. The counterfactual follows from the RCM's grounding in experiments, in which a causal effect can only be considered in relation to another causal effect (e.g., treatment versus control group). Ideally, the effect of an experiment would compare an individual participant's score on a variable when that subject received the treatment to the score for the same participant without the treatment. In most experiments, the same participant cannot realistically participate in both the treatment and control groups, because, for example, the effect of the treatment may carry over to the control condition. The counterfactual requires the consideration of a treatment effect for a person who was actually in the control condition. So the RCM (and other causal inference approaches) requires consideration of situations, contrary to fact, in which a person would have actually served in a condition that they did not actually serve. The historical precedent for this counterfactual idea is the potential yield concept described by Neyman (1923).

Because it is impossible to simultaneously observe the same person in two conditions, Holland (1986) calls this problem the fundamental problem of causal inference. However, if it is assumed that different persons have identical responses to treatment and control conditions, then one person can serve as the counterfactual case for another. Unit homogeneity is the assumption that the units (here persons) in the treatment and control group are so similar that they can be considered identical. If unit homogeneity can be assumed, then the treatment and control units are so similar before the experiment that the difference between units reflects the causal effect of the treatment after the experiment. It is unlikely that human subjects are similar enough to satisfy unit homogeneity, with the possible exception of some biological characteristics. In response to this problem, the average causal effect (ACE) is considered. If a large number of participants are randomly assigned to treatment and control groups, then the causal effect of a treatment can be ascertained by comparing the average of participants' scores in the treatment group to the average of the participants' scores in the control group. Randomization of units to conditions is used to ensure that assignment to conditions is unrelated to all other variables before the study. The average causal effect requires the stable unit treatment value assumption (SUTVA). The SUTVA is that the effects of a treatment are stable, such that one unit's potential outcomes do not depend on other unit's assignment and that assignment to conditions does not affect units in ways unrelated to the treatment. For example, SUTVA is violated if the control group participants resent the fact that treatment participants received the treatment and purposefully changed their behavior because of this resentment (resentful demoralization as described by Cook & Campbell, 1979). With SUTVA and successful randomization, the difference between the treatment and control means allows for causal inference to be made.

The RCM makes a crucial distinction between the equations for the causal relations among variables, the ACEs (Average Causal Effects), and the equations for observed data. This distinction is important because it clarifies how estimators based on observed data may be different from estimators in the causal model. Estimators of causal effects for observed data are called prima facie average causal effects (FACEs; prima facie means "on the face of it"). The difference in the average response in treatment versus control groups is a FACE when there is random assignment of units to conditions. The distinction between the ACE and the FACE is that the FACE can be computed from data, but it does not necessarily equal the ACE. The ACE requires information from the counterfactual and cannot be directly computed from data.

Observed and causal relations clarify the distinction between descriptive versus causal interpretation of results in the RCM. A descriptive interpretation of a mediation study of tobacco prevention, for example, would state that those persons whose norms against smoking increased after an intervention were less likely to smoke at a later date than persons whose norms against smoking stayed the same. This descriptive interpretation differs from a causal interpretation, which might state that changes in norms caused a change in smoking. The level of proof required for the causal interpretation is more detailed. The RCM clarifies the problems in making causal inference by the consideration of counterfactual situations.

The RCM was originally developed for the investigation of cases in which X does not represent random assignment to conditions (Rubin, 1974). In this situation, Rubin (1977) describes ignorability given a covariate, where ignorability means that X is independent of omitted variables once conditioned on another variable or variables. In this situation, the FACEs become covariate adjusted FACEs (C-FACEs). In this way, the RCM is very clear about the importance of how assignment occurred when considering causal inference. It is critical to specify an assignment mechanism for how units are assigned to conditions. The covariate represents a variable that accounts for the assignment mechanism. If the assignment mechanism is known, then accurate estimates of causal effects can be obtained under certain assumptions. The description of the RCM for mediation described later in this chapter is in terms of X as a randomized experiment because this often occurs in mediation studies and it simplifies aspects of the RCM application to mediation.

One other important aspect of the counterfactual idea is that appropriate causal interpretation can only be made when it is possible for individuals to be in either group (e.g., an individual could be in either the program or control group). As a result, effects of sex and race, for example, cannot be interpreted as causal effects in the RCM and related causal inference models because these variables cannot be manipulated. The model demonstrates that in most situations, only random assignment can lead to a causal interpretation of the effect of a treatment compared to a control group. Sobel (1998) and others (Pratt & Schlaifer, 1988) discuss situations in which it may be sensible to study the causal effect of variables such as sex, at least in part because the original assignment of sex at conception is likely to be random.

In summary, the RCM provides a general framework for understanding the limitations and strengths of possible causal inferences from any study including a mediation study. As described later in this chapter, the RCM and related methods have been extended to mediation models (Frangakis & Rubin, 2002; Holland, 1988a), for direct and indirect effects of epidemiological measures (Robins & Greenland, 1992), and for methods based on graph theory (Pearl, 2000).

13.4 Instrumental Variables

Several modern approaches to assessing causal mediation relations use instrumental variables. Instrumental variables methodology is a general approach to improve the interpretation of coefficients in a statistical model (Angrist & Krueger, 2001). Instrumental variables are more commonly used in economics and related fields in which experimental design cannot be easily used to rule out threats to conclusions from a research study. Instead, assumptions are made, and model-based corrected estimates are generated. As the situation approximates randomization, estimates approximate the true values. If assumptions are violated, estimates can be incorrect and even worse than uncorrected estimates (Stolzenberg & Relles, 1990). It is important to keep in mind that the instrumental variable methods are based on assumptions that may be violated (Shadish, Cook, & Campbell, 2002).

In economics, instrumental variables are used to deal with violation of regression assumptions including a nonzero correlation between an explanatory variable and an error term, correlated errors across equations, omitted variables, and violations of other assumptions. For example, instrumental variables provide better estimates of regression coefficients in multiple equation models with a nonzero correlation between errors across equations (Hanushek & Jackson, 1977, pp. 234–239). Other applications of instrumental variables included adjustment for latent variables and measurement error (Angrist & Krueger, 2001).

In the correlated errors across equations application of instrumental variables, an instrumental variable (also called an instrument) is constructed that is equal to the predicted scores from a regression equation. These predicted scores are then used as predictors in a second equation. To use the mediation example, the predicted scores of X on M, M', are used in a regression equation where Y is predicted by M'. The coefficient relating M' to Y is the instrumental variable estimator of the $\hat{b}$ coefficient. These coefficients are more accurate than ordinary least squares (OLS) estimates of the $\hat{b}$ coefficient if the correlated error is ignored in the OLS analysis (Hanushek & Jackson, 1977, pp. 234–239 for results from a simulation study). In general, the standard error of the instrumental variable estimator is larger than the standard error estimator relating M and Y without the instrument. In Hanushek and Jackson (1977) and other places, the derivation of the standard error of the instrumental variable effect is shown.

Controlling for omitted variables is a primary use of instrumental variable methods in mediation analysis. In this application of instrumental variables, the goal is to estimate a causal relation between a mediator and a dependent variable, such as the relation between schooling and income or the relation between military service and health. The original estimate of the relation between the mediator and outcome is likely to be inaccurate because of the potential influence of omitted variables that may alter the relation between M and Y. The instrumental variables solution is to use an instrumental variable, X, that reflects random assignment to a program that affects M but is related to Y only through its effect on M. Here the instrumental variable allows for the estimation of the relation of M and Y without bias from omitted variables. A good instrumental variable is related to M for clear reasons and unrelated to Y beyond its effect through M. Examples of this application of instrumental variables for mediation analysis are described next.

13.5 Instrumental Variables and Mediation

Recent applications of the RCM in the examination of mediating variables have focused on the effects of exposure to a treatment on an outcome measure for compliers. For example Angrist, Imbens, and Rubin (1996) investigated the effect of Vietnam War service on health by using random selection in the draft as an instrumental variable, serving in Vietnam as the mediating variable, and health as the dependent variable. The causal effect of military service on death rates for compliers was examined. The lottery for military service based on randomly selecting birth dates was used as an instrumental variable in the analysis. The selection of birth dates was random and was associated with increased military service. Using the draft as an instrumental variable allowed for an estimate of the causal effect of military service on death for compliers. The causal effect of the draft on death was substantial. Of subjects with low lottery numbers and more likely to be drafted, 2.04% died between 1974 and 1983 compared with 1.95% with high lottery numbers; the difference of 0.09% was an estimate of the complier average causal effect of draft status on mortality. The authors conducted sensitivity analysis of the assumptions required for the accuracy of the instrumental variables estimator of the relation between military service and health.

Angrist et al. (1996) and corresponding discussion papers described the instrumental variables approach for the effect of military service on health in terms of imperfect compliance. Compliance with the draft was not perfect, as some persons drafted did not serve in the military by staying in school, for example. One common way to evaluate randomized treatments in which compliance varies is to compare the difference in outcome between participants in the control and treatment groups for all participants present at the beginning of the study. This type of analysis has been called intent-to-treat (ITT) analysis because it estimates the group difference based on assignment to treatment or control groups, without consideration of the amount of the program actually received by program participants or control participants. However, in most research studies, persons participate in the intervention to different degrees and some subjects drop out before completing the treatment. Subjects in the control condition may actually receive some treatment such as persons with high lottery numbers volunteering for military service in the previous example. Although the ITT estimate is the treatment effect in the real world, the ITT approach may underestimate treatment effects, because, in fact, some participants may have gotten a minimal treatment or no treatment at all. Critics of ITT analysis argue for analyzing the effects of treatment on the treated (TOT), so that the treatment effect reflects only those persons who received the whole treatment. There are problems with the TOT effect as well, including the facts that it is often impossible to determine who will get the entire treatment before the study and it may be difficult to generalize effects beyond the unique group of TOT participants. The subset of participants in the treatment group who receive the entire treatment are unlikely to be a random sample of the treatment group (and control participants may take up the treatment), making them unique in some unknown ways. Another option is to use an instrumental variables approach to estimate the local average treatment effect (LATE) so that the amount of the treatment is taken into account. In general, the instrumental variables estimator may provide a more sensitive way than ITT or TOT to determine effects among the treated. As described by Angrist et al. (1996), the LATE is the treatment effect on compliers, persons induced to receive the whole treatment. This model generally assumes a binary compliance measure. Efron and Feldman (1991) addressed a continuous compliance measure and described analysis required to shed light on the relation of degree of compliance to the dependent variable in both treatment and control groups.

Neither the TOT nor the LATE estimator of treatment effects is likely to represent the effect of a treatment if it were made widely available. As a result, researchers have suggested that TOT and LATE estimators represent bounds for the average treatment effect under several assumptions if the goal is to extend the results of the single research study to the population. Under certain assumptions, the instrumental variables estimator is a valid LATE estimator of treatment-induced changes (Shadish et al., 2002). These assumptions, using the X, M, and Y mediation example, where M is compliance, are the following. (a) X is exogenous, which means that X is uncorrelated with unobserved characteristics of the persons, including pretreatment measures of Y (this assumption is most easily met by random assignment). (b) The effect of the instrument X (i.e., predicted values for M) on M is substantial. (c) The relation between X, M, and Y are independent across participants; that is, potential outcomes for one participant do not depend on assignment of other participants. This is the stable unit treatment alue (SUTVA) described earlier. (d) The effect of X on M is the same for all participants; that is, no one in the treatment group received less treatment than if they had, in fact, not received the treatment. This is related to the monotonicity assumption. An example of violating this assumption would occur if, for some reason, participants assigned to the treatment actually behaved in a way opposite to the treatment. (e) M completely mediates the effect of X on Y. This is called the exclusion restriction. However, complete mediation may be rare and unrealistic in many research contexts. Alternatively, it may be possible to design research studies and identify subgroups in which the assumption of complete mediation may be reasonable.

An analogous approach to instrumental variable analysis in a mediation context is found in studies in which the mediator is the single active ingredient in an intervention. In a clinical trial of a new drug, for example, the dosage of the drug can be treated as a mediator with random assignment to conditions as the instrumental variable (Rosenbaum, 2002b; see also Efron & Feldman, 1991). This approach estimates the biological efficacy of a treatment (LATE) compared with the programmatic effectiveness of a treatment (ITT). In this model, the exclusion restriction is that the effect of the treatment to the outcome is entirely due to effects on dose.

13.6 Instrumental Variable Estimation of the Mediation Effect

To use the mediation example, the estimates of the causal relation between M and Y are obtained by using X as an instrumental variable (Gennetian, Morris, Bos, & Bloom, 2005). Steps in this process are summarized in Table 13.1. The instrumental variable estimate of this causal effect reduces to $\hat{c}/\hat{a}$ from the single mediator equations in chapter 3. As described earlier, for the case of the mediation model, the idea is to use an instrument for the prediction of M and then use the predicted values of M to predict Y. The statistical significance of the coefficient relating predicted M to Y is the test of the $\hat{b}$ path for the mediated effect and is equal to $\hat{c}/\hat{a}$. Note that the instrumental variable must be related to M and not to Y, following the.

Table 13.1 Steps in Instrumental Variables Approach to Mediation
1. Use the X variable coding random assignment as the instrumental variable.
2. Estimate the regression of the mediating variable on the instrumental variable X and save the predicted scores on the mediators, M'.
3. Estimate the regression coefficient relating the predicted mediator scores from Step 2, M', on the dependent variable Y. This is an estimate of the $\hat{b}$ path for the mediated effect.

exclusion restriction. Furthermore, the stronger the relation of X to M, the better the instrument is, with the best instrument having a correlation of 1 with M; that is, the M variable is the same as the instrument. There are several limitations to this approach, the requirement of no relation of the instrumental variable with Y being one of the major limitations. Other limitations are the reasonableness of the assumptions described earlier. Shadish et al. (2002) reviewed the plausibility of the assumptions of instrumental variables approaches.

If there were multiple mediators, then a separate instrument would be required for each potential mediator. For the analogous case for the single mediator model, each mediator would be required to be randomly assigned to the units studied, which is rare in most research (West & Aiken, 1997). For example in drug prevention, social influences-based drug prevention programming may be randomly assigned to schools and, independently, resistance skills training would also be randomly assigned to schools. Both interventions, resistance skills and social influences prevention programming, are randomly assigned to schools. Two variables, one for each random assignment, would be used as separate instrumental variables.

The data from chapter 3 can be used to demonstrate a simple instrumental variable approach. Here the X variable coding random assignment to temperature is used as an instrumental variable. The relation of X to Y was nonsignificant when the mediator was included in the analysis, a result consistent with the exclusion restriction assumption but not exactly because the exclusion restriction refers to counterfactual values. The relation of X to M is assessed via linear regression, and the predicted scores for M, M', are saved and used in a regression equation relating M' to Y. The coefficient, $\hat{b}$, relating M' to Y is the estimator of the causal effect of M on Y. The regression equation for the prediction of M is M' = −20.70243 + 0.3386 X. When Y is regressed on M', the coefficient is 1.0643 (0.3967), t = 2.68. The ratio of $\hat{c}/\hat{a}$ = 0.3604/0.3386 = 1.0643, as expected because this is the value of $\hat{b}$. That $\hat{b} = \hat{c}/\hat{a}$ can be seen by solving algebraically for $\hat{b}$ in the equation $\hat{c} - \hat{c}' = \hat{a}\hat{b}$, where $\hat{c}'$ is zero based on the exclusion restriction (i.e., $\hat{c} = \hat{a}\hat{b}$ so $\hat{b} = \hat{c}/\hat{a}$ and $\hat{a} = \hat{c}/\hat{b}$). The predicted value of M based on X, M', represents the change in M from the randomization of units to X. The resulting relation of the instrumental variable M' to Y reflects the part of M that was changed by X that results in the change in Y.

13.7 The RCM and Mediation (Holland, 1988a)

For the case in which X represents random assignment to conditions, the causal interpretation of mediating variables (Holland, 1988a; Robins & Greenland, 1992) is improved for several reasons, including temporal precedence whereby the assignment to conditions precedes measurement of the mediating variable and the dependent variable. Holland applied the RCM to examine a mediating variable design called the encouragement design. In the encouragement design described by Holland, students are randomly assigned to one of two conditions, either to a group receiving encouragement to study or to a control group that does not receive such encouragement. Here the mediating process is that assignment to the encouragement condition affects the number of hours studied, which in turn affects test performance. This is similar to the compliance example (with continuous compliance), where here the compliance is encouragement to study.

Under the unit homogeneity, the usual regression coefficient for the group effect on test score, $\hat{c}$, and for the group effect on number of hours studied, $\hat{a}$, are valid estimators of the causal effect, because of the randomization of units to treatment. The relation between the mediating variable of the number of hours studied (M) and test score (Y) is more problematic because it does not consider potential outcomes. The regression coefficient, $\hat{b}$, may not be an accurate estimator of the causal effect because this relation is correlational, not the result of random assignment. The estimator $\hat{c}'$ is also not an accurate causal estimator of the direct effect because it reflects the relation of X to Y at different levels of M, and M is not randomly assigned. The missing information for the causal effects is whether the relation between the number of hours studied and test score would have been different for subjects in the treatment group if they had instead been assigned to the control group. That subjects in the treatment group are not directly comparable to subjects in the control group because they have not served in both groups is the counterfactual concept again. That is, what would be the participant's score if he or she had studied m hours if assigned to the control group compared with the same participant's score if he or she had studied m hours and was assigned to the treatment group? One other consideration in this causal approach is that the mediating variable must be a variable that could potentially be manipulated because it serves as both an effect of treatment assignment and a cause in its effect on the dependent variable.

13.8 Holland's Causal Mediation Model

Holland's causal model for the encouragement design uses a detailed notational system, consisting of two sets along with the three variables in the single mediator model. The two sets are U and K. The set U represents the units studied, which are participants in the study. Lower case u refers to an individual participant in the set of U participants. K represents the set of encouragement conditions. As in Holland (1988a) assume there are two conditions, either encouraged to study, t, or not, c, or K = {t,c}. The addition of the two sets U and K to the variables, X, M, and Y, clarifies the causal effects in the encouragement design. X represents random assignment to condition where X(u) = 1 if encouraged [the t group or X(u) = t] and X(u) = 0 if not encouraged [the c group or X(u) = c]. M codes number of hours of study, which depends on the participant, u, and the encouragement condition to which u is exposed, so that M is a function of the units u and experimental condition, x. That is, M = (u,x) has two possibilities: M(u,t) amount u studies if encouraged to study and M(u,c) amount u studies if not encouraged to study. Y represents the test score, which depends on the participant, u, on whether u is encouraged to study or not (x), and on the amount of time u studies (m). Y is a function of u, x, and m, so Y(u,t,m) is the test score for u if u is encouraged to study and u studies for m hours and Y(u,c,m) is the test score for u if u is not encouraged to study and u studies for m hours. Note that these two effects represent the test score for subject u who studies m hours for both treatment and control groups. But each participant is either in the treatment or control groups, not in both groups, so the researcher cannot obtain both Y(u,c,m) and Y(u,t,m), just Y(u,c, M(c)) or Y(u,t, M(t)). Note that M(c) refers to the mediator value in the control group and M(t) refers to the mediator value in the treatment group. In summary, ideally we would have the scores for every participant, u, in each possible condition, but we only have the score for each participant in the condition in which they actually served.

To summarize, the model for the encouragement design is a quintuple {U,K,X,M,Y} where X maps U to K, M is a function of (u,x), and Y is a function of (u,x,m). The values of M given u and x and Y given u, x and m are not directly observable for all combinations of u, x, and m and this makes causal inference difficult. According to the RCM, the notation M(u) and Y(u) for structural equation modeling is too simple because it does not reveal the causal structure of the problem where X and M are functions of counterfactual cases [i.e., M(u) should be M(u,x) and Y(u) should be Y(u,x,m) to represent the causal structure in terms of individual participants, u]. The terms X(u), M(u,x), and Y(u,x,m) in the causal model corresponding to the observed values of M and Y according to Holland (1988a, p. 462, with a notation of X for S and M for R) are as follows: M(u,X(u)) is the observed M response and Y(u,X(u)), M(u,X(u)) is the observed Y response. The dependence of M(u,x) and Y(u,x,m) on the unit, u, is how the RCM includes individual variation in response to causes. The value of a response (Y) depends both on causes that are measured, such as x and m, and other factors that affect the participant's (u's) responses.

13.9 Four Types of Unit-Level Causal Effects

There are four types of participant-level causal effects in Holland's extension of the RCM for encouragement designs: three different effects of encouragement (t) and one effect of studying (M). Two of the encouragement (t) effects are the causal effect of t on M and the causal effect of t on Y. The causal effect of t on M is the increment in the amount that unit u would study if encouraged to study over how much u would study if not encouraged. The causal effect of t on Y is the increment in the test score a participant (u) would receive if the participant (u) were encouraged to study over the test score the participant (u) would receive if the participant (u) were not encouraged to study. The causal effect of t on M corresponds to the *a* effect and the causal effect of t on Y corresponds to the *c* effect in the mediation model.

The third unit-level causal effect of encouragement is more complicated than the first two and represents how the RCM clarifies the mediation model. The third effect is the effect of t on Y for fixed M, which is the pure effect of encouragement on test scores because it is the increment in u's test score when u studies m hours and is encouraged to study, compared with u's test score when u studies m hours but is not encouraged to study. Only one of these scores is observed and the other is the counterfactual case. The effect of t on Y for fixed M demonstrates that the amount u studies is a self-selected treatment that can differ from the treatment that actually occurs. This effect corresponds to the *c'* parameter, but it is more complicated than the *c'* parameter, because the causal relation of t on Y for fixed M involves characteristics of the counterfactual for participants in each group. The effect of t on Y for fixed M describes the effect on test scores for the same number of hours of studying for the same subject in the encouragement and control conditions. This description of the *c'* effect makes it explicit that encouragement may have a different effect on test score even for the same subject and the same number of hours of studying, whereas the typical direct effect assumes a constant effect. It seems sensible to assume that this effect is zero in some situations, that is, that the encouragement design does not have an effect on test score if the numbers of hours studied are the same in the encouraged (t) and not encouraged (c) condition for the same subject.

The fourth unit-level causal effect corresponds to the effect of studying on test score and reflects the idea that amount of study is a self-selected treatment that can differ from the amount the student did study. For this unit level causal effect, the encouragement condition is fixed, x, and the causal effect of M on Y is the change in test score that results when the same individual u studies m versus m' hours. This effect is related to the *b* parameter and refers to how the change in M relates to the change in Y. Because the researcher does not have the same subject randomly assigned to all levels of M, it is not possible to determine this value with observed data in the RCM. That is, the researcher does not have information on the same participant's test score for m versus m' hours of study.

The four unit-level causal effects are never directly observable because of the fundamental problem of causal inference, but they may be used to define causal parameters that can be estimated or measured with data. Holland's theoretical analysis clarifies consideration of counterfactual situations, demonstrating how the self-selection of participants to level of the mediator makes interpretation of direct and mediated effects more complicated. Averaging each of the four types of unit-level causal effects over U results in the important causal parameters called ACEs, as described earlier in the description of the RCM. The four ACEs are (a) effect of t on M, (b) effect of t on Y, (c) effect of t on Y for fixed M, and (d) effect of M on Y for m versus m' values.

The ACEs must be distinguished from the FACEs, which are defined in terms of observable values of X, M, and Y. Because FACEs are based on observable data, the FACEs are associational parameters rather than causal parameters. They are primae facie ACEs rather than ACEs because they may or may not equal their corresponding ACEs, depending on whether certain assumptions are met.

13.10 Holland's ALICE Model

As described earlier, the first two ACEs correspond to parameters in a structural equation model, *a* and *c* (*c*, the total effect, is actually not in the structural model), respectively. The last two ACEs are not in mediation regression equations but correspond to the *c'* and *b* parameters. Holland describes a model for the encouragement design with which it is possible to estimate all four average causal effects, but it requires several assumptions, including Additive, Linear, and Constant Effects (ALICE). In the ALICE model, the effect of t on m and y for a given unit are additive, and the effect of m on y is linear. For the ALICE model, *p* is the constant number of hours that encouragement increases each student's amount of study, $f + pB_c$ is the constant linear improvement in test scores due to encouragement to study, *f* is the constant amount that encouragement increases the test scores of a student who always studies m hours, B_c is the constant amount that studying 1 hour more increases a student's test score. The causal effect of t on M is p. The causal effect of t on Y is $f + pB_c$. The causal effect of encouragement on test scores for a student who always studies m hours is f. The causal effect of M on Y for a person who studies m versus m' hours is $B_c(m - m')$.

The FACEs for the last two causal effects, f and $B_c(m - m')$, include an additional term that represents the average value of test scores for students when they are not encouraged to study and they do not study for all students who would study an amount m when they are not encouraged to study. Holland proposes a linear model for this quantity equal to $g + dm$, where a "positive d means that the more a student would study when not encouraged, the higher he or she would score on the test without studying and without encouragement. A negative d means that the more a student would study when not encouraged, the lower he or she would score without studying and without encouragement." (Holland, 1988a, p. 469). If "students who tend to study a lot tend to be those who do well even when they don't study, then d is positive but if those who study a lot are those who need to study, then d is negative." In other words the d parameter represents how a student's predisposition to studying is related to his or her test performance. Given these results, the a path corresponds to p, the b path corresponds to $b + d$, and the c' path corresponds to $c' - dp$. Note that a positive d reduces c' and a negative d increases c'. If d is equal to zero, where the tendency to study when not encouraged is unrelated to test score without studying and without encouragement, then the coefficients a, b, and c' reflect causal effects given the assumptions of the ALICE model.

An estimate the causal effect of encouraged activity is obtained by assuming that c' is zero and using an instrumental variables approach. The total effect of X on Y is then equal to $\hat{a}\hat{b}$ and the $\hat{b}$ coefficient is equal to $\hat{c}/\hat{a}$. This approach does not assume that d is zero but it does require the exclusion restriction that c' is equal to zero.

In summary, the causal inference problem is in the interpretation of the mediation relation between M and Y because levels of M are not randomly assigned. A researcher does not know the relation of M to Y for treated subjects if they were not given the treatment. Similarly, the researcher does not know the M to Y relation for controls if given the treatment. Similarly, the causal effect of X to Y adjusted for M is not known for either group.

Sobel (1998) extended the RCM in two ways. First, he outlined an instrumental variable procedure following Holland that does not make as strict a constant effects assumption (Sobel, in press). Second, he outlined the difficulties with causal inference for the case of multiple mediators. Causal interpretation with multiple mediators is more complex because of the unknown counterfactual relations of M to Y and X to Y adjusted for other mediators. Counterfactual relations for the multiple mediators as well as

Y must be considered. The assumption that the direct effect is zero in the multiple mediator model simplifies the interpretation of this model somewhat, but having no counterfactual relations among the multiple mediators is problematic. Theory and sequential randomization designs may be useful here to uncover causal relations among mediators. Random assignment of participants to receive different program components targeting different mediators in an instrumental variable approach may help clarify the mediating mechanisms operating in a multiple mediator study.

13.11 Principal Stratification and Other Extensions of the RCM

Frangakis and Rubin (2002) and Rubin (2004) described a new approach to dealing with the ambiguity regarding the relation of M to Y in the mediation model. The approach applies the notion of counterfactual or potential outcomes to the relation between M and Y and specifies stratifications of different types of units regarding how the relation between M and Y would change in response to the treatment X. These models specify different subsets of persons in terms of how they would respond under different conditions. Because the principal stratifications are in terms of potential outcomes, they are uncorrelated with treatment and can be used as a covariate in statistical analysis. The approach is based on an instrumental variables method in the RCM as in Angrist et al. (1996).

Rubin (2004) described an interesting example in which the effects of an anthrax vaccine were examined in macaques and humans. In the macaque sample, macaques were either vaccinated or not, a surrogate measure of immunogenicity (immunity to disease) was obtained, and then the macaques were exposed to anthrax virus and whether the macaque lived or died was recorded. The humans provided measures of vaccination or not and immunogenicity. The purpose of the study was to use the results from the macaques, which include measures of X, M, and Y, to infer the results of humans who have measures of only X and M. Rubin demonstrated that unobserved strata of units that may have different relations of vaccination to immunogenicity to disease introduces problems in the interpretation of direct and indirect effects. Three strata were described in the study: (a) macaques who have low immunogenicity whether vaccinated or not, (b) macaques who, if exposed to the vaccine, would change from low to high immunogenicity, and (c) macaques who would have high immunogenicity whether vaccinated or not. Rubin demonstrated that different patterns of response of the three strata in this case lead to different conclusions about direct and indirect effects than the conclusions reached based on observed data. The results from an analysis of the observed data would lead to different conclusions than the truth because information on potential outcomes based on types of individuals was not included in the analysis of observed data.

Frangakis and Rubin (2002) described a principal stratification example for patients with HIV infection and treatment to affect CD4 counts (CD4 is a measure of immunity) using four strata: (a) CD4 is low and unaffected by treatment, (b) CD4 is high and unaffected by treatment, (c) CD4 under new treatment would be higher than that with no treatment, and (d) CD4 under new treatment would be lower than with no treatment. Rubin (2004) and Frangakis and Rubin (2002) suggested that potential outcomes can be introduced into the analysis by imputation of potential outcomes, which can be used to generate principal strata. The imputation method produces the correct average estimate along with an estimate of the error of the estimate. Rubin described several additional assumptions and exclusion restrictions that will increase the accuracy of the imputation method. Principal stratification is a most promising approach to causal relations in mediation models. Although it will be critical to assess the application of the model to real data, the key benefit of these models is how it improves understanding of mediated effects. It will also be critical to evaluate these models as assumptions are violated.

Jo (2004) extended the RCM to the mediator case by focusing on the relation between the mediator and the outcome by conceptualizing the counterfactual as a latent, unobserved, variable. The strategy is to estimate potential values of mediator variables if control group participants were assigned to the treatment. The potential value of the mediator variable in the control group can be treated as a continuous latent variable. Treating the counterfactual case as a latent variable is consistent with descriptions of the counterfactual. Jo (2006) used a principal stratification approach in the mediation analysis of a program hypothesized to increase mastery, which then improves mental health outcomes. Four principal strata were used including children who never improve, children who get worse, children who improve, and children who always improve. In this model there was evidence that increases in mastery led to reduced depression.

13.12 Additional Causal Inference Approaches

This chapter has focused on the RCM approach to causal inference because of its clear application to mediation models and the limited space to develop other models. Other causal inference approaches also provide useful interpretations of mediation models. Pearl (2000) has developed an important approach to causal inference based on a method of identifying causal relations among variables on the basis of directional separation. The purpose of this approach is to determine which relations merit causal interpretation based on evidence from data. Directional separation (d-separation) refers to whether two variables are statistically independent after control for other variables. A variable is called a parent if it is a cause of another variable and if it is caused by another variable it is called a child. A cause of a parent is called a grandparent and so on. Ancestors are the causes of a variable and descendents are the variables that a variable causes. Two focal variables become independent if the research controls a common cause that would otherwise produce a relation between the two variables. Hayduk et al. (2003) demonstrate that the d-separation method is closely related to the concept of partial correlation.

Another important approach described by Greenland and Robins (1986) has much in common with the RCM. The method also specifies all the possible combinations of effects in a research study including the counterfactual cases that are not observed, with attention devoted to the case of X, M, and Y all binary. These researchers have developed an approach to estimating parameters of these models that includes both observed and counterfactual observations using a method called G-estimation, which has been programmed in a SAS macro (Witteman et al., 1998; see also Fischer-Lapp & Goetghebeur, 1999). The approach clarifies distinctions among different types of confounding and mediating variables.

13.13 Equivalent Models

Meehl and Waller (2002) outlined the major criticisms of recursive structural equation approaches, which include the mediation model as a special case. These criticisms refer to violations of the major assumptions of recursive structural equation models (Freedman, 1987; James, Mulaik, & Brett, 1982) which are (a) linear causal relations, (b) no reciprocal feedback, (c) no causal loops, (d) uncorrelated disturbances, (e) manifest variables being direct measures of causal factors rather than proxies, (f) model self-containment, that is, all relevant variables are included in the model, and (g) manifest variables being perfectly reliable (Meehl & Waller, 2002). As described in chapter 3, it is often not possible to test the validity of these assumptions. Some authors suggested that because these assumptions are unreasonable and often untestable, these models should not be applied (Berk, 2003; Freedman, 1987) or should at least be accompanied by much more additional detective work related to the variables in the model. In general, the criticisms demonstrate that estimates from structural equation models often do not represent causal relations, and it is incorrect to make causal interpretations from these models. This is the same distinction between descriptive and causal interpretations discussed in the RCM.

An example of such a criticism is that the mediation model methods based on the traditional regression and structural equation approach do not reflect a causal analysis of the relationships among variables. For example, if X (independent variable), M (mediator), and Y (dependent variable) are measured simultaneously, there are other equivalent models (e.g., X is the mediator of the M to Y relationship or M and Y both cause X) that could explain the data equally well, and it is not possible to distinguish these alternatives without more information (Duncan, 1975; MacKinnon, Krull, & Lockwood, 2000; Spirtes, Glymour, & Scheines, 1993). The different models may each adequately represent the data, but these equivalent models may suggest different conclusions than the final model obtained in a research project (MacCallum, Wegener, Uchino, & Fabrigar, 1993; Stelzl, 1986). Procedures for generating these equivalent models have been outlined (Lee & Hershberger, 1990). Similar criticisms of structural equation models have been made on the basis of mathematical and philosophical approaches to causality, and a computer program that will generate these equivalent models is available (Spirtes et al., 1993). Researchers typically address these equivalent models with randomization of units to levels of X, longitudinal data, and theory for the order of X, M, and Y. Nevertheless, consideration of equivalent models is critical in the evaluation of any mediation model. These equivalent models may actually provide insight into the true mediational process by forcing researchers to consider other, perhaps more accurate, representations of relations among variables. Several computer programs now allow the investigation of equivalent models. The AMOS program will test models by randomly switching the position of variables in the model. The TETRAD program will generate equivalent models as part of a principled search strategy (Scheines, Spirtes, Glymour, & Meek, 1994). The authors state that "All of its search procedures are `pointwise consistent`—they are guaranteed to converge almost certainly to correct information about the true structure in the large sample limit, provided that structure and the sample data satisfy various commonly made (but not always true!) assumptions."

13.14 Summary

The purpose of this chapter was to outline the RCM approach to causal inference in mediation models. The model demonstrates the problems in the interpretation of the relation between M and Y in mediation models, at least in part because this relation is not randomized but is self-selected in most applications. The main benefit of all these detailed causal approaches is the careful consideration of the limitations and strengths of different types of evidence for causal inference. However, there are criticisms of these detailed causal modeling approaches, which are best summarized in the title of an article by Berk (1991), "Toward a Methodology for Mere Mortals." With such extensive criteria for establishing causal relations, can any research study ever demonstrate a causal relation? The extra criteria may drastically reduce power to detect effects even in large samples. Another question is whether these criteria are necessary for obtaining useful research results that can be used to develop better research manipulations and to inform subsequent studies. At a minimum, the causal inference approaches force researchers to consider the assumptions under which mediation is investigated. For the most part, the sensitivity of the estimates to violation of assumptions is not generally known, and at least one study of other instrumental variable approaches demonstrated that they are not robust to violation of important assumptions (Stolzenberg & Relles, 1990). It would seem that analysis of sensitivity to violation of assumptions would differ greatly across research areas. More work is needed on approaches to assess robustness of results to confounding variables. Rosenbaum (2002b) describes a method to assess what the impact would have to be to alter inference about a relation (see also Frank, 2000 and Lin, Psaty, & Kronmal, 1998). At this point, these methods are complex and their application is challenging for most researchers. This chapter may help start more applications of these models. The next chapter provides some additional methods to help address some of the limitations described in this chapter.

13.15 Exercises

13.1. The simulation program described in chapter 4 can be extended to study the d parameter described in section 13.10. Add an additional simulation parameter called d to reflect the counterfactual relation between M and Y. In the section in which data are generated, include $c' - da$ instead of the c' parameter and $b + d$ instead of the b parameter. Conduct simulations with a positive value of delta of +2 and –2. How do the results change as a function of sample size? How do the results change as a function of the size of the b parameter?

13.2. For the single mediator model, summarize Holland's use of the RCM.

13.3. Apply the steps in Table 13.1 to your own data.

13.4. Discuss the reasonableness of the assumptions of the instrumental variable methods. Does it make sense to you that the predicted value of M by X is a valid way to assess the relation of M to Y? Why or why not?

13.5. List the equivalent models for the multiple mediator model described in chapter 5 and the path analysis model described in chapter 6.

13.6. The Angrist, Imbens, and Rubin (1996) paper assumed there are four types of persons in a compliance study: (a) complier—always complies with the treatment if in the program group, (b) never taker—never takes the treatment in the program group, (c) defier—would have received the treatment if had the control but would not have received the treatment if in the program group, and (d) always taker—always takes the treatment in the treatment group. It is often assumed that there are no defiers when applying these models. Do you think that assumption is always justified? What is one example for which that assumption is not justified?

14

Additional Approaches to Identifying Mediating Variables

> In the end, even the randomized experiment requires subjective decisions on the part of the researcher. This is why the independent replication of experiments in different locations using slightly different environmental or experimental conditions and therefore having different sets of ancillary assumptions is so important. As the causal hypothesis continues to be accepted in these new experiments, it becomes less and less reasonable to suppose incorrectly that auxiliary assumptions are conspiring to give the illusion of correct causal hypothesis.
>
> **—Bill Shipley, 2000, p. 53**

14.1 Overview

The purpose of this chapter is to describe additional methods to investigate mediating variables. Five major overlapping approaches are described in this chapter: (a) mediation designs, (b) mediation meta-analysis, (c) moderator and mediator models revisited, (d) qualitative methods, and (e) exploratory methods. A recurring theme of this book is that the identification of mediational processes is best addressed by programs of research that incorporate information from many different types of studies. These additional methods add evidence for mediational processes and help rule out alternative explanations of an observed mediation effect.

14.2 Mediation Designs

One of the best ways to investigate mediational processes is to conduct a program of research that includes research designs that directly test a mediation hypothesis (Shadish & Cook, 1999). The theme of the following discussion is that every study provides information on mediational processes. The quality of information about mediating processes differs across studies on the basis of the design of the study and assumptions of the analysis. This chapter describes the same general approach to design outlined in Shadish, Cook, and Campbell (2002; see also Cronbach, 1982). In general, the approach considers threats to the conclusions of a mediation analysis of a research study. There are two general aspects to validity of the conclusions from a research study. Internal validity refers to the extent to which the conclusions from a study are correct given other alternative explanations. Example alternative explanations are that observed changes are due to maturation of participants or nonrandom selection of participants in research groups. External validity is the second major aspect of design that refers to the extent to which the results from one study may be generalized to another group of persons, in a different context, at a different time. Research results may not be externally valid because they are unique to an age group or special context and as a result may not be obtained in a subsequent study with a sample having different characteristics.

In the following sections, less rigorous designs are described first followed by designs more likely to provide accurate information about mediational processes. Research designs in which an independent variable represents exposure to one or more experimental manipulations are given priority in the description of designs. To conserve space the independent variable is represented by X, the mediator by M, and the dependent variable by Y. The word *intervention* is used as a general term to describe any experimental manipulation or assignment to the conditions of a study.

Analysis for Correlational Studies of the M to Y and X to M Relations. Cross-sectional, correlational studies relating M to Y (and also X to M) can provide insight about whether M is related to Y (and whether X is related to M). In general, however, it is difficult to determine the direction of influence from cross-sectional studies (i.e., whether the M predicts Y or vice versa), as described in chapter 8. In addition, covariation between M and Y (or between X and M) may be due to another variable that is not measured but predicts both variables. Therefore, correlational studies provide limited information on the relation of M to Y or X to M because of the number of alternative explanations of any observed relations among variables.

Analysis of a Single Group Design. In this design all participants receive the same intervention, with assessment of M and Y before and after the intervention. The single group design allows for the assessment of change in M and Y. However, in the absence of a control or comparison group, it is difficult to establish whether any change in M or Y is due to the intervention. Several variables within the person and outside of the person could account for observed change across time (Cook & Campbell, 1979) and without a comparison group, these possibilities cannot be ruled out.

Measures of exposure to the intervention can be used to obtain some information on mediating variables (Weiss, 1997). One type of exposure study involves different exposure to the levels of X. In this situation, exposure is analogous to the dose of X. For example, assume that the intervention consists of a 10-session drug prevention program in which participants do not attend all sessions so that variation in session attendance may be considered a measure of the dose of the program. In this situation, X is a continuous measure of the amount of program exposure. An analysis of covariance adjusted for baseline values of M and Y or a difference score between baseline and follow-up analysis with program exposure as X may provide information on whether or not variation in exposure changed M which then changed drug use. Here, instead of an intervention effect for the c parameter in Equation 3.1 (and c' in Equation 3.2), the parameter codes an implementation effect. Although this analysis may appear to eliminate some problems associated with the lack of a control group, the results are still very difficult to interpret clearly. A positive relation between attendance (dose) and the dependent variable (and mediators) may be the result of other factors such as reporting bias. One common confounding influence is that motivation may strongly influence self-selection into program attendance. Furthermore, when amount of exposure is used to predict both the change in the mediator and the change in the outcome, the direction of the relation between the mediator and outcome is difficult to determine. A method based on instrumental variables described in chapter 13 may be relevant, but assumptions of this method may be violated such as the exclusion restriction, leading to inaccurate estimates of mediated effects. Continuous dose variables may be obtained from sources other than from the participant. For example, teachers may provide intervention exposure information based on participant attendance records. The same limitations of self-reported dosage apply to teacher exposure measures because the reports may be positively or negatively biased. In both cases of exposure, it may be possible to set up propensity scores for dosage as described by Rosenbaum (2002a; 2002b). In these models, the predictors of the propensity to receive a dosage are incorporated in the analysis. However, it may be difficult to accurately specify the propensity score model, and to date there have been few applications of the method for other than a binary X.

Another alternative is to evaluate mediated effects in a single group design and test comparison or control M or Y variables. These variables are selected so that they would be affected by the same response biases as targeted M and Y variables but are not expected to be affected by X. If the mediated effect is stronger for the targeted mediation relation than for the comparison variables, there is additional evidence for the mediation relation. For example, consider an intervention designed to reduce test anxiety. The targeted mediator is teaching students to learn to relax while taking the exam. The mediating measure of relaxation is a self-report of calmness during the exam. A comparison mediator could be self-report of happiness during the exam. A comparison Y variable could be a measure of social anxiety that is not expected to be affected by changes in relaxation during the exam. The evidence for mediation should be stronger for the relaxation mediator than for the happiness mediator if relaxation during the exam does lead to less test anxiety. If the only influence in the study is a response bias to respond favorably to all variables, then the evidence for mediation should be similar for both mediators and both dependent variables. The comparison variable approach suggests that researchers should routinely consider variables that address alternative explanations of any observed mediation effects.

Analysis of Multiple Interventions Without a Control Group. Another design without a control group is the situation in which more than one intervention is evaluated in a single study. For example, assume that three different interventions are delivered to three groups for which, ideally, each intervention targets one or more different mediators. Here, examination of the mediated effect across groups is of interest as a way to test the theory underlying each of the three programs. The significant mediated effects are ideally those predicted by theory before the study began. In this case, X represents group membership so it is not continuous (although it may be continuous if group membership reflects a quantitative variable). For a three-group study, one option is to specify two independent variables to code group membership, with contrast (or dummy) codes comparing pairs of groups. In the three-group case, there are separate X to M effects, a_1 and a_2, for each independent variable. For example, the code for a_1 could be 1 for group 1, –1 for group 2, and 0 for group 3. The other contrast code for a_1 could be 1 for group 1, 0 for group 2, and –1 for group 3. Ideally, these contrast codes would reflect meaningful comparisons among the groups. However, this design would have the same difficulties in interpretation that are common to all designs in which there is no control group to compare with the experimental groups. If there are no significant differences among the groups, it may be that none of the interventions worked or it could be that the interventions had equivalent effects. However, mediated effects can generally be compared across groups, and different hypothesized mediated effects across groups may provide more compelling evidence for specific mediational processes.

An example of multiple interventions without a control group is Project MATCH, which was a large scale evaluation in which three treatments were matched to alcohol-dependent persons based on client characteristics. The three treatments were a 12-Step program, a motivational interviewing program, and a cognitive behavioral therapy program. At the end of the study the programs were not significantly different on most measures, and there was no extensive evidence for a matching effect. The extent to which each program targeted specific mediators could be investigated (Longabaugh & Writz, 2001). Some of the mediators were working alliance between the client and therapist, amount of structure in treatment, amount of treatment offered, and treatment emphasis on psychology. The results of mediation analyses were equivocal, at least in part because modern approaches to assess mediation were not applied and the importance of investigating mediation was not widely known when the study was designed, so measures of many potential mediating variables were not included (Longabaugh & Writz, 2001, pp. 323–324). A further issue in this type of study is the number and conceptual overlap of the mediators. For example, all interventions may target one mediator but other interventions may target one or more different mediators, which may require more comprehensive models in an attempt to tease out the specific mediated effects for each intervention.

Analysis of a Single Intervention and a Control Group. The comparison of an intervention group and a control group is the most common type of research design. It is the design described in most of this book, and it has strengths and limitations as do all the other designs. Adding a control group with which to compare the intervention group improves the validity of the research conclusions from a study. The control group provides a measure of the effect if the intervention group was left untreated, as described in chapter 13. Ideally the program would be based on theory such that the program components target specific mediators so that each mediated effect can be tested. It is also ideal if measures of mediators are included that should not be affected by the intervention but should be affected by other explanations of mediation effects—the aforementioned comparison variables. For example, a measure of response bias may be useful to demonstrate that it does not serve as a mediator of the effect of an intervention on a self-report outcome measure.

An example of the program versus control group mediation design is the Midwestern Prevention Project (MPP), based on social cognitive theory. The MPP (Pentz et al., 1989) targeted two potential mediators of drug use (a) perceptions of friends' reactions to drug use and (b) beliefs about the positive consequences of drug use. The program consisted of 10 sessions to correct normative expectations and change beliefs. Forty-two middle schools were assigned to either the control or treatment group. Mediation analysis allowed the investigators to evaluate whether both, one, any, all, or none of the mediator variables explained the program effect. For example, there was evidence that changes in perceptions of friends' tolerance mediated the program effects on drug use.

Mediation analyses are important whether there was an intervention effect on the outcome or not. Using a drug prevention example, if the intervention effect was explained by one or more of the mediators, there should be increases in mediators, indicating that the program did in fact change the mediator (action theory), which would affect the outcome for the experimental group (conceptual theory). In this case, perceptions of friends' tolerance of drug use decreased (action theory), indicating that the program was effective in changing the mediator and the decrease in friends' tolerance decreased drug use (conceptual theory), supporting the social cognitive theory of the program. Analogous results were obtained for positive consequences. An ideal subsequent study would attempt to manipulate perception of friends' tolerance in isolation and observe resulting effects on drug use.

When critical mediating processes are identified, then the intervention can be improved by focusing on the most effective components and removing ineffective or even counterproductive components. If none of the mediated effects were significant, yet the program was effective in reducing drug use, this would inform the researcher that some other, unmeasured, mediational processes (e.g., attention that the experimental group received) may explain the effect. In any case, applying mediation analysis to the program can guide future research (MacKinnon, 1994).

Analysis of Multiple Interventions and a Control Group. An ideal study has several interventions based on different theories regarding Y along with a control group. Using drug prevention as an example, one program might target social norms, another program might focus on teaching resistance skills, and a third program might attempt to increase knowledge of the health consequences of drug use. A fourth group, a control group, would be included to control for the general changes in the outcome and mediator variables over time. Again, X would be changed to reflect contrasts among groups. One ideal strategy is to select dummy codes such that each intervention group is compared with the control group. In this case of four groups, three dummy codes would be used in the mediation model.

A multiple program design can be informative, but one potential problem is that program components are often related and work together to affect the outcome or have interactive effects on the outcome. For example, it is possible that none of the aforementioned interventions—the social norms program, the resistance skills program, or the knowledge of health consequences program—is able to affect the outcome independently, but they are effective when combined in one program. Perhaps knowledge of health consequences helps the adolescent want to improve resistance skills and knowing the real social norms makes knowledge of health consequences easier to absorb. To better understand the processes by which programs have their effects, more complicated designs can be used. However, multiple program designs can be informative especially if there are theoretical reasons to believe that one program would be more effective or work in a different way than another program. Finally, this design can also be used to examine competing theories of the outcome. In fact, mediation analyses are most compelling when alternative theories predict different mediational pathways for program effects on drug use. For example, Hansen and Graham (1991) found evidence for the efficacy of the norm-setting mediator but not the resistance skills mediator after experimental manipulation of both norms and skills in a drug prevention study. Similarly, social influence approaches have been more successful than affective based programs such as improving self-esteem (Flay, 1985).

Although a control group improves the validity of the study, how units are assigned to groups is critical. For example, if adolescents self-selected into the experimental group and the control group were taken from the remaining population, covariates such as socioeconomic status (SES) and baseline drug use may explain any changes in drug use. These and other nonequivalencies between the control and experimental groups can potentially bias the measure of a program effect. Measuring any potential covariates before program implementation can potentially reduce some of the bias that can occur as a result of nonrandomized assignment to groups. It may be possible to use these covariates to obtain more accurate estimates of effects using propensity scoring methods (Rosenbaum, 2002b). Propensity scores for each person are obtained by using background and other variables to predict group membership. The effect of the experimental manipulation is examined at each level of the propensity score. Under certain assumptions, such as accurate propensity scores, these methods yield accurate tests of conditions, but there are difficulties with this approach (McCaffrey, Ridgeway, & Morral, 2004). Nevertheless, the ideal situation is to randomly assign a large number of units to the experimental and control groups to minimize nonequivalence on any covariates.

Examination of Intervention Components. Once an intervention is found to be successful, it is reasonable to conduct further research to identify the most powerful components of the intervention. Two designs are discussed here: dismantling and constructive research strategies (West & Aiken, 1997; West, Aiken, & Todd, 1993). With the dismantling strategy, the full intervention is compared with a version of the intervention in which at least one component is removed. In this strategy, the presumption is that the component that is removed may not contribute any positive change in the desired Y or may even produce change in the undesired direction. With the constructive research strategy, the full manipulation or a reduced version of the manipulation is compared with a version(s) of the program that has the additional component(s). In this case, the interest is in examining the increase in the effects of the added components above and beyond the effects of the base program. It is important to consider that the original program may be so effective that additional program components are unlikely to improve effects if the new components affect the same mediating variables addressed in the original program. The same methods of analysis would hold for both strategies, with strategies being distinguishable only by which program is designated as the full program and the research question. Both strategies are used to answer questions about the incremental success of individual program components (Kazdin, 1998). Such designs are useful in terms of cost-benefit analyses to make decisions about adding and deleting program components (West & Aiken, 1997). They also facilitate decisions about components to be included in an intervention instituted by an agency after the intervention trial phase of the program (Sussman, 2001).

Separate program components may each have an impact on only one mediating variable. In this case, program components are orthogonal. However, a single program component is likely to affect more than one mediator and a single mediator may be influenced by more than one program component. When a single program component is intended to influence a single mediator but has unintended influences on other mediators, sequential random assignment to program components may clarify results. For example, in the first week of a program, subjects are randomly assigned to receive the first component or not. During the second week, subjects receiving the first component are randomly assigned to receive the second component or not, and so on. The analysis of this design would be similar to the method described for the analysis of multiple program groups with a control group. In this case, contrasts between groups may be useful to clarify the importance of added components.

As it is possible for program components to overlap, program mediators may be nonorthogonal as well. There are examples of correlated mediators in most research areas. For example, a drug prevention intervention that only targets drug refusal self-efficacy may also have an impact on norms regarding drugs. However, change in both of these mediators would be difficult to interpret in the single component framework. In this hypothetical example, the program may affect both mediators or change in social norms may lead to change in perceived parental approval. In this case, a constructive research strategy comparing a self-efficacy only component, a social norm plus a self-efficacy component, and an equivalent no-treatment group might offer a solution for disentangling this problem of interpreting intervention effects with correlated mediators and correlated components.

Mediation Links in Multiple Mediator Models. A multiple mediator analysis will typically lead to a smaller number of significant mediators. As described in chapter 13, because the relations among the mediators and the relations from the mediators to the outcome are correlational, there are many potential models for the true relations among the variables, including one in which the dependent variable affects the mediator. In this context, if a mediator that does not provide a significant mediated effect, it suggests that this mediator may not be important. The lack of a significant effect should be further examined for the source of the lack of significance. If the link from X to M is nonsignificant, this suggests that the independent variable is not related to the mediator, but if the effects of X on Y were significant, then there is evidence that this mediator was not a significant mediator of the program. It is also possible that the mediator was not measured well enough for an effect to be statistically significant. If there was another dependent variable with the same reliability for which the mediator was statistically significant, then it is less likely that poor measurement would explain the lack of a mediated effect on the first dependent variable. This specificity of the mediated effect for one dependent variable but not another increases the likelihood that a real mediator has been found. Similarly, if one potential mediating variable does not mediate a relation but another mediator does, this increases the likelihood that the mediator is a real one. In some situations it may be useful to include mediators that assess plausible alternative explanations (for examples for fear appeals, see Leventhal, 1971). These comparison mediators, or mediators that, if significant, would represent alternative explanations of the results, may be especially useful to disentangle more complicated multiple mediator models. For example, in a program designed to change norms, a mediator reflecting skills should not be statistically significant. A measure of acquiescence bias (increased likelihood of agreeing with all statements) should not serve as a mediator unless participants do indeed tend to respond yes to all questions and that is the explanation of program effects.

If the relation of X to M is significant but the M to Y relation is not, then the possible function of the mediator in a chain of mediation should be examined by considering and estimating additional models whereby the mediator is a link in such a chain. If the mediator is not significantly related to other mediators, then it may not be part of a chain of mediators, however. An alternative explanation is that the mediator is not related to the dependent variable. The single mediator model described earlier is easily expanded to include a chain of mediating variables. In fact, most mediating variables are actually part of a longer theoretical mediational chain (Cook & Campbell, 1979). For example, a research study may measure each of the four constructs in a theoretical chain from exposure to a prevention program, to comprehension of the program, to short-term attitude change, to change in social norms, and, finally, to change in the dependent variable. Typically, researchers measure an overall social norms mediator rather than all mediators in the chain, even though a more detailed chain is theorized.

The single mediator methods can also be extended to multiple mediators and multiple outcomes with correspondingly more mediated effects as described in chapter 6. Multiple mediator models are often justified because most independent variables have effects through multiple mediating processes. The true causal relations are difficult to disentangle in this model because of the number of potential alternative relations among variables. One solution to the problems inherent in the causal interpretation of multiple as well as single mediator models is to view the identification of mediating variables as a sustained research effort requiring a variety of experimental and nonexperimental approaches to identifying mediating variables. The analysis of multiple mediators in one study informs the design of randomized experiments to contrast alternative mediating variables, leading to refined understanding of mediating processes (West & Aiken, 1997). Meta-analytical studies provide information about the consistency of mediating variable effects across many situations (Cook et al., 1992).

Double Randomization. In this design, participants are randomly assigned to an intervention targeting a certain mediator and after assignment to intervention conditions and after the intervention has affected the mediator, there is random assignment within groups to an intervention that will change the same mediator. Triple and quadruple randomization may be applied in the same manner. Given certain assumptions described in chapter 13, valid estimates of program effects on the mediator and the dependent variable can be obtained and valid estimates of the mediator effects on the outcome can be obtained because participants were randomly assigned to levels of the mediator within each group. This type of design may not be realistic in many studies, for which the goal of the research is to deliver a single powerful program. However, the delivery of most interventions has an inherent ordering because not all interventions can be delivered at once. The timing of the delivery of these components could be incorporated in these models in a way to provide more accurate information about program mediators and components.

In some designs it may be possible to investigate a mediational process by a randomized experiment to investigate the X to M relation and a second randomized experiment to investigate the M to Y relation (MacKinnon, Lockwood, Hoffman, West & Sheets, 2002; Spencer, Zanna, & Fong, 2005; West & Aiken, 1997). Spencer et al. (2005) recently summarized two experiments reported by Word, Zanna, and Cooper (1974) that executed this design in a study of self-fulfilling prophecy for racial stereotypes. In study 1, White participants were randomly assigned to interview a Black or White confederate. Using measures from the participants, Black applicants received less immediacy, higher rates of speech errors, and shorter interviews than White applicants. This part of the study demonstrated that race of applicant (X) significantly affected interview quality (M). In Study 2, confederate White interviewers interviewed the participants. The confederate interviewers either gave interviews like White applicants were given in Study 1, or they interviewed applicants with less immediacy, higher rates of speech errors, and shorter amounts of interviewer time, like Black applicants received. Here the M variable, type of interview, was randomized and the behavior of the applicants, the Y variable, was measured. The results of Study 2 indicated that participants treated like Blacks in Study 1 performed less adequately and were more nervous in the interview than participants treated like Whites in Study 1. So randomized experimental evidence was obtained for the relation of race (X) on interview quality (M) and the relation of interview quality (M) on applicant performance (Y).

A hypothetical example in prevention research would be an intervention to increase exercise to reduce obesity among adolescents. An experimental investigation would study the X to M relation by randomly assigning persons to a norm change manipulation to increase exercise, measured by the number of steps taken each day. The M to Y relation would be randomized by randomly assigning persons to increase the number of steps exactly equal to the effect of the intervention in the X to M study. Such a study may be unrealistic because of the difficulty of directly assigning persons to increase the number of steps.

Although double randomization experiments do much to reduce alternative explanations of the mediation hypothesis, it may be difficult to implement the design in practice. Generally the most difficult aspect of the design is randomly assigning participants to the levels of the mediator so that the M to Y part of the relation can be studied experimentally. It is also interesting to note that a statistical mediation analysis may be relevant in the M to Y study because the manipulation to directly change M may not be perfectly successful.

Designs to Replicate and Extend a Mediational Hypothesis. This section describes five different types of experimental designs to investigate mediational hypothesis outlined by Mark (1986). In general these designs are used to seek further evidence for a mediational hypothesis using a randomized design. The first type of design is a direct observation method to directly observe the mediational process by measuring the mediator and conducting mediation analysis. This approach has been the primary approach of this book. Both the statistical methods described in this book and qualitative methods may be used to directly investigate the process. One assumption of this approach discussed in chapter 13 is that the relation of M to Y represents a real causal relation so that other studies that directly change M will lead to a change in Y.

The second experimental design is called a blockage design. In this design, a manipulation is used to block the mediational process. If the intervention to block the mediation process removes the mediation relation, then there is evidence for the mediational process. For example, consider a mediation hypothesis that exercise increases endorphins, which then decreases depression. A blockage study would have persons randomly assigned to either an experimental group that receives a drug that blocks the production of endorphins or to a control group that does not receive the drug to block endorphins. Reduced depression should be observed in the control group but not in the group that received the drug if exercise reduces depression by increasing endorphins. Another hypothetical example of the blockage design is from a study to investigate the extent to which an intervention to reduce drug use works by changing social norms through contact among friends. Persons receiving the intervention may be randomly assigned to a condition in which contact among friends was eliminated or to a control condition that allowed regular contact among friends. If social norms among friends is the mediator of the drug prevention program, then reduced drug use should be observed in the control group but not in the group in which norm change was not possible because of lack of contact among friends.

A third type of mediation replication study is called an enhancement study. This design is similar to the blockage study except that mediation effects are expected to be enhanced in certain groups. For example, consider that a research study of medical care evaluations found more beneficial effects for patients in locations where there was more discussion of patients and problems (Maxwell, Bashook, & Sandlow, 1986). However, the level of discussion was not randomly assigned in the original investigation so the relation between discussion and the outcome is correlational. Imagine a follow-up study in which the amount of discussion was randomly assigned to each location, perhaps by paying medical personal to spend more time discussing patients. If the discussion is an important mediational process, then the largest beneficial effects should be obtained in the group randomly assigned to receive the most discussion. A similar study was conducted by Klesges, Vasey, and Glasgow (1986) in which participation was considered an important mediator of antismoking campaigns. Klesges et al. designed strategies to increase participation in some locations. A hypothetical enhancement design to investigate whether social support is an important mediator of addiction treatment may randomly assign participants to a condition for which social support is enhanced by increasing contact with persons or to another group that would have standard contact among persons.

A fourth type of model is the purification approach whereby repeated mediation studies are used to develop the best possible intervention. In purification studies important mediators are typically selected and replication studies with these mediators are conducted to increase powerful components and remove ineffective components. The analog in the biological research is studies to identify the active ingredient in a medicine. The purification approach requires a program of research that may be unrealistic in research contexts in which individual studies are excessively cumbersome or expensive to conduct. For example, in drug prevention studies, among the roughly 10 types of mediators targeted, there is evidence that changes in perceived positive consequences of drug use, social norms, and intentions to avoid drugs are important mediators. A purification approach would include programs of studies to help identify the critical ingredients of successful drug prevention.

A fifth approach, called pattern matching (Trochim, 1985), is the general approach of this book. The idea is to conduct research in many different contexts, in different types of interventions, at different times, and with different samples of participants to validate a mediational hypothesis. Pattern matching may be observed for multiple variables whereby a mediation relation is observed for one dependent variable but not another; for example, changes in beliefs about positive consequences of alcohol use is a mediator for program effects on alcohol but not for tobacco use. Similarly, a variable may function as a mediator and another variable that shares similar measurement biases may not; for example, beliefs about positive consequences of alcohol use is a mediator, but beliefs about negative consequences is not. Pattern matching for different settings also provides further evidence for a mediation theory, for example, an intervention designed to change norms should be more effective in settings in which norm change is more likely to occur. Another example of setting is demonstration of a mediation relation in animal research that is also present among humans. Different types of manipulations that target the same mediator should also lead to the same change on an outcome variable if the mediation theory is correct. Mediation relations may be expected to occur in some samples and not others, which may provide further evidence for a mediation relation. Overall, the goal of the pattern matching is to design studies whereby the process has different patterns of prediction. Pattern matching may be most appropriate in situations for which it is easier to conduct a variety of studies. For example, research in college settings may be well suited to study variations in intervention design and specified mediation relations but may not be ideal for assessing mediated relations in older persons or other groups of persons who may be ideal to test the external validity of mediation relations.

Summary of Mediation Designs. The design of a mediation study leads to different information about mediation relations. It is the quality of information that varies across research studies. The ideal design would include random assignment to conditions, theoretically specified mediating mechanisms targeted that differ across interventions, longitudinal measurement, and good measures of mediating and outcome variables. The use of comparison mediators, mediators that should not change but address alternative mediational hypotheses, and randomization of the levels of the mediator may also improve the conclusions from a research study. Replication studies also provide additional evidence that an observed relation is not due to chance, especially when the mediated effect is replicated by different researchers, in different contexts, and for different measures (Rosenbaum, 2001). It is important to note also that many of the designs to investigate mediation will yield data useful for a statistical mediation analysis.

14.3 Combining Moderators and Mediators

As described in chapter 10, moderator variables alter the strength of the relation between two other variables and can also alter the strength of the relations in a mediation model. In the context of program evaluation, it is possible that the program did not have a consistent mediation effect across particular subgroups (e.g., age, gender, ethnicity, SES, or program implementation) or across preintervention variables that affect mediators as well as outcome variables (Morgan-Lopez, Castro, Chassin, & MacKinnon, 2003; Tein, Sandler, MacKinnon, & Wolchik, 2004). Moderator effects may provide further evidence for mediational processes if mediated effects differ across subgroups that differ on the baseline measure of the mediating variable. For example, more evidence of the effects of social norms as a mediator may be obtained if the size of the mediated effect depends on the baseline level of social norms. In particular, if the mediated effect is largest for those persons low on the mediator at baseline, this provides some additional evidence for the importance of that mediator. These mediated baseline by treatment interactions were described in chapter 10. However, these methods are problematic because the possible self-selection of treatment such that a moderator effect may represent different motivations among participants in a research study.

Combining variable-oriented with person-oriented methods is an example of the investigation of moderators and mediators. Recent developments in structural equation modeling with multiple time points allow for identification of classes of persons based on the change in the dependent variable over time (Nagin, 1999, 2005; Muthén & Muthén, 2004). These models mix person-oriented relations to form classes with variable-oriented relations among variables (i.e., mixture models). One way that these mixture models could be especially useful is in identifying persons based on trajectories, identifying mediation models within these groups, and then testing equality of mediation across groups. These types of models require care because the mediation effect is conditional on the classes obtained. The methods may also be especially susceptible to violations of assumptions such as non-normal data (Bauer & Curran, 2003).

An alternative mixture model approach would be to attempt to explain the classes of trajectories obtained with a mediating variable. The trajectories reflect classes of persons with similar trajectories of the variable across time. For example, consider an intervention that changes the trajectory class of heavy users of some drug. A mediation analysis may address which mediating variables changed by the intervention led to the change in the trajectory class of heavy users. This is similar to identifying classes based on predictor variables but here the focus would be to determine classes based on mediational processes. It is likely that the mediating variables themselves would also have to be changing over time to explain trajectories over time. These types of models are important for future development including investigation of whether these models may be particularly susceptible to the violation of assumptions.

14.4 Meta Analysis

One way to investigate mediational process is to conduct a systematic review of studies relevant to action and conceptual theory in a research area. In some situations, it is possible to quantify effect sizes for relations among variables such that a qualitative review can be combined with quantitative information about the consistency and size of effects across many studies. Meta-analysis (Hedges & Olkin, 1985), the methodology for combining of quantitative information across many studies, is an active area of methods development and substantive application for several reasons. Meta-analysis provides an objective way to combine information across many studies that has the promise of making research reviews into scientific studies in their own right. Meta-analyses can also show gaps in the research literature on certain topics. Although the characteristics of each study may differ, the combination of results from many studies may reveal consistent effects difficult to identify in a typical research review. In this way, the consistency of effects across many studies is explicitly investigated as urged by Shipley in the quote at the beginning of this chapter. Consistent results across many studies may also make it easier for effective interventions to be more widely disseminated because they help convince nonscientists to provide resources for treatments. For example, Shadish and Baldwin (2003) suggested that effective marriage and family counseling programs be classified as meta-analytically supported treatments (MASTs).

Generally, meta-analysis consists of five stages as summarized in Cook et al. (1992): (a) specification of the research problem, (b) identification of relevant research studies, (c) retrieval of data such as effect sizes from research studies, (d) analysis of data from studies and interpretation of results, and (e) public presentation in a research document. The common purpose of most meta-analyses is to synthesize effect sizes relating an independent variable to a dependent variable across many studies. The independent variable may be a type of intervention such as psychotherapy (Shadish, Matt, Navarro, & Phillips, 2000) or drug prevention (Tobler, 1986). The independent variable may also be exposure to advertisement (Brown & Stayman, 1992) or age (Verhaeghen & Salthouse, 1997). Examples of dependent variables are science achievement (Becker, 1992) and effect size for marriage and family therapy (Shadish & Baldwin, 2003). Meta-analysis is also used to find surrogate endpoints (Buyse, Molenberghs, Burzykowski, Renard, & Geys, 2000). Meta-analysis studies may also consider potential moderator variables such as research design, sample composition, and demographic variables.

Cook et al. (1992) argued that meta-analysis is useful for explanations of how or why variables are related in addition to whether results suggest consistent effects for a relation between an independent and dependent variable. In particular, several researchers have suggested that meta-analysis of mediating variables may be useful for identifying mediating processes by which an independent variable affects a dependent variable(Becker & Schram, 1994; Cook et al., 1992; Harris & Rosenthal, 1985; Shadish, 1996). The rationale here is that it may be reasonable to combine information across different studies to conduct a meta-analysis of relations among more than just an independent and a dependent variable. In the context of an intervention or treatment, the purpose of mediational meta-analysis is to determine the extent to which studies support conceptual and action theory for the intervention or treatment. That is, to identify successful mediating mechanisms by focusing both on how successful the programs are at changing mediators as well as the relation from the mediators to the outcome.

Because mediation involves at least two paths represented by the relations between X and M and M and Y, there are several challenges introduced in meta-analysis for mediational processes. Unlike meta-analysis of relations between an independent variable and a dependent variable, in which each individual study may provide one or more effect sizes, the studies of the relation between X and M may differ from the studies that examined the relation of M to Y. As a result, information for a mediational meta-analysis may consist of (a) within-study relations for the independent variable, mediator, and dependent variable. which are all collected in the same study and (b) across-study information, which is combined information on different parts of mediational relations from different studies. The potential limitations of across-study relations in meta-analysis reflect problems in comparing coefficients for X to M and M to Y obtained in different studies with different samples and other characteristics. There is also information on mediation relations within each study and also relations between studies where the studies are the unit of analysis. For example, whether an article is published or not is an example of a between-study variable. The sample size for between-study analysis of the published or not variable is the number of studies in the meta-analysis. An example of a within-study relation is the correlation between teacher expectancy and feedback in each study. The sample size for these relations is more complicated because the correlation obtained from each study is based on the sample size in that study. Both within and between relations could be examined in the same meta-analysis.

One example of the across-study approach was Harris and Rosenthal's (1985) examination of mediators of how expectations of high performance enhance performance in others, as discussed in chapter 4. Harris and Rosenthal conducted a meta-analysis of 135 studies of the expectancy phenomenon and documented at least 1 of 31 different behavioral variables related to the following four hypothesized explanations for the effect: (a) change in the social climate, (b) increased feedback from teachers, (c) more material taught, and (d) the tendency to give students more opportunities to respond. Some of the studies in the meta-analysis reported the results of a manipulation, and other studies reported correlations. The correlations were averaged across the studies. For climate, feedback, material taught, and response opportunities, the correlations for the $\hat{a}$ paths from teacher expectancy were 0.20, 0.13, 0.26, and 0.19 and for the $\hat{b}$ paths related to student performance were 0.36, 0.07, 0.33, and 0.20, respectively. A massive amount of research results were combined in this study.

Verhaeghen and Salthouse (1997) investigated a model for relations among age and five cognitive variables—speed of processing, primary working memory, episodic memory, reasoning, and spatial ability—from which the 15 correlations (Verhaeghen & Salthouse, 1997, Table 5) among these variables were obtained from 91 studies. Some studies produced more than one correlation for a relation, and the number of correlations for each of the 15 relations differed; for example, there were correlations from 22 studies for speed-working memory and 50 studies provided information for the age-speed relation. The correlations across studies were combined using a method described by Hedges and Olkin (1985). The method converts correlations to Fisher's z, the average Fisher's z is computed, and the z is then converted back to a correlation. The study combined an enormous amount of information from many different studies and generally showed that speed of processing and primary working memory were substantial mediators of the relation between age-related differences and other measures.

Shadish and colleagues (Shadish, 1996; Shadish & Sweeney, 1991; Shadish, Matt, Navarro, & Phillips, 2000) have provided leadership in the development and application of mediational meta-analysis. One primary focus of Shadish et al.'s work on mediational meta-analysis has been the meta-analysis of mediating mechanisms of psychotherapy. Shadish and Sweeney (1991) conducted a between-study analysis of data from 71 randomized studies comparing a treated group with a control group at posttest. The following data were collected from each of the 71 studies: behavioral orientation, treatment standardization, treatment implementation, behavior-dependent variable, dissertation status, and effect size. These data provided the information for a path analysis model. Of importance, the relation of behavioral orientation of therapy had a nonsignificant over-all effect but had an indirect effect through its effects on mediators. Later Shadish (1996) provided an example of an opposing mediational process such that behavioral orientation of therapy increases the likelihood of using behavior-dependent variables, which led to increased effect sizes. Studies of behavioral therapy are more likely to match participants to treatment before randomization, which led to reduced effects. There was evidence that both of these mediation effects were statistically significant but opposite in direction, leading to an overall nonsignificant effect. Cook et al. (1992) stated "it remains to be seen whether this (between-studies) strategy will prove to be useful in meta-analysis."

In summary, there are two types of data for mediational meta-analysis. One type of meta-analysis includes values of the $\hat{a}$ coefficient from stud-ies that may or may not also provide a $\hat{b}$ coefficient, or between-study comparisons. An alternative is to combine estimates of both $\hat{a}$ and $\hat{b}$ and consequently the mediated effect within studies. There are two types of relations investigated in mediation analysis, the within-study relations among variables exemplified by Harris and Rosenthal (1985) and Premack and Hunter (1988) and the between-study relations exemplified by Shad-ish (1996; Shadish & Sweeney, 1991).

There are several limitations to mediational meta-analysis. Probably the most important difficulty of meta-analytic studies of mediational processes is that relatively few studies include any mediation analysis, and thus few studies report information on relations for mediating vari-ables. Second, different studies often measure different mediators, and even when the same mediator is the focus of measurement, the actual measures are rarely the same. In some respects, the different measures of the same construct improve the generalizability of the results. There are also meta-analytic methods to assess whether it is reasonable to combine effect size measures from different studies as well as methods to allow for treating effects as random effects, which further increases the likeli-hood that results will generalize to other studies. Similarly, the number of relations obtained from each study may differ, creating a missing data problem for those studies that do not include measures of all variables of interest. Third, the values for paths from different studies may differ in many ways, other than simply sampling variability, making the interpretation of mediation effects somewhat suspect. It is also possible that for some studies unadjusted relations among variables are shown rather than results adjusted for other variables in the model, for example, the relation between M and Y adjusted for X. Fourth, the specified model may not be accurate, which is the same problem as with path analysis models described earlier in chapter 1. For any model, there may be many alternative models that may fit the data as well as or better than the specified model. Nevertheless, mediational meta-analysis provides a useful way to combine information across many studies. The inclusion of quantitative information with a qualitative review is likely to reveal more interesting results. As for any mediational analyses, it is important that individual studies report relations among variables that could be used for subsequent mediational analysis. At a minimum, values of $\hat{a}$, $\hat{b}$, $\hat{c}$, and $\hat{c}'$ along with their standard errors should be reported. Ideally the covariance matrix among variables is made available either in the article itself or by contacting authors of the article. Although there are problems with mediational meta-analysis, the promise of the method is substantial because it combines and organizes information from a variety of studies.

One of the ways in which methods in this book may improve mediation meta analysis is based on formulas for the standard error of the mediated effect. If the t values for paths in the model are available, it is possible to test the significance and create confidence limits for the mediated effect using any of the standard errors described in chapter 4 including the asymmetric confidence limits based on the distribution of the product. To illustrate this procedure using the Brown and Stayman (1992) article, the coefficient for the relation between advertisement cognitions and advertisement attitude was 0.52 ($t = 21.53$). The relation between advertisement attitude and brand attitude was 0.57 ($t = 25.58$). By using the multivariate delta standard error in Equation 3.7 rather than the distribution of the product because the t values are large, the lower confidence limit was 0.2611 and the upper confidence limit was 0.3316 for a mediated effect equal to 0.2964. The multilevel mediation models described in chapter 9 may be useful in that models for the between-study relations can be combined with models for the within-study relations as done by the Becker and colleagues in their meta-analysis (Becker, 1992; Becker & Schram, 1994).

Another important part of meta-analysis studies is the investigation of moderator variables, where the size of an effect depends on the level of a third variable. Meta-analytic studies that investigate moderators of effect sizes are more common than those for mediators of effects, at least in part because some moderators, such as sex and age, are more often measured. Once important moderator variables are identified in a meta-analysis, it is reasonable to then examine mediators that explain why the moderator effect is present. Application of models that included moderators and mediators can be applied to these studies.

14.5 Qualitative Approaches

Scientific innovations and explanations often arise from qualitative methods such as intuition, clinical skill, ethnography, and historical observation. Mediational theories start out as a qualitative idea that is translated into testing hypotheses using the methods described in this book. As the investigation of mediational processes becomes more precise from initial relations to complicated causal inference models, the actual results of a study may become less relevant to the real world, even though the veracity of the mediating mechanisms may be more clearly demonstrated. Qualitative methods are a useful addition to a quantitative mediation study to study processes in detail and provide a method to learn about unexpected effects (Maxwell, 2004). For example, providing an open-ended question about how an experimental intervention affects individuals may provide valuable information about the meaning and interpretation of the intervention by participants in the study. In particular, qualitative methods may provide valuable information if the process of an intervention differs from the researcher's expectation.

A recent paper on the evaluation of a HIV/AIDS prevention intervention illustrates the usefulness of open-ended questions (Dworkin, Exner, Melendez, Hoffman, & Ehrhardt, 2006). Interviews of study participants were conducted at the 1-year follow-up assessment. Open-ended questions were asked about how the study affected the participants' lives. Qualitative evidence for mediation was observed for several mediators, including increased susceptibility to HIV/sexually transmitted diseases, greater social support, openness to discuss sexual matters, and empowerment.

Cronbach (1982) most clearly stated this view of research when he argued that rigid experimental designs including those discussed throughout this book are rarely how actual evaluations of social and educational programs are conducted. The evaluation of these programs requires an ongoing interpretation and reinterpretation of the many effects of the intervention, effects that may have unexpected and unintended influences. A rigid design may be very ineffective in this context; these evaluations require vigilance by researchers to extract the most information from a research study. For example, Cronbach described how the evaluation of clinical observation of effective therapies also provides more information about mediational processes.

There are several useful approaches that incorporate qualitative information in a mediation analysis. As described by Crabtree and Miller (1999), qualitative data come from many disciplines and research traditions. Qualitative studies are generally of three types: (a) observational, (b) interview, and (c) material culture—based on materials such as newspapers and other documents. Observations include field studies in which the observer is also a participant in the study. As a participant, the researcher is in an ideal position to experience the intervention. A field observer attempts to identify the meaning of the processes in a research study with data obtained from diaries, recordings, and structured information such as checklists or unstructured information such as general impressions of persons in a research study. Interviews may be structured or unstructured and may consist of life histories, free associations, and open-ended surveys. In key informant interviews a small number of persons identified as critical to the research are interviewed in detail. Key informants may be considered experts in the description of the process of a research study. Material culture studies use archival information and documentation to identify themes and meanings. For example, the content of newspaper articles may be examined for attention to particular topics such as violence or drug overdose.

Thought listing, where participants write down their thoughts during the study, is a popular qualitative method for assessing mediation in marketing, social, and cognitive psychology. The contents of the listed thoughts are then organized and scored, and these scores are evaluated as mediators of effects. For example, in a study of the effects of warnings on alcohol advertisements, participants wrote down their thoughts as they waited to respond to a subsequent survey. These listed thoughts were then categorized by independent raters.

Focus groups are another source of important qualitative information on mediators. Participants in focus groups are generally selected on the basis of their interest in the topic of the focus group and representiveness of views on the topic. The moderator of the focus group is critical; acting as a moderator often requires skill both in the content of the focus group and understanding the appropriate methodology for successful focus groups such as ensuring that all members of the focus group are allowed to contribute. Focus groups are also used in the identification of potential mediators, as described in chapter 2.

The overall purpose of qualitative methods is to identify the meanings and ideas among participants in a research study, including the research participants and researchers themselves. In the case of mediation studies, responses to open-ended questions may provide unique insight into how and why (or why not) persons were affected by an intervention. Qualitative methods may uncover additional important information that complements quantitative information. In this regard, the addition of a qualitative component is especially useful for mediation studies because a purpose of qualitative methods is to identify what happens in the process by which an independent variable affects a dependent variable (Swanson & Chapman, 1994). However, there are limitations to qualitative methods. Weaknesses of qualitative methods are sampling that is not representative, imprecise measurement of constructs, and bias, which can lead to erroneous conclusions (Diaconis, 1985).

14.6 Exploratory Methods

The statistical methods used in this book can also be used to explore a data set for potential mediating variables. These analyses may include plots of mediation relations, estimation of potential mediation relations, and the qualitative methods described earlier. If possible, the variables in this study should be grouped into three types: independent variables, mediators, and dependent variables. If the independent variable is randomly assigned, then the independent variable may be considered the first variable in the mediation sequence. The two parts of the mediation relation may be explored in this situation, including the M to Y relation and the X to M relation. In the first phase of an exploratory analysis, the intervention effects on the potential mediator and dependent variables represent tests of the $\hat{a}$ coefficient and also the total effect test, $\hat{c}$. In the exploratory context, it is useful to test individual mediating variable effects on each outcome measure. This can represent a large number of tests. The researcher may want to control for experiment-wise error rates because of the large number of tests. Both the single mediator and multiple mediator models are useful in this context. An important next step for exploratory models is the consideration of equivalent models described in chapter 13. It is important to consider the possibility that the dependent variable is actually the cause of the mediator and other equivalent models for the data at hand.

The next stages in the exploratory analysis consider the other assumptions of the mediation model as described in chapter 3. First, the possibility of moderator variables not among the mediators or outcome should be considered, followed by consideration of the possibility that each mediator or outcome may interact with the program such that program effects differ across levels of the mediator or outcome. Plots of relations among variables in the mediation model may be especially helpful to understand relations among variables and perhaps identify subgroups of persons for whom the relations differ. A great deal of information and analyses may be generated in an exploratory analysis. Ideally specific hypotheses are generated on the basis of the exploratory results. Similarly, it may be most useful to focus on smaller numbers of the variables in a controlled study. A primary goal of the exploratory analysis is to identify mediation relations to be explored in a subsequent study.

14.7 Summary

The purpose of this chapter was to describe alternatives to identifying mediational processes besides the statistical approach addressed in most of this book. The most widely used method is the development of designs to identify mediational processes. It is clear that this is the best approach for many reasons not only from a causal inference perspective as described in chapter 13 but also because of the importance of studies that replicate results. Similarly, the borrowing of information across many studies in a meta-analysis would seem to be an ideal application for mediation. However, one problem with existing meta-analyses is that the measures used in each study may differ drastically, making comparisons across studies difficult. However, the review of studies, especially with detailed interpretation of action and conceptual theory, improves understanding of mediating mechanisms within and across behaviors.

Qualitative methods provide valuable information and often form the basis for theory. Clinical judgments about how interventions work form the basis of treatment and prevention studies. Qualitative studies and exploratory studies can be used to develop methods to test with quantitative methods in a new study. The combination of person- and variable-oriented methods would seem to be an ideal method to triangulate on important mediational processes.

Most of the methods described in this book focus on one study. In reality, the research enterprise consists of a series of studies that vary in design and goals. Experimental results are combined with intuition, clinical skill, and luck to find a true phenomenon. Single study methods have the capability of extracting the maximum amount of information from a single research study. Nevertheless, replication studies are critical for the identification of mediational processes. These replication studies should ideally include variation in assignment of units to conditions and vary the context in which a treatment is delivered, especially in observational studies of treatment effects (Rosenbaum, 2002b).

14.8 Exercises

14.1. Write out the coding matrix for the following study:
  a. Subjects are randomly assigned to one of three groups, control, cognitive therapy, and psychoanalytic therapy. The degree to which there is a therapeutic alliance between the client and the therapist is measured at the end of therapy, and it was hypothesized that therapeutic alliance is the mediating mechanism by which depression is reduced.
14.2. How does randomization improve the interpretation of a mediation study?

14.3. Provide evidence for and against the idea that all information on mediating mechanisms is qualitative.

14.4. Given that you could only conduct one research study, in general, what research design would you use? Describe the research design in a substantive area of research.

14.5. Describe the research studies that you would conduct, given that you have resources to conduct a program of research to investigate mediation relations. Describe the program of research in a substantive area.

14.6. Compare and contrast the investigation of mediation relations in a research area in which the maximum amount of information must be extracted from one or a few studies (such as a randomized community health intervention) and a research area in which it is easy to conduct multiple replication and extension studies (such as a study of mediation of a social psychological processes with college student participants).

15

Conclusions and Future Directions

> This should not be interpreted as meaning that randomization is necessary for drawing causal inferences. In many cases, appropriate untestable assumptions will be well supported by intuition, theory, or past evidence. In such cases, we should not avoid drawing causal inferences and hide behind the cover of uninteresting descriptive statements. Rather we should make causal statements that explicate the underlying assumptions and justify them as well as possible.
>
> **—Paul Holland and Donald Rubin, 1983, p. 19**

15.1 Overview

The purpose of this chapter is to summarize the material covered in this book in the context of recommendations for investigating mediational processes in confirmatory and exploratory research. Future statistical, methodological, and theoretical research is then outlined.

15.2 Goals

The main goal of this book was to describe methods to assess mediation. The book began with a description of the different types of relations among variables in the three-variable model, and then focused on mediation relations. Mediation relations are characterized by a variable that is intermediate in the sequence from an independent variable to a dependent variable. These processes were distinguished from moderator or confounder relations. In most cases, statistical methodology cannot distinguish among these different possibilities, and theory or prior research is used to justify the relation. Many examples of the mediator model in applied and basic research were described. Methods to investigate mediation in the single mediator model using ordinary least squares regression were then described along with the assumptions required for such methods to be accurate. Approaches to addressing these assumptions were covered in the rest of the book. Considerable space was devoted to covariance structure models, which represent a general method to assess mediated effects in many research situations. Methods to assess mediation in longitudinal studies were used to illustrate the assumptions and limitations of cross-sectional analyses. Several special topics in mediation analysis were then described including multilevel models, models with categorical outcomes, and resampling methods. Models with both moderators and mediators, described in chapter 10, provide a general approach to assess how mediation relations differ across people. Models for causal inference of the mediation relation were described, as were experimental and nonexperimental designs for the assessment of mediation. These methods provide a very general and adaptable approach to assessing mediation that differs, depending on research topic and design.

15.3 Two Components of Mediation

A mediation relation is composed of two relations, a relation between X and M and a relation between M and Y (Sobel, 1990). Much of this book was devoted to identifying estimators of the mediated effect and standard error based on the product of the paths relating X to M and M to Y in a wide variety of situations. This approach has several benefits over the causal steps approaches of Baron and Kenny (1986) and Judd and Kenny (1981a). Judd and Kenny (1981b) and Baron and Kenny (1986) required a statistically significant relation between X and Y for mediation to exist. However, the requirement that X has a substantial relation with Y is not necessary for mediation. There are substantive and simulation examples in which mediation is present when this criterion is not satisfied. In addition, the requirement for a statistically significant relation between X and Y reduces power to detect mediated effects, especially in complete mediation models. In some research situations, there may be a compelling reason for keeping this criterion as a way to reduce the sheer number of mediation analyses in an exploratory analysis of many dependent variables. However, researchers should be aware that mediated effects may be missed with this requirement. In particular, models in which the mediated and direct effects have opposite signs may be missed.

Similarly, the Judd and Kenny (1981a) and Baron and Kenny (1986) requirement that there be a reduction in the coefficient for the relation of X to Y when M is included in the statistical model is not necessary and can lead to missing inconsistent, or opposing mediation effects. By definition in ordinary least squares regression, if there is either a consistent or inconsistent mediation effect, the coefficient $\hat{c}$ will differ from $\hat{c}'$ in the single mediator model because $\hat{c} - \hat{c}' = \hat{a}\hat{b}$. The requirement of a reduction in $\hat{c}'$ from $\hat{c}$ occurs only for consistent relations in a mediation model, that is, when $\hat{a}\hat{b}$ and $\hat{c}'$ have the same sign. However, the requirement of a drop in the value of the unadjusted and adjusted coefficients may prohibit the identification of iatrogenic (opposing) mediation effects (MacKinnon, Krull, & Lockwood, 2000). In fact, the additional requirements of causal step methods regarding the X to Y relation and the drop in adjusted and unadjusted coefficients may have limited mediation analysis to only consistent mediation models; yet inconsistent mediation models may be present in many situations. In any research study, it is important to consider the possibility that opposing mediation effects may be present.

The requirement that the relation of X to Y adjusted for M ($\hat{c}'$), the direct effect, is nonsignificant is also not necessary. A nonsignificant relation of X to Y adjusted for M, $\hat{c}'$, and a significant mediated effect are consistent with complete mediation. In most social science research, complete mediation is unlikely. There are many substantive examples for which $\hat{a}\hat{b}$ and $\hat{c}'$ are both statistically significant. As described in chapter 13, however, causal interpretation of mediation relations is more defensible when the direct effect ($\hat{c}'$) is zero.

To summarize, the relation of X to M and the relation of M to Y (adjusted for X) are the primary mediation relations. These two relations are applicable to all mediation models described in this book, including complicated covariance structure models. The specification of these relations and estimation of these relations may differ depending on the design and measurements in the study. Categorical dependent variables require special estimation strategies, for example. These two relations and the sign of the mediated and direct effect are useful for differentiating consistent and inconsistent mediation models.

15.4 Assumptions of the Mediation Model

There are several additional criteria for identifying mediation relations besides the X to M and M to Y adjusted for X criteria. First, the functional form of the mediation relations is assumed to be linear in most treatments of mediation in this book. It is possible to specify and test nonlinear relations among variables, however. Second, if X, M, and Y are measured simultaneously, the temporal precedence of the variables is unclear, and other models may fit the data as well as the X to M to Y model (e.g., X to Y to M or M to Y to X). In the case of X representing a randomized treatment, X clearly comes before M and Y. The temporal order of M and Y is difficult to defend with cross-sectional data. Theory or previous empirical research may provide the basis for the M to Y relation. Mediation analysis requires some justification for the assumption about the temporal ordering of variables.

Longitudinal data can be used to investigate the temporal precedence of variables. Evidence for a relation of M to Y for example, can be obtained if M at time 2 adds to the prediction of Y at time 3, after adjustment for the effect of Y at time 2. Such effects are more convincing if there is no evidence for the opposite relation from Y to M. It is important to note that theoretical or empirical justification for temporal precedence is required for longitudinal data as well as for cross-sectional data. That a variable is measured before another variable, such as M measured before Y, does not mean that M is a cause of Y. A measure of Y at an earlier time point may actually cause M.

Other assumptions relate to the timing and level of the mediated effect. The design of the study is assumed to be sufficient to investigate the timing of the relations among X, M, and Y (Collins & Graham, 2002). If relations occur at a long time interval but measurements are taken at shorter intervals, then mediation relations may be missed. Similarly, the level of analysis is assumed to be correct to identify mediational processes. For example, if a mediation process present at the individual level is studied at the level of school, then conclusions about mediation may be incorrect. Mediation analysis also assumes that the correct variables in the micromediational chain were investigated. If the variables selected for study are in very different locations in the chain of mediation with multiple steps between them, then mediated effects may be too small to detect and massive sample sizes are necessary. Violation of each of these assumptions, accurate timing, correct level of analysis, and the correct mediational chain tend to reduce power to detect a mediated effect and can introduce bias.

Another important assumption is that no influences that would affect the mediation model are omitted. A variety of omitted variables may explain an observed mediation relation including unmeasured moderators and mediators. A model that is unaffected by omitted influences is called a self-contained system of variables. Given the interrelations among many variables, it is likely that few models are self-contained. Perhaps the best a researcher can do is to measure as many of these potential variables and include them in the model, consider the possible effects of unmeasured omitted variables, and hope that these omitted relations have random or small effects on the mediating process. Mediation studies by different researchers and in different contexts can reduce omitted influence explanations of a mediation model.

Another assumption of a mediation relation is that the observed mediation relation does, in fact, represent the true underlying relations among variables. As described in chapter 13 for the counterfactual assumption, there are many ways in which the M to Y relation (and also the X to Y relation adjusted for M) may not reflect a true relation. Replication studies that include experimental manipulations designed to precisely alter mediating variables can provide more convincing evidence about a mediation relation. Testing predictions of a mediation relation in other contexts gives further evidence for the veracity of mediation relations.

Measurement error can invalidate observed relations among variables. Methods to improve reliability include detailed psychometric research programs. For some variables, such as intelligence, extensive psychometric studies have been conducted. However, for many variables, measurement validity and reliability are not well known. Although latent variable models theoretically lead to more reliable measures, they have been criticized because latent variables are unobserved and may be more difficult to use as predictors in future data sets (as are true scores from reliability theory or from item response analysis). Information on the reliability and validity of measures in a mediation model is central to accurate interpretation of these models. In addition to measurement error, correlations among errors across mediation equations and between errors and predictors may be assumed to be zero; that is, the model is correctly specified.

Many of the methods described in this book assume normal distributions for variables in the mediation model. There are strategies, such as resampling methods, that accommodate some violations of distributions. Methods based on the distribution of the product of random variables lead to more accurate statistical tests for the mediated effect.

15.5 Recommendations for Mediation Studies

As for most research studies, the quality of a research project is a function of decisions made before the study is conducted. In general, design is more important than statistical adjustments. In the case of a mediation study, the identification of how a dependent variable will be affected by change in mediators is a central task. The timing of how changes in X affect M that then affect Y must be hypothesized. Decisions about the timing of relations among variables specify the number and when longitudinal measurements should be taken. Decisions must also be made about what variables in a mediational chain will be measured. Similarly, the level of mediating processes such as biological, individual, social, community, or a combination of these levels must be determined. Potential moderator variables should be specified if different mediation effects are expected across subgroups defined by categorical or continuous moderator variables. Depending on the context of the research study, potential moderator effects may be characteristics that are not likely to change such as age, gender, and location, and person characteristics unlikely to change such as tendency to take risks, depression, and educational achievement. Moderator effects that may differ across levels of baseline outcome and mediator variables should also be considered.

As described in chapter 2, decisions about the relation between the mediators and the dependent variable are based on conceptual theory and prior empirical evidence. Measures of effect size relating mediators to the dependent variables are helpful in selecting mediators especially for applied research. Action theory decisions must also be made about how an experimental intervention will affect the targeted mediators. These decisions are difficult in treatment or prevention research because the mediators with the largest effects are often the hardest to change with an intervention. Again measures of effect size relating an intervention to the mediator are helpful for making action theory decisions. In most cases, prior empirical research and theory relating mediators to outcomes is incomplete and the researcher must make some decisions regarding the ideal mediators and program components. In the ideal research study, different theories predicting different effective mediators are compared. Theory is important because good theory is applicable to situations outside the situations for which it was developed. In treatment and prevention research, several competing mediating variables are often available. Because the theories are tested on the same data set, the superiority of one theory over another suggests that the theory may be a better description of the mediating mechanisms operating in the research study.

A sample size should be selected that will have sufficient statistical power to detect a real mediated effect. For the most part, prior research on mediational processes has been underpowered. If the asymmetric confidence interval method is used to test for mediation in the single mediator model, sample sizes of approximately 500 are necessary to detect small effects for both the X to M and X to Y adjusted for M relations. More detailed power calculations can be conducted with increased information about effect sizes in the mediation model. If a more complicated multiple mediator model is used, larger sample sizes may be necessary to detect small effect size relations among variables. Longitudinal designs increase power to detect effects by reducing unexplained variability, but effects may decay over time.

Before the research study, the validity and reliability of measures of program exposure, mediators, and outcomes must be established. In many cases, however, the research literature will not contain sufficient background for every proposed measure. As mediator studies often include novel or new theoretical interpretations, at least some of the mediators will require new psychometric development. In this case, the researcher ideally conducts psychometric studies before the larger study to assess the measurement properties of the mediators. Otherwise, failure to find a statistically significant mediator may be the result of inadequate measurement. Even if the measures are not new, many different measurement decisions must be made before the study. One decision is whether to measure a construct narrowly or to measure the most general form of the construct, e.g., self-efficacy for health behaviors in general versus self-efficacy for refusing drug offers in a drug prevention study. Often both narrow and general measures are included in a research study. Qualitative measures of mediators should also be considered. At least some open-ended questions of mediating mechanisms should be obtained from study participants.

There are four overlapping steps in the identification and measurement of the mediators in a research study. To use the evaluation of a prevention program as an example, the first step in this process is the identification of mediating variables targeted by each component of the intervention. A table with mediators along the left side and components along the top with entries indicating which mediator is targeted by each component is useful to clarify this process. The second step once these mediators are identified, is the specification of multiple measures of each mediating variable in the existing measurement protocol (usually a questionnaire, but alternatives to self-report are often important). In some situations, a single measure may be sufficient, such as a biological mediator, but in general more measures lead to better psychometric properties (but consider the possibility that testing more mediators may lead to finding significance effects by chance alone). Researchers should consider including measures of variables that help address alternative explanations of research results. An example of such a comparison mediator would be a measure designed to determine the tendency for participants to respond in a biased way to please (or displease) the researchers. If the response bias measure is a significant mediator of program effects, then there is evidence that response bias may be an alternative explanation of observed mediation effects. Specificity of mediated effects could be investigated by including mediators that are consistent with one theory but not with another theory. In the third step, after measures of each mediator are specified, psychometric analyses are used to identify the extent to which the measurement of the mediator is adequate. Generally, reliability measures of 0.7 or greater are adequate, but individual researchers must make decisions about the adequacy of their measures. Confirmatory factor analysis provides a way to identify whether the mediators specified represent unique constructs or if there is evidence of excessive overlap among the measures. This process is iterative and can be quite time consuming, but it helps researchers clarify the meaning of the mediators targeted and the measures selected for the mediators. In the fourth step, decisions made about the measurement of mediators are documented in a report. Similar analyses are conducted for major dependent and independent variables if necessary. Often these types of analyses are conducted on baseline data before an intervention has been delivered to one of the research groups.

For many reasons as described in chapter 13, random assignment of units to conditions improves the causal interpretation of a mediation analysis. As a result, in the ideal study X represents randomization to experimental groups. Researchers should also consider randomization of different components of an intervention or double randomization of components so additional information on mediators and program components can be obtained. In some cases, it will be unethical or impossible to randomly assign persons to conditions. In this situation it will be helpful to consider measures of alternative explanations of any observed results and potential instrumental variables. Some of these alternative explanations include baseline nonequivalence and differential group trajectories. In any research study, it is critical to obtain information on how assignment to conditions was done.

As described in several places in this book, longitudinal data are ideal for the examination of mediation because both cross-sectional and longitudinal mediation relations can be investigated. Theory regarding the timing of the relations among X, M, and Y should be used to determine when repeated measures are taken. Pragmatically, more repeated measures usually mean a better outcome and at least four repeated measures enable the application of more detailed longitudinal models such as the latent growth models described in chapter 8. The delivery of the intervention at some point after a baseline measurement will allow for an assessment of group equivalence at baseline. Additional measures before an experimental manipulation would improve assessment of effects because a baseline for longitudinal change can be determined. At this point, the usefulness of continuous time differential equation models for mediation has not yet been determined. However, ideally, analysis of longitudinal data would include a continuous time model that may be more easily generalizable to other research studies.

Many studies include multiple mediators. To simplify analyses, the first step of the mediation analysis should evaluate one mediator at a time using the most comprehensive model. Often theory about mediators focuses on single mediators so that investigating one mediator at a time tests specific hypotheses about mediated effects. Nonsignificant as well as significant tests of potential mediators should be reported as lack of significant mediation can be as important as statistically significant mediation. Generally it is wise to first examine potential moderator effects in single mediator models. If there are many mediators and moderators investigated, some control for experiment-wise error rates may be warranted to protect against finding significant effects that are not truly present. As a second step, multiple mediator models should be estimated. In general,

it is prudent to include all measured mediators in the multiple mediator model rather than only including significant mediators identified in
the first step. In the third step, a final multiple mediator model should be
estimated by fixing paths to zero to form the most parsimonious model.
There are limitations to the third step because it is possible that important
relations may be left out, leading to biased estimates.

Programs of research are required for the identification of mediational
processes. In many respects, the problems with identifying mediational
processes are not statistical or methodological but conceptual and theoretical. As described in the quote at the beginning of chapter 14, consistent
evidence for mediational processes across different contexts with different researchers is the goal for demonstrating real mediated effects. Specificity of evidence for one mediator and not others bolsters evidence for
that mediator.

In summary, the ideal mediation study has clearly specified mediational processes based on competing theories and prior mediation analysis. The study includes random assignment of units to conditions in a
longitudinal design with the timing of observations based on theory. The
ideal study would also have at least four longitudinal measurements so
that advanced longitudinal methods can be applied. Each measure in the
study would be valid and reliable on the basis of considerable empirical
research. The mediation effects are then replicated in different contexts
and by different researchers to establish a real mediational process.

15.6 Exploratory Mediator and Moderator Analysis

Exploratory analysis is used to identify possible relations that can be evaluated in other data sets and in future studies. Because limited theory or
an unspecified model drives the analysis, the likelihood of Type I errors
increases because the chances of finding a significant mediator increases
owing to the number of statistical tests. The steps outlined earlier for the
ideal mediation study apply to the case of an exploratory study except that
the detailed expectations from theory and prior research are not available. Rather than confirming predictions, exploratory mediation analysis
consists of testing a large number of mediators and moderators as well as
testing mediators at the different levels of the moderators. Tests for all of
these mediators and moderators are then used to specify hypotheses for
future studies. Qualitative methods described in chapter 14 also have an
important role in the generation of research questions and ideas.

The most likely situation in which an exploratory mediator and moderator analysis would be conducted is after a series of hypothesized
mediation and moderation relations are tested using methods described
in this book. The following steps are described for a longitudinal study of

randomized intervention, but they will also apply to other types of studies. Three general analyses are outlined: (a) moderator analysis, (b) mediator analysis, and (c) combined moderator and mediator analysis. In an exploratory analysis, these three general analyses could be conducted in any order, although the moderator, mediator, and moderator/mediator sequence is likely to be more consistent with the priorities for the most research studies. In addition, it may be wise to investigate moderator variables first as these may qualify any mediation effects investigated later. Note that the timing of measurement and variables measured may limit these analyses. In most situations, it is difficult to investigate change in the mediator as an explanation of change in an outcome if there is no longitudinal measurement of variables. In general, a variable that does not change from baseline to follow-up cannot be a mediator because it appears to be unaffected by the independent variable, but this is not always true; in developmental studies no change in a variable may reflect a reduction from the normal growth in variables. A variable that is measured only at baseline can be included in the analysis only as a moderator, although these effects may reflect mediation, if the effect of the program depends on where the participant scored on the baseline variable.

To keep some organization to the moderator analysis, moderators reflecting unchangeable characteristics of individuals such as demographic variables are examined first. In a second step, moderator effects related to baseline mediator and outcome measures are examined, as these results reflect important program effects. In a third step, other moderator effects should be considered such as personality measures of impulsivity or sociopathy. The overall results of the moderator analysis should then be organized and investigated with contrasts and plots of the data. A final model including all or a subset of important moderators should then be estimated to understand how the moderators may act together. These results should be further investigated with contrasts and plots to understand the significant mediators in the study.

In the mediation analysis stage, mediation analysis of all possible mediators should be conducted. These analyses should include documenting whether the $\hat{a}$ path was statistically significant or the $\hat{b}$ path was statistically significant, as these two paths reflect the action and conceptual theory of the intervention, respectively. In an exploratory study, researchers should consider many variables so as to not overlook unexpected mediating variables. The results of mediator analysis should be summarized including plots and contrasts. Two different multiple mediator models should be considered here. One multiple mediator model should include all mediators or a subset of them to understand how the mediators are related in a comprehensive model. Another multiple mediator model should consider the possible chains of mediation that may be present. As the number of mediators increases, the number of potential orderings of mediators get very large, so some decisions to reduce this number should be considered.

The third phase consists of models with both moderators and mediators in the same analysis. The simplest approach to this analysis may be to include only moderators and mediators that were statistically significant in individual analyses or some other reasonable decision of which mediators and moderators to include. Given the large number of potential tests, some control over experiment-wise error rates is warranted. As described earlier, in some contexts, researchers may want to start with models that have both moderation and mediation. Given the complexity of these analyses, building up of results from moderator to mediator analysis followed by models with both moderators and mediators seems most sensible.

In most studies, if all mediators, moderators, and their combinations are considered, the number of analyses is prohibitive. So even in an exploratory analysis, it may be necessary to limit analyses on the basis of theory or practical considerations. An alternative to the exploratory analysis described earlier is to use a program such as TETRAD mentioned in chapter 13 to conduct a search for models given a set of possible variables.

15.7 Sensitivity Analysis

Once a mediation analysis is completed it is useful to consider how violation of assumptions may have affected results. These types of analyses are known as sensitivity analyses (Angrist, Imbens, & Rubin, 1996). Usually, sensitivity analyses assess the influences of situations outside the observed data set. Sensitivity analyses provide another way to evaluate the veracity of the numerous assumptions of mediation analysis. The influence of measurement error may be assessed by estimating model relations after systematically adding measurement error to a variable or group of variables. The influence of measurement error on mediation results can be investigated by estimating a model with a larger coefficient for error variance or actually adding random error to each observation. A change in mediated effect estimates reflects the extent to which increasing measurement error may affect results. Similarly, the extent to which a confounder affects results may be considered by including an artificially constructed variable that has a specific correlation with the mediating variable and the dependent variable and assessing how this would affect results either using analytical formulas for mediation model quantities or by generating data and evaluating the analysis results (Rosenbaum, 2002b; Frank, 2000). Often, an artificially constructed confounder that is strongly related to the variables in the mediation model does not change conclusions regarding a mediation analysis. Bias in observed relations owing to nonrandom missing data or selection bias may be evaluated using methods by systematically removing or adding observations. The influence of confounders, measurement error, and missing data is evaluated on effect size measures as well as whether the mediated effect is statistically significant or not. Mediation analysis with resampling methods may be useful to address alternative interpretation of results in terms of violation of distributional assumptions. The extent to which the relation between the mediator and the dependent variable may be assessed by considering the specificity of the relation as well as its consistency with theory and qualitative results. Consideration of model results as consistent with theory or not is also useful but should not be used to deny new or counterintuitive mediation results. Finally, the replication of mediators with new data and new contexts provides more credibility to conclusions about mediating mechanisms. Mediating mechanisms that are present in different areas of research, different samples of participants, and across different methodologies provide more definitive assessment of mediation.

15.8 Future Research

A goal of this book was to describe the state of the knowledge of mediation analysis. In the process of doing this, several weaknesses and areas of needed methodology have been identified. The need for future research falls in overlapping categories of statistical, methodological, and theoretical aspects of mediation analysis.

Regarding statistical developments, it will be illustrative to demonstrate analytically how the different formulas for the standard error of the mediated effect are related. Similarly, the accuracy of general methods for the derivation of the standard error of functions of coefficients based on the covariance among parameter estimates should continue to be examined in analytical and simulation studies. In particular, the best effect size measures for mediation are yet to be determined. Confidence interval methods in multilevel models require evaluation. For these and other questions, it is important to evaluate methods with both analytical and statistical simulation studies.

Values for the distribution of the product of t statistics may also improve the accuracy of the distribution of the product calculations; the ratio of regression estimate to its standard error is a t statistic. Similarly, statistical theory and computational methods for the distribution of three or more random variables are necessary for obtaining confidence limits for more complicated mediated effects. Resampling methods for assessing mediation effects have shown considerable promise and have been used for more complicated mediation effects. More elaborate resampling methods may also prove useful including the iterated bootstrap and bootstrapping asymmetric confidence limits based on the distribution of the product. Different variations of the permutation test described in chapter 11 may be useful for mediation analysis.

Bayesian approaches to investigating mediation relations show promise—at least in part because they incorporate additional information to inform mediation analysis. Models for linear and nonlinear relations among variables in a mediation model would also be useful. In particular, generalized additive models that allow for any relation among variables in the mediation model (Brown, 1993) would appear to be straightforward to apply to mediation models. For these models, any relation among variables would be modeled rather than the strict linear (or hypothesized nonlinear) relations now included in mediation models.

Another important area of statistical development is person-centered approaches to mediation. Methods to identify person-centered versions of mediation like the Collins, Graham, and Flaherty (1998) methods described in chapter 8 may help clarify mediational processes. In contrast to the variable-centered model, person-oriented models consider the question of what pattern of responses is consistent or inconsistent with mediation. Models with both person-oriented and variable-oriented mediation may also prove useful. Models that include moderation and mediation in the same analysis need further development. An example of combining moderation and mediation is the mixture models in which trajectories of types of individuals are identified and mediational processes for these trajectories explain the trajectories. This model is like a model with mediation and moderation, but the classes of persons are determined with a statistical method based on similar trajectories rather than moderator variables of sex, for example, that have two distinct categories. Type I and Type II errors and confidence limit coverage rates will continue to be an important way to evaluate new methods.

Important methodological developments include a clearer description of causal inference approaches to mediation. In particular, the similarities and differences of different approaches to causal inference such as directed graph approaches (Pearl, 2000) and the RCM (Rubin, 1974) described in chapter 13 would help clarify the meaning of both approaches to mediation analysis. Application of instrumental variable methods with more than one instrumental variable and mediator may help answer questions about true relations in multiple mediator models or lead to reduced confidence in mediation relations. Perhaps the most important methodological contribution of future research will be the application of these methods to studying real mediation situations. Models are often very clear and helpful when described in ideal situations but may not be helpful for practical interpretation of data. The discussion of causal models in chapter 13 may suggest to some researchers that it is not worth the effort to conduct mediation analysis because it is so difficult to make causal inferences. However, the information mediational analyses may provide is too important about how variables are related to dismiss as impossible.

The adequacy of alternative longitudinal mediation models has not been determined. Continuous time longitudinal models have the potential to provide more generalizable models of mediation relations. Longitudinal mediation models hold the promise of specifying the timing of interventions and timing of relations among variables. In general, the different conceptual foundations and statistical performance of mediation longitudinal models requires more clarification. No single longitudinal framework for assessing mediation can be considered ideal now.

Theory is the glue that holds the investigation of mediation together. There are potentially an infinite number of variables to measure and samples to study. Theory provides a way to approach this unwieldy problem by limiting the total number of possibilities to consider. There is a need for theories for specific mediational hypotheses. The timing of relations between variables in the model should be a new criterion for good theory. Ideally, competing theories will be specified with clear alternative predictions regarding a mediation study. Ideally a program of research would investigate the same mediational processes in a variety of substantive areas. It is likely that the development of methods to assess mediational processes will lead to more detailed theories regarding these processes and the development of mediation methods will lead to more detailed theories. One benefit of understanding the importance of mediation in general is that it forces researchers to think about specific mediational processes. The increased conceptual attention to theoretical mediational processes may be of more benefit than any statistical mediation analyses.

For health promotion and disease prevention and treatment programs, mediation analysis has the potential to identify critical components, thereby reducing costs and increasing scientific understanding of health behavior. The methods described in this book are applicable to all prevention and treatment programs and can be applied to data that have already been collected. Mediation analyses are likely to increase the amount of information extracted from these studies.

15.9 Summary

The purpose of this book was to describe the rationale for assessing mediation and to describe methods to assess mediated effects. The ultimate goal of the book is to increase the number of studies applying mediation analysis as summarized in figure 15.1. The book targeted mediators of knowledge of statistical methods to assess mediation, the norm that mediation is important, comprehension of reasons for mediation analy-

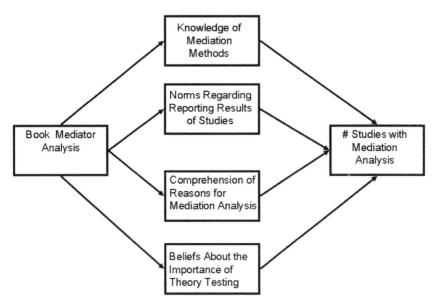

Figure 15.1. A mediation model for this book.

sis, and the importance of theory testing. The hypothesis was that if persons understand why mediation is important, know how to conduct the analysis, and understand limitations of the methods then more rigorous mediation studies will be conducted. Attention to the limitations of mediation analysis is especially important because it helps generate alternative explanations of results. These alternative interpretations are then addressed in each study and inform subsequent research design. In particular, experimental studies of mediation processes are important. For example, health promotion and disease prevention program research is an ideal application for mediation analysis because these studies are designed to change mediators, replication and extension studies are often feasible, and the dependent variable is often clearly defined. Limitations of current methods also stimulate future methodological and statistical developments. Another goal of the book was to change the norm regarding reporting research results so that mediation results, especially estimates of mediation effects are routinely reported. Consideration of how an intervention achieved its effects or failed to achieve effects increases the amount of information from a research study. Another goal of the book was to emphasize the importance of theory testing. There are often a large number of potential mediators to examine in a research study. Theory provides a way to organize prior research and make clear predictions for future studies. Of course, mediation analysis is also useful when theory is not available and interventions to change an outcome in any way possible are desired. It is unclear whether the mediators in Figure 15.1 are the critical mediators for increasing the number of studies investigating mediation. However, these mediators hold promise for increasing the study of variables that are intermediate in the sequence relating an independent variable to a dependent variable.

References

Abelson, R. P. (1985). A variance explanation paradox: When a little is a lot. *Psychological Bulletin, 97,* 129–133.

Aguinis, H. (2004). *Regression analysis for categorical moderators.* New York: Guilford Press.

Aiken, L. S., & West, S. G. (1991). *Multiple regression: Testing and interpreting interactions.* Newbury Park, CA: Sage.

Allen, M. J., & Yen, W. M. (1979). *Introduction to measurement theory.* Monterey, CA: Brooks/Cole.

Allison, P. D. (1995a). The impact of random predictors on comparisons of coefficients between models: Comment on Clogg, Petkova, and Haritou. *American Journal of Sociology, 100,* 1294–1305.

Allison, P. D. (1995b). Exact variance of indirect effects in recursive linear models. *Sociological Methodology, 25,* 253–266.

Alwin, D. F., & Hauser, R. M. (1975). The decomposition of effects in path analysis. *American Sociological Review, 40,* 37–47.

Ambler, T. (2001). Mediators and moderators. *Journal of Consumer Psychology, 10,* 98–100.

Amemiya, T. (1981). Qualitative response models: A survey. *Journal of Economic Literature, 19,* 1483–1536.

Angrist, J. D., Imbens, G. W., & Rubin, D. B. (1996). Identification of causal effects using instrumental variables (with comments). *Journal of the American Statistical Association, 91,* 444–472.

Angrist, J. D., & Krueger, A. B. (2001). Instrumental variables and the search for identification: From supply and demand to natural experiments. *Journal of Economic Perspectives, 15,* 69–85.

Arbuckle, J. L., & Wothke, W. (1999). Amos users' 4.0 (Version 3.6) [Computer software]. Chicago: Smallwaters Corporation.

Arminger, G. (1986). Linear stochastic differential equation models for panel data with unobserved variables. *Sociological Methodology, 16,* 187–212.

Aroian, L. A. (1947). The probability function of the product of two normally distributed variables. *Annals of Mathematical Statistics, 18,* 265–271.

Aroian, L. A., Taneja, V. S., & Cornwell, L. W. (1978). Mathematical forms of the distribution of the product of two normal variables. *Communications in Statistics: Theory and Methods, A7,* 165–172.

Ashby, W. R. (1956). *An introduction to cybernetics.* New York: Wiley.

Bachman, J. G., Johnston, L. D., O'Malley, P. M., & Humphrey, R. H. (1988). Explaining the recent decline in marijuana use: Differentiating the effects of perceived risks, disapproval, and general lifestyle factors. *Journal of Health and Social Behavior, 29,* 92–112.

Bagozzi, R. P., & Heatherton, T. F. (1994). A general approach to representing multifaceted personality constructs: Application to state self-esteem. *Structural Equation Modeling, 1,* 35–67.

Bandura, A. (1977). *Social learning theory.* Englewood Cliffs, NJ: Prentice-Hall.

Baranowski, T., Anderson, C., & Carmack, C. (1998). Mediating variable framework in physical activity interventions: How are we doing? How might we do better? *American Journal of Preventive Medicine, 15*, 266–297.

Baranowski, T., Lin, L. S., Wetter, D. W., Resnicow, K., & Hearn, M. D. (1997). Theory as mediating variables: Why aren't community interventions working as desired? *Annals of Epidemiology, 7*(Suppl. 7), s89–s95.

Barcikowski, R. S. (1981). Statistical power with group mean as the unit of analysis. *Journal of Educational Statistics, 6*, 267–285.

Baron, R. M., & Kenny, D. A. (1986). The moderator-mediator variable distinction in social psychological research: Conceptual, strategic, and statistical considerations. *Journal of Personality and Social Psychology, 51*, 1173–1182.

Bauer, D. J., & Curran, P. J. (2003). Distributional assumptions of growth mixture models: Implications for overextraction of latent trajectory classes. *Psychological Methods, 8*, 338–363.

Bauer, D. J., Preacher, K. J., & Gil, K. M. (2006). Conceptualizing and testing random indirect effects and moderated mediation in multilevel models: New procedures and recommendations. *Psychological Methods, 11*, 142–163.

Becker, B. J. (1992). Models of science achievement: Forces affecting male and female performance in school science. In T. D. Cook, H. Cooper, D. S. Cordray, H. Hartmann, L. V. Hedges, R. J. Light, et al. (Eds.), *Meta-analysis for explanation: A casebook* (pp. 209–281). New York: Sage.

Becker, B. J., & Schram, C. M. (1994). Examining explanatory models through research synthesis. In H. Cooper & L. V. Hedges (Eds.), *Handbook of research synthesis* (pp. 357–381). New York: Russell Sage.

Begg, C. B., & Leung, D. H. Y. (2000). On the use of surrogate end points in randomized trials. *Journal of the Royal Statistical Society (Series A—Statistics in Society), 163*, 15–28.

Bem, D. J. (1972). Self-perception theory. In L. Berkowitz (Ed.), *Advances in experimental social psychology* (Vol. 6, pp. 1–62). New York: Academic Press.

Bennett, J. A. (2000). Mediator and moderator variables in nursing research: Conceptual and statistical differences. *Research in Nursing and Health, 23*, 415–420.

Bentler, P. M. (1980). Multivariate analysis with latent variables: Causal modeling. *Annual Review of Psychology, 31*, 419–456.

Bentler, P. M. (1997). *EQS for Windows (Version 5.6)* [Computer software]. Encino, CA: Multivariate Software.

Bentler, P. M., & Speckart, G. (1979). Models of attitude-behavior relations. *Psychological Review, 86*, 452–464.

Bentler, P. M., & Speckart, G. (1981). Attitudes "cause" behaviors: A structural equation analysis. *Journal of Personality and Social Psychology, 40*, 226–238.

Bentler, P. M., & Weeks, D. G. (1982). Multivariate analysis with latent variables. In P. R. Krishnaiah & L. Kanal (Eds.), *Handbook of statistics* (Vol. 2, pp. 747–771). Amsterdam: North Holland Publishing Company.

Berk, R. A. (1991). Toward a methodology for mere mortals. *Sociological Methodology, 21*, 315–324.

Berk, R. A. (2003). *Regression analysis: A constructive critique.* Thousand Oaks, CA: Sage.

Billings, R. S., & Wroten, S. P. (1978). Use of path analysis in industrial/organizational psychology: Criticisms and suggestions. *Journal of Applied Psychology, 63*, 677–688.

Bishop, Y. M. M., Fienberg, S. E., & Holland, P. W. (1975). *Discrete multivariate analysis: Theory and practice.* Cambridge, MA: MIT Press.

Blalock, H. M. (1969). *Theory construction: From verbal to mathematical formulations.* Englewood Cliffs, NJ: Prentice-Hall.

Blalock, H. M. (Ed.) (1971). *Causal models in the social sciences.* Chicago: Aldine-Atherton.

Blalock, H. M. (1991). Are there really any constructive alternatives to causal modeling? *Sociological Methodology, 21,* 325–335.

Blank, S., Seiter, C., & Bruce, P. (1999). *Resampling stats in Excel (Version 1.1).* Arlington, VA: Resampling Stats.

Blau, P. M., & Duncan, O. D. (1967). *The American occupational structure.* New York: Wiley.

Bobko, P., & Rieck, A. (1980). Large sample estimators for standard errors of functions of correlation coefficients. *Applied Psychological Measurement, 4,* 385–398.

Boker, S. M., & Nesselroade, J. R. (2002). A method for modeling the intrinsic dynamics of intraindividual variability: Recovering the parameters of simulated oscillators in multi-wave panel data. *Multivariate Behavioral Research, 37,* 127–160.

Bollen, K. A. (1987). Total, direct, and indirect effects in structural equation models. *Sociological Methodology, 17,* 37–69.

Bollen, K. A. (1989). *Structural equations with latent variables.* New York: Wiley.

Bollen, K. A. (2002). Latent variables in psychology and the social sciences. *Annual Review of Psychology, 53,* 605–634.

Bollen, K. A., & Curran, P. J. (2004). Autoregressive latent trajectory (ALT) models: A synthesis of two traditions. *Sociological Methods and Research, 32,* 336–383.

Bollen, K. A., & Stine, R. (1990). Direct and indirect effects: Classical and bootstrap estimates of variability. *Sociological Methodology, 20,* 115–140.

Bollen, K. A., & Stine, R. A. (1993). Bootstrapping goodness-of-fit measures in structural equation models. In K. A. Bollen & J. S. Long (Eds.), *Testing structural equation models* (pp. 111–135). Newbury Park, CA: Sage.

Bonate, P. L. (2000). *Analysis of pretest-posttest designs.* Boca Raton, FL: Chapman & Hall.

Botvin, G. J. (2000). Preventing drug abuse in schools: Social and competence enhancement approaches targeting individual-level etiologic factors. *Addictive Behaviors, 25,* 887–897.

Botvin, G. J., Baker, E., Renick, N. L., Filazzola, A. D., & Botvin, E. M. (1984). A cognitive-behavioral approach to substance abuse prevention. *Addictive Behaviors, 9,* 137–147.

Botvin, G. J., Dusenbury, L., Baker, E., James-Ortiz, S., Botvin, E. M., & Kerner, J. (1992). Smoking prevention among urban minority youth: Assessing effects on outcome and mediating variables. *Health Psychology, 11,* 290–299.

Botvin, G. J., Eng, A., & Williams, C. L. (1980). Preventing the onset of cigarette smoking through life skills training. *Preventive Medicine, 9,* 135–143.

Brookmeyer, R. (Ed.) (1989). Statistical and mathematical modeling of the AIDS epidemic [Special issue]. *Statistics in Medicine, 8,* 1–139.

Brown, C. H. (1993). Analyzing preventive trials with generalized additive models. *American Journal of Community Psychology, 21,* 635–664.

Brown, S. P., & Stayman, D. M. (1992). Antecedents and consequences of attitude toward the ad: A meta-analysis. *Journal of Consumer Research, 19,* 34–51.

Brown, T. L., LeMay, H. E., & Bursten, B. E. (2000). *Chemistry: The central science* (8th ed.). Upper Saddle River, NJ: Prentice Hall.

Browne, M. W. (1984). Asymptotically distribution-free methods for the analysis of covariance structures. *British Journal of Mathematical and Statistical Psychology, 37*, 62–83.

Bryk, A. S., & Raudenbush, S. W. (1992). *Hierarchical linear models: Applications and data analysis methods*. Newbury Park, CA: Sage.

Burr, J. A., & Nesselroade, J. R. (1990). Change measurement. In A. von Eye (Ed.), *Statistical methods in longitudinal research* (Vol. I, pp. 3–34). New York: Academic Press.

Burstein, L. (1980). The analysis of multilevel data in educational research and evaluation. In D. C. Berliner (Ed.), *Review of research in education* (Vol. 8, pp. 158–233). Washington, DC: American Educational Research Association.

Burstein, L. (1985). Units of analysis. *International Encyclopedia of Education*. London: Pergamon Press.

Buyse, M., & Molenberghs, G. (1998). Criteria for the validation of surrogate endpoints in randomized experiments. *Biometrics, 54*, 1014–1029.

Buyse, M., Molenberghs, G., Burzykowski, T., Renard, D., & Geys, H. (2000). The validation of surrogate endpoints in meta-analyses of randomized experiments. *Biostatistics, 1*, 49–67.

Campbell, D. T., & Kenny, D. A. (1999). *A primer on regression artifacts*. New York: Guilford.

Campbell, N. A., Reece, J. B., Taylor, M. R., & Simon, E. J. (2006). *Biology: Concepts and connections* (5th ed.). San Francisco: Pearson/Benjamin Cummings.

Chassin, L., Pillow, D. R., Curran, P. J., Molina, B. S. G., & Barrera, M. (1993). Relation of parental alcoholism to early adolescent substance use: A test of three mediating mechanisms. *Journal of Abnormal Psychology, 102*, 3–19.

Chen, H. T. (1990). *Theory-driven evaluations*. Newbury Park, CA: Sage.

Cheong, J., MacKinnon, D. P., & Khoo, S. T. (2003). Investigation of mediational processes using parallel process latent growth curve modeling. *Structural Equation Modeling, 10*, 238–262.

Chernick, M. R. (1999). *Bootstrap methods: A practitioner's guide*. New York: Wiley.

Choi, S., Lagakos, S. W., Schooley, R. T., & Volberding, P. A. (1993). CD4+ lymphocytes are an incomplete surrogate marker for clinical progression in persons with asymptomatic HIV infection taking zidovudine. *Annals of Internal Medicine, 118*, 674–680.

Cliff, N. (1983). Some cautions concerning the application of causal modeling methods. *Multivariate Behavioral Research, 18*, 115–126.

Clogg, C. C., Petkova, E., & Cheng, T. (1995). Reply to Allison: More on comparing regression coefficients. *American Journal of Sociology, 100*, 1305–1312.

Clogg, C. C., Petkova, E., & Shihadeh, E. S. (1992). Statistical methods for analyzing collapsibility in regression models. *Journal of Educational Statistics, 17*, 51–74.

Cochran, W. G. (1957). Analysis of covariance: Its nature and uses. *Biometrics, 13*, 261–281.

Cochran, W. G., & Cox, G. M. (1957). *Experimental designs* (2nd ed.). New York: Wiley.

Cohen, J. (1988). *Statistical power analysis for the behavioral sciences* (2nd ed.). Hillsdale, NJ: Lawrence Erlbaum Associates.

Cohen, J., & Cohen, P. (1983). *Applied multiple regression/correlation analysis for the behavioral sciences.* Hillsdale, NJ: Lawrence Erlbaum Associates.

Cohen, J., Cohen, P., West, S. G., & Aiken, L. S. (2003). *Applied multiple regression/ correlation analysis for the behavioral sciences* (3rd ed.). Mahwah, NJ: Lawrence Erlbaum Associates.

Cole, D. A., & Maxwell, S. E. (2003). Testing mediational models with longitudinal data: Questions and tips in the use of structural equation modeling. *Journal of Abnormal Psychology, 112,* 558–577.

Collins, L. M., & Graham, J. W. (2002). The effect of the timing and spacing of observations in longitudinal studies of tobacco and other drug use: temporal design considerations. *Drug and Alcohol Dependence, 68,* S85–S96.

Collins, L. M., Graham, J. W., & Flaherty, B. P. (1998). An alternative framework for defining mediation. *Multivariate Behavioral Research, 33,* 295–312.

Conger, A. J. (1974). A revised definition for suppressor variables: A guide to their identification and interpretation. *Educational and Psychological Measurement, 34,* 35–46.

Cook, T. D., & Campbell, D. T. (1979). *Quasi-experimentation: Design and analysis issues for field settings.* Chicago: Rand McNally.

Cook, T. D., Cooper, H., Cordray, D. S., Hartmann, H., Hedges, L. V., Light, R. J., Louis, T. A., & Mosteller, F. (1992). *Meta-analysis for explanation: A casebook.* New York: Sage.

Coyle, S. L., Boruch, R. F., & Turner, C. F. (Eds.) (1991). *Evaluating AIDS prevention programs.* Washington, DC: National Academy Press.

Crabtree, B. F., & Miller, W. L. (1999). *Doing qualitative research* (2nd ed.). Thousand Oaks, CA: Sage.

Craig, C. C. (1936). On the frequency function of xy. *Annals of Mathematical Statistics, 7,* 1–15.

Crocker, L., & Algina, J. (1986). *Introduction to classical and modern test theory.* New York: Harcourt, Brace, Jovanovich.

Cronbach, L. J. (1982). *Designing evaluations of educational and social programs.* San Francisco: Jossey-Bass.

Cronbach, L. J., & Furby, L. (1970). How should we measure "change" or should we? *Psychological Bulletin, 74,* 68–80.

Cudeck, R. (1991). Comment on "Using causal models to estimate indirect effects." In L. M. Collins & J. L. Horn (Eds.), *Best methods for the analysis of change: Recent advances, unanswered questions, future directions* (pp. 260–263). Washington DC: American Psychological Association.

Cuijpers, P. (2002). Effective ingredients of school-based drug prevention programs: A systematic review. *Addictive Behaviors, 27,* 1009–1023.

Curran, P. J., & Bollen, K. A. (2001). The best of both worlds: Combining autoregressive and latent curve models. In L. M. Collins & A. G. Sayer (Eds.), *New methods for the analysis of change* (pp. 107–136). Washington, DC: American Psychological Association.

Curran, P. J., & Hussong, A. M. (2003). The use of latent trajectory models in psychopathology research. *Journal of Abnormal Psychology, 112,* 526–544.

Darlington, R. B. (1990). *Regression and linear models.* New York: McGraw-Hill.

Darwin, C. (1876). *The effects of cross- and self-fertilisation in the vegetable kingdom.* London: John Murray.

Davis, J. A. (1985). *The logic of causal order.* Sage University Paper Series on Quantitative Applications in the Social Sciences (07-055), Beverly Hills, CA: Sage.

Dawber, T. R. (1980). *The Framingham study: The epidemiology of atherosclerotic disease.* Cambridge, MA: Harvard University Press.

Day, N. E., & Duffy, S. W. (1996). Trial design based on surrogate end points—Application to comparison of different breast screening frequencies. *Journal of the Royal Statistical Society, Series A (Statistics in Society), 159,* 49–60.

de Leeuw, J. (1992). Series editor's introduction to Hierarchical Linear Models. In A. S. Bryk & S. W. Raudenbush (Eds.), *Hierarchical linear models: Applications and data analysis methods* (pp. xiii–xvi). Newbury Park, CA: Sage.

Diaconis, P. (1985). Theories of data analysis: From magical thinking through classical statistics. In D. C. Hoaglin, F. Mosteller, & J. W. Tukey (Eds.), *Exploring data tables, trends, and shapes* (pp. 1–35). New York: Wiley.

Dodge, K. A., Bates, J. E., & Pettit, G. S. (1990). Mechanisms in the cycle of violence. *Science, 250,* 1678–1683.

Donaldson, S. I. (2001). Mediator and moderator analysis in program development. In S. Sussman (Ed.), *Handbook of program development for health behavior research and practice* (pp. 470–496). Thousand Oaks, CA: Sage.

Donaldson, S. I., Graham, J. W., & Hansen, W. B. (1994). Testing the generalizability of intervening mechanism theories: Understanding the effects of adolescent drug use prevention interventions. *Journal of Behavioral Medicine, 17,* 195–216.

Dryfoos, J. G. (1990). *Adolescents at risk: Prevalence and prevention.* New York: Oxford.

Duncan, O. D. (1966). Path analysis: Sociological examples. *American Journal of Sociology, 72,* 1–16.

Duncan, O. D. (1975). *Introduction to structural equation models.* New York: Academic Press.

Duncan, O. D., Featherman, D. L., & Duncan, B. (1972). *Socioeconomic background and achievement.* New York: Seminar Press.

Duncan, T. E., Duncan, S. C., Strycker, L. A., Li, F., & Alpert, A. (1999). *An introduction to latent variable growth curve modeling: Concepts, issues, and applications.* Mahwah, NJ: Lawrence Erlbaum Associates.

Dworkin, S. L., Exner, T., Melendez, R., Hoffman, S., & Ehrhardt, A. A. (2006). Revisiting "success": Posttrial analysis of gender-specific HIV/STD prevention intervention. *AIDS and Behavior, 10,* 41–51.

Dwyer, J. H. (1983). *Statistical models for the social and behavioral sciences.* New York: Oxford.

Dwyer, J. H. (1992). Differential equation models for longitudinal data. Application: Blood pressure and relative weight. In J. H. Dwyer, M. Feinleib, P. Lippert, & H. Hoffmeister (Eds.), *Statistical models for longitudinal studies of health* (pp. 71–98). New York: Oxford University Press.

Echt, D. S., Liebson, P. R., Mitchell, L. B., Peters, R. W., Obias-Manno, D., Barker, A. H., et al. (1991). Mortality and morbidity in patients receiving encainide, flecainide or placebo: The cardiac arrhythmia suppression trial. *The New England Journal of Medicine, 324,* 781–788.

Eddy, J. M., & Chamberlain, P. (2000). Family management and deviant peer association as mediators of the impact of treatment condition on youth antisocial behavior. *Journal of Consulting and Clinical Psychology, 68,* 857–863.

Eden, T., & Yates, F. (1933). On the validity of Fisher's *z* test when applied to an actual example of non-normal data. *Journal of Agricultural Science, 23,* 6–17.

Edgington, E. S. (1995). *Randomization tests* (3rd ed.). New York: Marcel-Dekker.

Efron, B. (1987). Better bootstrap confidence intervals. *Journal of the American Statistical Association, 82,* 171–185.

Efron, B. (2000). The bootstrap and modern statistics. *Journal of the American Statistical Association, 95,* 1293–1296.

Efron, B., & Feldman, D. (1991). Compliance as an explanatory variable in clinical trials. *Journal of the American Statistical Association, 86,* 9–17.

Efron, B., & Tibshirani, R. J. (1993). *An introduction to the bootstrap.* New York: Chapman & Hall.

Eisenberg, L., & Hall, K. (1994). *101 back-to-school jokes.* New York: Scholastic.

Fairchild, A., & MacKinnon, D. P. (2005). *Tests of significance for a person-centered approach to mediation.* Unpublished manuscript.

Fay, M. P., & Follmann, D. A. (2002). Designing Monte Carlo implementations of permutation or bootstrap hypothesis tests. *American Statistician, 56,* 63–70.

Ferrer, E., & McArdle, J. J. (2003). Alternative structural models for multivariate longitudinal data analysis. *Structural Equation Modeling, 10,* 493–524.

Fischer-Lapp, K., & Goetghebeur, E. (1999). Practical properties of some structural mean analyses of the effect of compliance in randomized trials. *Controlled Clinical Trials, 20,* 531–546.

Fishbein, M., & Ajzen, I. (1975). *Belief, attitude, intention, and behavior: An introduction to theory and research.* Reading, MA: Addison-Wesley.

Fisher, R. A. (1934). *Statistical methods for research workers* (5th ed.). Edinburgh, Scotland: Oliver and Boyd Lt.

Fisher, R. A. (1960). *The design of experiments* (7th ed.). New York: Hafner.

Fiske, S. T., Kenny, D. A., & Taylor, S. E. (1982). Structural models for the mediation of salience effects on attribution. *Journal of Experimental Social Psychology, 18,* 105–127.

Flay, B. R. (1985). Psychosocial approaches to smoking prevention: A review of findings. *Health Psychology, 4,* 449–488.

Flay, B. R. (1987). Social psychological approaches to smoking prevention: Review and recommendations. *Advances in Health Education and Promotion, 2,* 121–180.

Fleming, T. R., & DeMets, D. L. (1996). Surrogate end points in clinical trials: Are we being misled? *Annals of Internal Medicine, 125,* 605–613.

Folmer, H. (1981). Measurement of the effects of regional policy instruments by means of linear structural equation models and panel data. *Environment and Planning A, 13,* 1435–1448.

Foshee, V. A., Bauman, K. E., Arriaga, X. B., Helms, R. W., Koch, G. G., & Linder, G. F. (1998). An evaluation of Safe Dates, an adolescent dating violence prevention program. *American Journal of Public Health, 88,* 45–50.

Fox, J. (1980). Effect analysis in structural equation models: Extensions and simplified methods of computation. *Sociological Methods and Research, 9,* 3–28.

Frangakis, C. E., & Rubin, D. B. (2002). Principal stratification in causal inference. *Biometrics, 58,* 21–29.

Frank, K. A. (2000). Impact of a confounding variable on a regression coefficient. *Sociological Methods and Research, 29,* 147–194.

Freedheim, D. K., & Russ, S. W. (1992). Psychotherapy with children. In C. Walker & M. Roberts (Eds.), *Handbook of clinical child psychology* (2nd ed., pp. 765–781). New York: Wiley.

Freedman, D. A. (1987). As others see us: A case study in path analysis (with discussion). *Journal of Educational Statistics, 12,* 101–223.

Freedman, D. A. (1991). Statistical models and shoe leather. *Sociological Methodology, 21,* 291–313.

Freedman, L. S. (2001). Confidence intervals and statistical power of the 'validation' ratio for surrogate or intermediate endpoints. *Journal of Statistical Planning and Inference, 96,* 143–153.

Freedman, L. S., Graubard, B. I., & Schatzkin, A. (1992). Statistical validation of intermediate endpoints for chronic diseases. *Statistics in Medicine, 11,* 167–178.

Freedman, L. S., & Schatzkin, A. (1992). Sample size for studying intermediate endpoints within intervention trials or observational studies. *American Journal of Epidemiology, 136,* 1148–1159.

Fritz, M. S., & MacKinnon, D. P. (2007). Required sample size to detect the mediated effect. *Psychological Science, 18,* 223–239.

Frost, R. (1920). *Mountain interval.* New York: Henry Holt.

Gennetian, L. A., Morris, P. A., Bos, J. M., & Bloom, H. S. (2005). Constructing instrumental variables from experimental data to explore how treatments produce effects. In H. S. Bloom (Ed.), *Learning more from social experiments* (pp. 75–114). New York: Sage.

Ginsberg, A. (1954). Hypothetical constructs and intervening variables. *Psychological Review, 61,* 119–131.

Gleser, L. J. (1996). Comment on "Bootstrap confidence intervals" by T. J. DiCiccio and B. Efron. *Statistical Science, 11,* 219–221.

Goldberg, L., Elliot, D., Clarke, G. N., MacKinnon, D. P., Moe, E., Zoref, L., et al. (1996). Effects of a multidimensional anabolic steroid prevention intervention: The Adolescents Training and Learning to Avoid Steroids (ATLAS) program. *Journal of the American Medical Association, 276,* 1555–1562.

Goldberger, A. S. (1972). Structural equation methods in the social sciences. *Econometrica, 40,* 979–1001.

Gollob, H. F., & Reichardt, C. S. (1991). Interpreting and estimating indirect effects assuming time lags really matter. In L. M. Collins & J. L. Horn (Eds.), *Best methods for the analysis of change: Recent advances, unanswered questions, future directions* (pp. 243–259). Washington DC: American Psychological Association.

Good, P. (2000). *Permutation tests: A practical guide to resampling methods for testing hypotheses* (2nd ed.). New York: Springer-Verlag.

Goodman, L. A. (1960). On the exact variance of products. *Journal of the American Statistical Association, 55,* 708–713.

Gorgas, W. C. (1915). *Sanitation in Panama.* New York: D. Appleton.

Graff, J., & Schmidt, P. (1982). A general model for decomposition of effects. In K. G. Jöreskog & H. Wold (Eds.), *Systems under indirect observation: Causality, structure, prediction* (pp. 131–148). Amsterdam: North-Holland.

Greenland, S., & Morgenstern, H. (2001). Confounding in health research. *Annual Review of Public Health, 22,* 189–212.

Greenland, S., & Robins, J. M. (1986). Identifiability, exchangeability, and epidemiological confounding. *International Journal of Epidemiology, 15,* 413–419.

Griffin, M. A., Mathieu, J. E., & Jacobs, R. R. (2001). Perceptions of work contexts: Disentangling influences at multiple levels of analysis. *Journal of Occupational and Organizational Psychology, 74,* 563–579.

Guralnik, D. B. (Ed.) (1970). *Webster's new world dictionary of the American language* (2nd ed.). New York: The World Publishing Company.

Haggard, E. A. (1958). *Intraclass correlation and the analysis of variance.* New York: Dryden Press.

Haggstrom, G. W. (1983). Logistic regression and discriminant analysis by ordinary least squares. *Journal of Business & Economic Statistics, 1,* 229–238.

Hall, D. T., & Foster, L. W. (1977). A psychological success cycle and goal setting: Goals, performance, and attitudes. *Academy of Management Journal, 20,* 282–290.

Hamilton, D. (1987). Sometimes $R^2 > r^2_{yx1} + r^2_{yx2}$: Correlated variables are not always redundant. *American Statistician, 41,* 129–132.

Hannon, L. (1997). AFDC and homicide. *Journal of Sociology and Social Welfare, 24,* 125–136.

Hansen, W. B. (1992). School-based substance abuse prevention: A review of the state of the art in curriculum, 1980–1990. *Health Education Research, 7,* 403–430.

Hansen, W. B., & Graham, J. W. (1991). Preventing alcohol, marijuana, and cigarette use among adolescents: Peer pressure resistance training versus establishing conservative norms. *Preventive Medicine, 20,* 414–430.

Hansen, W. B., & McNeal, R. B. (1996). The law of maximum expected potential effect: Constraints placed on program effectiveness by mediator relationships. *Health Education Research: Theory and Practice, 11,* 501–507.

Hansen, W. B., & McNeal, R. B. (1997). How DARE works: An examination of program effects on mediating variables. *Health Education and Behavior, 24,* 165–176.

Hanushek, E. A., & Jackson, J. E. (1977). *Statistical methods for social scientists.* New York: Academic Press.

Harlow, L. L., Mulaik, S. A., & Steiger, J. H. (Eds.) (1997). *What if there were no significance tests?* Mahwah, NJ: Lawrence Erlbaum Associates.

Harris, M. J., & Rosenthal, R. (1985). Mediation of interpersonal expectancy effects: 31 meta-analyses. *Psychological Bulletin, 97,* 363–386.

Hawkins, J. D., Catalano, R. F., & Miller, J. Y. (1992). Risk and protective factors for alcohol and other drug problems in adolescence and early adulthood: Implications for substance abuse prevention. *Psychological Bulletin, 112,* 64–105.

Hayduk, L. A. (1987). *Structural equation models with LISREL: Essentials and advances.* Baltimore: Johns Hopkins University Press.

Hayduk, L. A., Cummings, G., Stratkotter, R., Nimmo, M., Grygoryev, K., Dosman, D., et al. (2003). Pearl's d-separation: One more step into causal thinking. *Structural Equation Modeling, 10,* 289–311.

Hayduk, L. A., & Wonnacott, T. H. (1980). 'Effect equations' or 'effect coefficients': A note on the visual and verbal presentation of multiple regression interactions. *Canadian Journal of Sociology, 5,* 399–404.

Heath, T. (2001). Mediators and moderators. *Journal of Consumer Psychology, 10,* 94–97.

Hebb, D. O. (1966). *A textbook of psychology* (2nd ed.). Philadelphia: Saunders.

Heck, R. H. (2001). Multilevel modeling with SEM. In G. A. Marcoulides & R. E. Schumacker (Eds.), *New developments and techniques in structural equation modeling* (pp. 89–127). Mahwah, NJ: Lawrence Erlbaum Associates.

Hedeker, D., Gibbons, R. D., & Flay, B. R. (1994). Random-effects regression models for clustered data with an example from smoking prevention research. *Journal of Consulting and Clinical Psychology, 62*, 757–765.

Hedges, L. V., & Olkin, I. (1985). *Statistical methods for meta-analysis*. Orlando, FL: Academic Press.

Heller, K., Price, R. H., Reinharz, S., Riger, S., & Wandersman, A. (with D'Aunno, T. A.) (1984). *Psychology and community change: Challenges of the future* (2nd ed.). Homewood, IL: Dorsey Press.

Henney, J. E. (1999). *Remarks by: Jane E. Henney, M.D. Commissioner of Food and Drugs*. International Conference on Surrogate Endpoints and Biomarkers—National Institutes of Health, Retrieved November 21, 2001, from http://www.fda.gov/oc/speeches/surrogates8.html

Herson, J. (1975). Fieller's theorem vs. the delta method for significance intervals for ratios. *Journal of Statistical Computing and Simulation, 3*, 265–274.

Hill, A. B. (1965). The environment and disease: Association or causation? *Proceedings of the Royal Society of Medicine, 58*, 295–300.

Hill, A. B. (1971). *Principles of medical statistics* (9th ed.). New York: Oxford.

Hinshaw, S. P. (2002). Intervention research, theoretical mechanisms, and causal processes related to externalizing behavior patterns. *Development and Psychopathology, 14*, 789–818.

Hofmann, D. A., & Gavin, M. B. (1998). Centering decisions in hierarchical linear models: Implications for research in organizations. *Journal of Management, 24*, 623–641.

Holbert, R. L., & Stephenson, M. T. (2003). The importance of indirect effects in media effects research: Testing for mediation in structural equation modeling. *Journal of Broadcasting & Electronic Media, 47*, 556–572.

Holland, P. W. (1986). Statistics and causal inference (with comments). *Journal of the American Statistical Association, 81*, 945–970.

Holland, P. W. (1988a). Causal inference, path analysis, and recursive structural equation models. *Sociological Methodology, 18*, 449–484.

Holland, P. W. (1988b). Comment: Causal mechanism or causal effect: Which is best for statistical science? *Statistical Science, 3*, 186–188.

Holland, P. W., & Rubin, D. B. (1983). On Lord's paradox. In H. Wainer & S. Messick (Eds.), *Principals of modern psychological measurement: A festschrift for Frederick M. Lord* (pp. 3–25). Hillsdale, NJ: Lawrence Erlbaum Associates.

Hollon, S. D., Evans, M. D., & DeRubeis, R., J. (1990). Cognitive mediation of relapse prevention following treatment for depression: Implications of differential risk. In R. E. Ingram (Ed.), *Contemporary psychological approaches to depression: theory, research, and treatment* (pp. 117–136). New York: Plenum.

Holmbeck, G. N. (1997). Toward terminological, conceptual, and statistical clarity in the study of mediators and moderators: Examples from the child-clinical and pediatric psychology literatures. *Journal of Consulting and Clinical Psychology, 65*, 599–610.

Horst, P. (1941). The role of prediction variables which are independent of the criterion. *Social Science Research Council Bulletin, 48*, 431–436.

Hosmer, D. W., & Lemeshow, S. (2000). *Applied logistic regression* (2nd ed.). New York: Wiley.

Howe, G. W., Reiss, D., & Yuh, J. (2002). Can prevention trials test theories of etiology? *Development and Psychopathology, 14*, 673–694.

Hox, J. J. (2002). *Multilevel analysis: Techniques and applications.* Mahwah, NJ: Lawrence Erlbaum Associates.

Hoyle, R. H., & Kenny, D. A. (1999). Sample size, reliability, and tests of statistical mediation. In R. H. Hoyle (Ed.), *Statistical strategies for small sample research* (pp. 195–222). Thousand Oaks, CA: Sage.

Hoyle, R. H., & Smith, G. T. (1994). Formulating clinical research hypotheses as structural equation models: A conceptual overview. *Journal of Consulting and Clinical Psychology, 62*, 429–440.

Hu, L., & Bentler, P. M. (1999). Cutoff criteria for fit indexes in covariance structure analysis: Conventional criteria versus new alternatives. *Structural Equation Modeling, 6*, 1–55.

Huey, S. J., Henggeler, S. W., Brondino, M. J., & Pickrel, S. G. (2000). Mechanisms of change in multisystemic therapy: Reducing delinquent behavior through therapist adherence and improved family and peer functioning. *Journal of Consulting and Clinical Psychology, 68*, 451–467.

Huitema, B. E. (1980). *The analysis of covariance and alternatives.* New York: Wiley.

Hull, C. L. (1937). Mind, mechanism, and adaptive behavior. *Psychological Review, 44*, 1–32.

Hull, C. L. (1943). *Principles of behavior.* New York: Appleton-Century-Crofts.

Hume, D. (1748). *An enquiry concerning human understanding.* London.

Hyman, H. H. (1955). *Survey design and analysis: Principles, cases and procedures.* Glencoe, IL: Free Press.

Jackson, K. M., & Sher, K. J. (2003). Alcohol use disorders and psychological distress: A prospective state-trait analysis. *Journal of Abnormal Psychology, 112*, 599–613.

James, L. R., & Brett, J. M. (1984). Mediators, moderators, and tests for mediation. *Journal of Applied Psychology, 69*, 307–321.

James, L. R., James, L. A., & Ashe, D. K. (1990). The meaning of organizations: The role of cognition and values. In B. Schneider (Ed.), *Organizational climate and culture* (pp. 40–84). San Francisco: Jossey-Bass.

James, L. R., Mulaik, S. A., & Brett, J. M. (1982). *Causal analysis: Assumptions, models, and data.* Beverly Hills, CA: Sage.

James, L. R., Mulaik, S. A., & Brett, J. M. (2006). A tale of two methods. *Organizational Research Methods, 9*, 233–244.

Jessor, R., & Jessor, S. L. (1980). A social-psychological framework for studying drug use. In D. J. Lettieri, M. Sayers, & H. W. Pearson (Eds.), *National Institute on Drug Abuse Monograph 30. Theories on drug abuse: Selected contemporary perspectives* (pp. 102–109). Washington, DC: U.S. Government Printing Office.

Jo, B. (2004, May). *Causal inference in mediation models.* Paper presented at the 12th annual meeting of the Society for Prevention Research, Quebec City, Quebec, Canada.

Jo, B. (2006). *Causal inference in randomized trials with mediational processes.* Unpublished paper.

Jöreskog, K. G. (1970). A general method for analysis of covariance structures. *Biometrika, 57,* 239–251.

Jöreskog, K. G. (1973). A general method for estimating a linear structural equation system. In A. S. Golberger & O. D. Duncan (Eds.), *Structural equation models in the social sciences* (pp. 85–112). New York: Seminar Press.

Jöreskog, K. G. (1979). Statistical estimation of structural models in longitudinal-developmental investigations. In J. R. Nesselroade & P. B. Baltes (Eds.), *Longitudinal research in the study of behavior and development* (pp. 303–352), New York: Academic.

Jöreskog, K. G., & Sörbom, D. (2001). *LISREL (Version 8.5)* [Computer software]. Chicago: Scientific Software International.

Judd, C. M., & Kenny, D. A. (1981a). *Estimating the effects of social interventions.* Cambridge, England: Cambridge University Press.

Judd, C. M., & Kenny, D. A. (1981b). Process analysis: Estimating mediation in treatment evaluations. *Evaluation Review, 5,* 602–619.

Judd, C. M., Kenny, D. A., & McClelland, G. H. (2001). Estimating and testing mediation and moderation in within-subject designs. *Psychological Methods, 6,* 115–134.

Kant, I. (1965). *Critique of pure reason* (N. M. Smith, Trans.). New York: St. Martins Press. (Original work published 1781)

Kaplan, D. (2000). *Structural equation modeling: Foundations and extensions.* Thousand Oaks, CA: Sage.

Kazdin, A. E. (1989). Childhood depression. In E. J. Mash & R. A. Barkley (Eds.), *Treatment of Childhood Disorders* (pp. 135–166). New York: Guilford Press.

Kazdin, A. E. (1998). *Research design in clinical psychology* (3rd ed.). Boston: Allyn & Bacon.

Kazdin, A. E. (2000). Developing a research agenda for child and adolescent psychotherapy. *Archives of General Psychiatry, 57,* 829–835.

Kazdin, A. E., & Nock, M. K. (2003). Delineating mechanisms of change in child and adolescent therapy: Methodological issues and research recommendations. *Journal of Child Psychology and Psychiatry, 44,* 1116–1129.

Kazdin, A. E., & Weisz, J. R. (Eds.) (2003). *Evidence-based psychotherapies for children and adolescents.* New York: Guilford Press.

Keesling, J. W. (1972, June). *Maximum likelihood approaches to causal analysis.* Unpublished doctoral dissertation, University of Chicago.

Kendall, P. L., & Lazarsfeld, P. F. (1950). Problems of survey analysis. In R. K. Merton & P. F. Lazarsfeld (Eds.), *Continuities in social research: Studies in the scope and method of "The American Soldier"* (pp. 133–196). Glencoe, IL: Free Press.

Kenny, D. A. (1979). *Correlation and causality.* New York: Wiley.

Kenny, D. A., Bolger, N., & Korchmaros, J. D. (2003). Lower level mediation in multilevel models. *Psychological Methods, 8,* 115–128.

Kenny, D. A., Kashy, D. A., & Bolger, N. (1998). Data analysis in social psychology. In D. T. Gilbert, S. T. Fiske, & G. Lindzey (Eds.), *The handbook of social psychology* (4th ed., Vol. 1, pp. 233–265). New York: Oxford University Press.

Keppel, G., & Wickens, T. D. (2004). *Design and analysis: A researcher's handbook* (4th ed.). Upper Saddle River, NJ: Pearson/Prentice Hall.

Kerckhoff, A. C. (1974). *ASA Rose Monograph Series. Ambition and attainment: A study of four samples of American boys.* Washington DC: American Sociological Association.

Kish, L. (1965). *Survey sampling.* New York: Wiley.

Klein, A., & Moosbrugger, H. (2000). Maximum likelihood estimation of latent interaction effects with the LMS method. *Psychometrika, 65,* 457–474.

Klesges, R. C., Vasey, M. M., & Glasgow, R. E. (1986). A worksite smoking modification competition: Potential for public health impact. *American Journal of Public Health, 76,* 198–200.

Kline, R. B. (1998). *Principles and practice of structural equation modeling.* New York: Guilford Press.

Kline, R. B. (2004). *Beyond significance testing: Reforming data analysis methods in behavioral research.* Washington, DC: American Psychological Association.

Komro, K. A., Perry, C. L., Williams, C. L., Stigler, M. H., Farbakhsh, K., & Veblen-Mortenson, S. (2001). How did Project Northland reduce alcohol use among young adolescents? Analysis of mediating variables. *Health Education Research, 16,* 59–70.

Kraemer, H. C. (2003, November). *Finding structural needles in statistical haystacks: Methods for identifying mediators and moderators.* Mediators & Moderators Workshop, Western Psychiatric Institute and Clinic at the University of Pittsburgh School of Medicine, Pittsburgh, PA.

Kraemer, H. C., Kiernan, M., Essex, M., & Kupfer, D. (2004). *Moderators and mediators in biomedical research: The MacArthur and the Baron and Kenny approaches.* Unpublished manuscript.

Kraemer, H. C., Stice, E., Kazdin, A., Offord, D., & Kupfer, D. (2001). How do risk factors work together? Mediators, moderators, and independent, overlapping, and proxy risk factors. *American Journal of Psychiatry, 158,* 848–856.

Kraemer, H. C., Wilson, G. T., Fairburn, C. G., & Agras, W. S. (2002). Mediators and moderators of treatment effects in randomized clinical trials. *Archives of General Psychiatry, 59,* 877–883.

Krantz, D. H. (1999). The null hypothesis testing controversy in psychology. *Journal of the American Statistical Association, 44,* 1372–1381.

Kreft, I. G. G. (1996). *Are multilevel techniques necessary? An overview, including simulation studies.* Retrieved Month XX, 200X, from http://www.calstatela.edu/faculty/ikreft/quarterly/quarterly.html

Kreft, I. G. G., de Leeuw, J., & Aiken, L. S. (1995). The effect of different forms of centering in hierarchical linear models. *Multivariate Behavioral Research, 30,* 1–21.

Kristal, A. R., Glanz, K., Tilley, B. C., & Li, S. (2000). Mediating factors in dietary change: Understanding the impact of a worksite nutrition intervention. *Health Education and Behavior, 27,* 112–125.

Krull, J. L., & MacKinnon, D. P. (1999). Multilevel mediation modeling in group-based intervention studies. *Evaluation Review, 23,* 418–444.

Krull, J. L., & MacKinnon, D. P. (2001). Multilevel modeling of individual and group level mediated effects. *Multivariate Behavioral Research, 36,* 249–277.

Last, J. M. (1988). *A dictionary of epidemiology* (2nd ed.). New York: Oxford University Press.

Last, J. M., & Wallace, R. B. (1992). *Maxcy-Rosenau-Last public health and preventive medicine* (13th ed.). East Norwalk, CT: Appleton & Lange.

Lazarsfeld, P. F. (1955). Interpretation of statistical relations as a research operation. In P. F. Lazarsfeld & M. Rosenberg (Eds.), *The language of social research: A reader in the methodology of social research* (pp. 115–125). Glencoe, IL: Free Press.

Lee, S., & Hershberger, S. (1990). A simple rule for generating equivalent models in covariance structure modeling. *Multivariate Behavioral Research, 25,* 313–334.

Lehmann, D. (2001). Mediators and moderators. *Journal of Consumer Psychology, 10,* 90–92.

Leigh, J. P. (1983). Direct and indirect effects of education on health. *Social Science and Medicine, 17,* 227–234.

Leventhal, H. (1971). Fear appeals and persuasion: The differentiation of a motivational construct. *American Journal of Public Health, 61,* 1208–1224.

Lewis, B. A., Marcus, B. H., Pate, R. R., & Dunn, A. L. (2002). Psychosocial mediators of physical activity behavior among adults and children. *American Journal of Preventive Medicine, 23,* 26–35.

Lin, D. Y., Psaty, B. M., & Kronmal, R. A. (1998). Assessing the sensitivity of regression results to unmeasured confounders in observational studies. *Biometrics, 54,* 948–963.

Ling, R. (1982). Review of the book: *Correlation and causation,* by D. A. Kenny. *Journal of the American Statistical Association, 77,* 489–491.

Lipsey, M. W. (1993). Theory as method: Small theories of treatments. In L. B. Sechrest & A. G. Scott (Eds.), *Understanding causes and generalizing about them: New directions for program evaluation* (pp. 5–38). San Francisco: Jossey-Bass.

Lockwood, C. M., & MacKinnon, D. P. (1998). Bootstrapping the standard error of the mediated effect. In *Proceedings of the Twenty-Third Annual SAS Users Group International Conference* (pp. 997–1002). Cary, NC: SAS Institute.

Lomnicki, Z. A. (1967). On the distribution of products of random variables. *Journal of the Royal Statistical Society, Series B (Methodological), 29,* 513–524.

Longabaugh, R., & Writz, P. W. (Eds.) (2001). *Project MATCH Hypotheses: Results and causal chain analyses.* U.S. Department of Health and Human Services. Washington, DC: U.S. Government Printing Office.

Lord, F. M. (1963). Elementary models for measuring change. In C. W. Harris (Ed.), *Problems in measuring change* (pp. 21–38). Madison, WI: University of Wisconsin Press.

Lord, F. M., & Novick, M. R. (1968). *Statistical theories of mental test scores.* Reading, MA: Addison-Wesley.

Ludbrook, J., & Dudley, H. (1998). Why permutation tests are superior to *t* and *F* tests in biomedical research. *American Statistician, 52,* 127–132.

MacCallum, R. C., & Austin, J. T. (2000). Applications of structural equation modeling in psychological research. *Annual Review of Psychology, 51,* 201–226.

MacCallum, R. C., Wegener, D. T., Uchino, B. N., & Fabrigar, L. R. (1993). The problem of equivalent models in applications of covariance structure analysis. *Psychological Bulletin, 114,* 185–199.

MacCorquodale, K., & Meehl, P. E. (1948). On a distinction between hypothetical constructs and intervening constructs. *Psychological Review, 55,* 95–107.

MacKinnon, D. P. (1994). Analysis of mediating variables in prevention and intervention research. In A. Cazares & L. A. Beatty (Eds.), *Scientific methods for prevention/intervention research* (NIDA Research Monograph Series 139, DHHS Publication No. 94-3631, pp. 127–153). Washington, DC: U.S. Department of Health and Human Services.

MacKinnon, D. P. (2000). Contrasts in multiple mediator models. In J. S. Rose, L. Chassin, C. C. Presson, & S. J. Sherman (Eds.), *Multivariate applications in substance use research: New methods for new questions* (pp. 141–160). Mahwah, NJ: Lawrence Erlbaum Associates.

MacKinnon, D. P. (2001). Mediating variable. In N. J. Smelser & P. B. Baltes (Eds.), *International encyclopedia of the social and behavioral sciences* (pp. 9503–9507). Oxford, England: Pergamon.

MacKinnon, D. P., & Dwyer, J. H. (1993). Estimating mediated effects in prevention studies. *Evaluation Review, 17*, 144–158.

MacKinnon, D. P., Dwyer, J. H., & Arminger, G. (1992). DIFFLONG: A program to calculate the parameters of differential equation models for longitudinal data. Appendix in J. H. Dwyer, M. Feinleib, P. Lippert, & H. Hoffmeister (Eds.), *Statistical models for longitudinal studies of health* (pp. 96–97). New York: Oxford University Press.

MacKinnon, D. P., Fritz, M. S., Williams, J., & Lockwood, C. M. (2007). Distribution of the product confidence limits for the indirect effect: Program PRODCLIN. *Behavior Research Methods, 39*, 384–389.

MacKinnon, D. P., Goldberg, L., Clarke, G. N., Elliot, D. L., Cheong, J., Lapin, A., et al. (2001). Mediating mechanisms in a program to reduce intentions to use anabolic steroids and improve exercise self-efficacy and dietary behavior. *Prevention Science, 2*, 15–28.

MacKinnon, D. P., Johnson, C. A., Pentz, M. A., Dwyer, J. H., Hansen, W. B., Flay, B. R., & Wang, E. Y. I. (1991). Mediating mechanisms in a school-based drug prevention program: First-year effects of the Midwestern Prevention Project. *Health Psychology, 10*, 164–172.

MacKinnon, D. P., Krull, J. L., & Lockwood, C. M. (2000). Equivalence of the mediation, confounding, and suppression effect. *Prevention Science, 1*, 173–181.

MacKinnon, D. P., & Lockwood, C. M. (2001, May). *An approximate randomization test for the mediated effect.* Abstract presented at the annual meeting of the Western Psychological Association, Maui, HI.

MacKinnon, D. P., Lockwood, C. M., Brown, C. H., Wang, W., & Hoffman, J. M. (2006). *The intermediate variable effect in logistic and probit regression.* Manuscript submitted for publication.

MacKinnon, D. P., Lockwood C. M., Hoffman, J. M., West, S. G., & Sheets, V. (2002). A comparison of methods to test mediation and other intervening variable effects. *Psychological Methods, 7*, 83–104.

MacKinnon, D. P., Lockwood C. M., & Williams, J. (2004). Confidence limits for the indirect effect: Distribution of the product and resampling methods. *Multivariate Behavioral Research, 39*, 99–128.

MacKinnon, D. P., Taborga, M. P., & Morgan-Lopez, A. A. (2002). Mediation designs for tobacco prevention research. *Drug and Alcohol Dependence, 68*, S69-S83.

MacKinnon, D. P., Warsi, G., & Dwyer, J. H. (1995). A simulation study of mediated effect measures. *Multivariate Behavioral Research, 30*, 41–62.

MacKinnon, D. P., Weber, M. D., & Pentz, M. A. (1989). How do school-based drug prevention programs work and for whom? *Drugs and Society, 3*, 125–143.

Malone, P. S., Lansford, J. E., Castellino, D. R., Berlin, L. J., Dodge, K. A., Bates, J. E., & Pettit, G. S. (2004). Divorce and child behavior problems: Applying latent change score models to life event data. *Structural Equation Modeling, 11*, 401–423.

Manly, B. F. J. (1997). *Randomization and Monte Carlo methods in biology* (2nd ed.). London: Chapman & Hall.

Mark, M. M. (1986). Validity typologies and the logic and practice of quasi-experimentation. In W. M. K. Trochim (Ed.), *Advances in quasi-experimental design and analysis* (pp. 47–66). San Francisco: Jossey-Bass.

Marsh, H. W., Wen, Z., & Hau, K. T. (2004). Structural equation models of latent interactions: Evaluation of alternative estimation strategies and indicator construction. *Psychological Methods, 9*, 275–300.

Maxwell, J. A. (2004). Causal explanation, qualitative research, and scientific inquiry in education. *Educational Researcher, 33*, 3–11.

Maxwell, J. A., Bashook, P. G., & Sandlow, L. J. (1986). Combining ethnographic and experimental methods in educational evaluation: A case study. In D. M. Fetterman & M. A. Pittman (Eds.), *Educational evaluation: Ethnography in theory, practice, and politics* (pp. 121–143). Newbury Park, CA: Sage.

Mays, V. M., Albee, G. W., & Schneider, S. F. (1989). *Primary prevention of AIDS: Psychological approaches*. Newbury Park, CA: Sage.

McAlister, A. L., Perry, C., & Maccoby, N. (1979). Adolescent smoking: Onset and prevention. *Pediatrics, 63*, 650–658.

McArdle, J. J. (2001). A latent difference score approach to longitudinal dynamic structural analysis. In R. Cudeck, S. du Toit, & D. Sörbom (Eds.), *Structural equation modeling: Present and future. A festschrift in honor of Karl Jöreskog* (pp. 341–380). Lincolnwood, IL: Scientific Software International.

McArdle, J. J., & Hamagami, F. (2001). Latent difference score structural models for linear dynamic analyses with incomplete longitudinal data. In L. M. Collins & A. G. Sayer (Eds.), *New methods for the analysis of change* (pp. 139–175). Washington, DC: American Psychological Association.

McArdle, J. J., & McDonald, R. P. (1984). Some algebraic properties of the reticular action model for moment structures. *British Journal of Mathematical and Statistical Psychology, 37*, 234–251.

McArdle, J. J., & Nesselroade, J. R. (2003). Growth curve analysis in contemporary psychological research. In J. Schinka & W. Velicer (Eds.), *Comprehensive handbook of psychology, Vol. II: Research methods in psychology* (pp. 447–480). New York: Pergamon Press.

McCaffrey, D. F., Ridgeway, G., & Morral, A. R. (2004). Propensity score estimation with boosted regression for evaluating causal effects in observational studies. *Psychological Methods, 9*, 403–425.

McCaul, K. D., & Glasgow, R. E. (1985). Preventing adolescent smoking: What have we learned about treatment construct validity? *Health Psychology, 4*, 361–387.

McCullagh, P., & Nelder, J. A. (1989). *Generalized linear models* (2nd ed.). New York: Chapman & Hall.

McDonald, R. P. (1997). Haldane's lungs: A case study in path analysis. *Multivariate Behavioral Research, 32*, 1–38.

McFatter, R. M. (1979). The use of structural equation models in interpreting regression equations including suppressor and enhancer variables. *Applied Psychological Measurement, 3*, 123–135.

McGraw, K. O., & Wong, S. P. (1996). Forming inferences about some intraclass correlation coefficients. *Psychological Methods, 1*, 30–46.

McGuigan, K., & Langholz, B. (1988). *A note on testing mediation paths using ordinary least-squares regression.* Unpublished manuscript.

McGuire, W. J. (1999). *Constructing social psychology: Creative and critical processes.* Cambridge, England: Cambridge University Press.

McLeod, D. M, Kosicki, G. M., & McLeod, J. M. (2002). Resurveying the boundaries of political communication effects. In J. Bryant & D. Zillmann (Eds.), *Media effects: Advances in theory and research* (2nd ed., pp. 215–267). Mahwah, NJ: Lawrence Erlbaum Associates.

McLeod, J. M., & Reeves, B. (1980). On the nature of mass media effects. In S. B. Withey & R. P. Abeles (Eds.), *Television and social behavior: Beyond violence and children* (pp. 17–54). Hillsdale, NJ: Lawrence Erlbaum Associates.

Meehl, P. E., & Waller, N. G. (2002). The path analysis controversy: A new statistical approach to strong appraisal of verisimilitude. *Psychological Methods, 7,* 283–300.

Meeker, W. Q., Jr., Cornwell, L. W., & Aroian, L. A. (1981). The product of two normally distributed random variables. In W. J. Kennedy & R. E. Odeh (Eds.), *Selected Tables in Mathematical Statistics* (Vol. VII, pp. 1–256). Providence, RI: American Mathematical Society.

Meeker, W. Q., & Escobar, L. A. (1994). An algorithm to compute the cdf of the product of two normal random variables. *Communications in Statistics: Simulation and Computation, 23,* 271–280.

Meinert, C. L. (with Tonascia, S.) (1986). *Monographs in epidemiology and biostatistics: Vol. 8. Clinical trials: design, conduct, and analysis.* New York: Oxford University Press.

Mensinger, J. L. (2005). Disordered eating and gender socialization in independent-school environments: A multilevel mediation model. *Journal of Ambulatory Care Management, 28,* 30–40.

Merrill, R. M. (1994). *Treatment effect evaluation in nonadditive mediation models.* Unpublished doctoral dissertation, Arizona State University, Tempe.

Merrill, R. M., MacKinnon, D. P., & Mayer, L. S. (1994). *Estimation of moderated mediation effects in experimental studies.* Unpublished manuscript.

Mill, J. S. (1843). *A system of logic.* London: John W. Parker.

Miller, L., & Downer, A. (1988). AIDS: What you and your friends need to know—A lesson plan for adolescents. *Journal of School Health, 58,* 137–141.

Mood, A. M., Graybill, F. A., & Boes, D. C. (1974). *Introduction to the theory of statistics* (3rd ed.). New York: McGraw-Hill.

Mooney, C. Z., & Duval, R. D. (1993). *Bootstrapping: A non-parametric approach to statistical inference.* Newbury Park, CA: Sage.

Morgan-Lopez, A. A., Castro, F. G., Chassin, L., & MacKinnon, D. P. (2003). A mediated moderation model of cigarette use among Mexican American youth. *Addictive Behaviors, 28,* 583–589.

Morgan-Lopez, A. A., & MacKinnon, D. P. (2001, June). *A mediated moderation model simulation: Mediational processes that vary as a function of second predictors.* Abstract presented at the 9th annual meeting of the Society for Prevention Research, Washington, DC.

Mosteller, F., & Tukey, J. W. (1977). *Data analysis and regression: A second course in statistics.* Reading, MA: Addison-Wesley.

Moulton, B. R. (1986). Random group effects and the precision of regression estimates. *Journal of Econometrics, 32,* 385–397.

MTA Cooperative Group (1999). Moderators and mediators of treatment response for children with attention-deficit/hyperactivity disorder. *Archives of General Psychiatry, 56,* 1088–1096.

Mulaik, S. A. (1972). *The foundations of factor analysis.* New York: McGraw-Hill.

Muller, D., Judd, C. M., & Yzerbyt, V. Y. (2005). When moderation is mediated and when mediation is moderated. *Journal of Personality and Social Psychology, 89,* 852–863.

Multiple Risk Factor Intervention Trial Research Group (1990). Mortality rates after 10.5 years for participants in the Multiple Risk Factor Intervention Trial. *Journal of the American Medical Association, 263,* 1795–1801.

Murray, D. M. (1998). *Design and analysis of group-randomized trials.* New York: Oxford University Press.

Murray, D. M., Catellier, D. J., Hannan, P. J., Treuth, M. S., Stevens, J., Schmitz, K. H., et al. (2004). School-level intraclass correlation for physical activity in adolescent girls. *Medicine & Science in Sports & Exercise, 36,* 876–882.

Murray, D. M., Luepker, R. V., Pirie, P. L., Grimm, R. H., Bloom, E., Davis, M. A., et al. (1986). Systematic risk factor screening and education: A community-wide approach to prevention of coronary heart disease. *Preventive Medicine, 15,* 661–672.

Murray, D. M., Rooney, B. L., Hannan, P. J., Peterson, A. V., Ary, D. V., Biglan, A., Botvin, G. J., Evans, R. I., Flay, B. R., Futterman, R., Getz, J. G., Marek, P. M., Orlandi, M., Pentz, M. A., Perry, C. L., & Schinke, S. P. (1994). Intraclass correlation among common measures of adolescent smoking: Estimates, correlates, and applications in smoking prevention studies. *American Journal of Epidemiology, 140,* 1038–1050.

Muthén, B. (1984). A general structural equation model with dichotomous, ordered categorical, and continuous latent variable indicators. *Psychometrika, 49,* 115–132.

Muthén, B. O., & Curran, P. J. (1997). General longitudinal modeling of individual differences in experimental designs: A latent variable framework for analysis and power estimation. *Psychological Methods, 2,* 371–402.

Muthén, B. O., & Satorra, A. (1995). Complex sample data in structural equation modeling. *Sociological Methodology, 25,* 267–316.

Muthén, L. K., & Muthén, B. O. (1998–2004). *Mplus 3.0: User's guide.* Los Angeles: Author.

Nagin, D. S. (1999). Analyzing developmental trajectories: A semiparametric, group-based, approach. *Psychological Methods, 4,* 139–157.

Nagin, D. S. (2005). *Group-based modeling of development.* Cambridge, MA: Harvard University Press.

Neale, M. C., Boker, S. M., Xie, G., & Maes, H. H. (2002). *Mx: Statistical modeling* (6th ed.). Richmond, VA: Department of Psychiatry, Virginia Commonwealth University.

Neyman, J. (1923). On the application of probability theory to agricultural experiments: Essay on principles (with discussion). Section 9 (D. M. Dabrowska & T. P. Speed, Trans.). *Statistical Science, 5,* 465–480.

Niles, H. E. (1922). Correlation, causation, and Wright's theory of "path coefficients." *Genetics, 7,* 258–273.

Niles, H. E. (1923). The method of path coefficients: An answer to Wright. *Genetics, 8,* 256–260.

Noreen, E. W. (1989). *Computer-intensive methods for testing hypotheses: An introduction.* New York: Wiley.

Olkin, I., & Finn, J. D. (1995). Correlations redux. *Psychological Bulletin, 118,* 155–164.

Olkin, I., & Siotani, M. (1976). Asymptotic distribution of functions of a correlation matrix. In S. Ikeda (Ed.), *Essays in probability and statistics* (pp. 235–251). Tokyo: Shinko Tsusho.

Ouimette, P. C., Finney, J. W., & Moos, R. H. (1999). Two-year posttreatment functioning and coping of substance abuse patients with posttraumatic stress disorder. *Psychology of Addictive Behaviors, 13,* 105–114.

Overton, R. C. (2001). Moderated multiple regression for interactions involving categorical variables: A statistical control for heterogeneous variance across two groups. *Psychological Methods, 6,* 218–233.

Palmer, R. F., Graham, J. W., White, E. L., & Hansen, W. B. (1998). Applying multilevel analytic strategies in adolescent substance use prevention research. *Preventive Medicine, 27,* 328–336.

Pearl, J. (2000). *Causality: models, reasoning, and inference.* Cambridge, England: Cambridge University Press.

Pearson, K. (1911). *The grammar of science* (3rd ed.). London: Adam & Charles Black.

Pentz, M. A., Dwyer, J. H., MacKinnon, D. P., Flay, B. R., Hansen, W. B., Wang, E. Y. I., et al. (1989). A multicommunity trial for primary prevention of adolescent drug abuse: Effects on drug use prevalence. *Journal of the American Medical Association, 261,* 3259–3266.

Peterson, A. V., Kealey, K. A., Mann, S. L., Marek, P. M., & Sarason, I. G. (2000). Hutchinson Smoking Prevention Project: Long-term randomized trial in school-based tobacco use prevention—results on smoking. *Journal of the National Cancer Institute, 92,* 1979–1991.

Petrosino, A. (2000). Mediators and moderators in the evaluation of programs for children. *Evaluation Review, 24,* 47–72.

Pitman, E. J. G. (1937). Significance tests which may be applied to samples from any populations. *Journal of the Royal Statistical Society Supplement, 4,* 119–130.

Popper, K. R. (1959). *The logic of scientific discovery* (in German). New York: Basic Books.

Pratt, J. W., & Schlaifer, R. (1988). On the interpretation and observation of laws. *Journal of Econometrics, 39,* 23–52.

Preacher, K. J., Curran, P. J., & Bauer, D. J. (2006). Computational tools for probing interactions in multiple linear regression, multilevel modeling, and latent curve analysis. *Journal of Educational and Behavioral Statistics, 31,* 437–448.

Preacher, K. J., & Hayes, A. F. (2004). SPSS and SAS procedures for estimating indirect effects in simple mediation models. *Behavior Research Methods, Instruments, & Computers, 36,* 717–731.

Premack, S. L., & Hunter, J. E., (1988). Individual unionization decisions. *Psychological Bulletin, 103,* 223–234.

Prentice, R. L. (1989). Surrogate endpoints in clinical trials: Definition and operational criteria. *Statistics in Medicine, 8,* 431–440.

Prochaska, J. O., DiClemente, C. C., & Norcross, J. C. (1992). In search of how people change: Applications to addictive behaviors. *American Psychologist, 47,* 1102–1114.

Prussia, G. E., & Kinicki, A. J. (1996). A motivational investigation of group effectiveness using social-cognitive theory. *Journal of Applied Psychology, 81,* 187–198.

Pynoos, R. S., & Nader, K. (1989). Prevention of psychiatric morbidity in children after disaster. In D. Shaffer, I. Philips, & N. B. Enzer (Eds.), *Prevention of mental disorder, alcohol, and other drug use in children and adolescents* (Office for Substance Abuse Prevention Monograph 2, DHHS Publication No. (ADM) 89-1646, pp. 25–271). Washington, DC: U.S. Government Printing Office.

Rao, C. R. (1973). *Linear statistical inference and its applications.* New York: Wiley.

Raudenbush, S. W., & Sampson, R. (1999). Assessing direct and indirect effects in multilevel designs with latent variables. *Sociological Methods & Research, 28,* 123–153.

Rice, J. A. (1988). *Mathematical statistics and data analysis.* Monterey, CA: Brooks/Cole Company.

Robins, J. M., & Greenland, S. (1992). Identifiability and exchangeability for direct and indirect effects. *Epidemiology, 3,* 143–155.

Robinson, W. S. (1950). Ecological correlations and the behavior of individuals. *American Sociological Review, 15,* 351–357.

Rogosa, D. R. (1988). Myths about longitudinal research. In K. W. Schaie, R. T. Campbell, W. M. Meredith, & S. C. Rawlings (Eds.), *Methodological issues in aging research* (pp. 171–209). New York: Springer.

Rosenbaum, P. R. (1984). The consequences of adjustment for a concomitant variable that has been affected by the treatment. *Journal of the Royal Statistical Society, A, 147,* 656–666.

Rosenbaum, P. R. (2001). Replicating effects and biases. *American Statistician, 55,* 223–227.

Rosenbaum, P. R. (2002a). Covariance adjustment in randomized experiments and observational studies. *Statistical Science, 17,* 286–327.

Rosenbaum, P. R. (2002b). *Observational studies* (2nd ed.). New York: Springer.

Rosenberg, M. (1968). *The logic of survey analysis.* New York: Basic Books.

Rosenthal, R. (1987). Pygmalion effects: Existence, magnitude, and social importance: A reply to Wineburg. *Educational Researcher, 16,* 37–41.

Rosenthal, R., & Fode, K. L. (1963). The effect of experimenter bias on the performance of the albino rat. *Behavioral Science, 8,* 183–189.

Rosetti, C. G. (1872). *Sing-song: A nursery rhyme book.* London: G. Routledge.

Rosnow, R. L., & Rosenthal. R. (1989). Statistical procedures and the justification of knowledge in psychological science. *American Psychologist, 44,* 1276–1284.

Rothman, K. J., & Greenland, S. (1998). *Modern epidemiology* (2nd ed.). Philadelphia: Lippincott, Williams & Wilkins.

Rozeboom, W. W. (1956). Mediation variables in scientific theory. *Psychological Review, 63,* 249–264.

Rubin, D. B. (1974). Estimating causal effects of treatments in randomized and nonrandomized studies. *Journal of Educational Psychology, 66,* 688–701.

Rubin, D. B. (1977). Assignment to treatment group on the basis of a covariate. *Journal of Educational Statistics, 2,* 1–26.

Rubin, D. B. (2004). Direct and indirect causal effects via potential outcomes. *Scandinavian Journal of Statistics, 31,* 161–170.

Russell, D. W., Kahn, J. H., Spoth, R., & Altmaier, E. M. (1998). Analyzing data from experimental studies: A latent variable structural equation modeling approach. *Journal of Counseling Psychology, 45,* 18–29.

Salthouse, T. A. (1984). Effects of age and skill in typing. *Journal of Experimental Psychology: General, 113,* 345–371.

Sampson, C. B., & Breunig, H. L. (1971). Some statistical aspects of pharmaceutical content uniformity. *Journal of Quality Technology, 3,* 170–178.

Sampson, R. J., Morenoff, J. D., & Gannon-Rowley, T. (2002). Assessing "neighborhood effects": Social processes and new directions in research. *Annual Review of Sociology, 28,* 443–478.

Sampson, R. J., Raudenbush, S. W., & Earls, F. (1997). Neighborhoods and violent crime: A multilevel study of collective efficacy. *Science, 277,* 918–924.

Sandler, I. N., Wolchik, S. A., MacKinnon, D. P., Ayers, T. S., & Roosa, M. W. (1997). Developing linkages between theory and intervention in stress and coping processes. In S. A. Wolchik & I. N. Sandler (Eds.), *Handbook of children's coping: Linking theory and intervention* (pp. 3–40). New York: Plenum Press.

SAS (Version 6.12) [Computer software]. (1989). Cary, NC: SAS Institute.

Scariano, S. M., & Davenport, J. M. (1987). The effects of violations of independence assumptions in the one-way ANOVA. *The American Statistician, 41,* 123–129.

Scheines, R., Spirtes, P., Glymour, C., & Meek, C. (1994). *TETRAD II: Tools for discovery.* Hillsdale, NJ: Lawrence Erlbaum Associates.

Scott, A. J., & Holt, D. (1982). The effect of two-stage sampling on ordinary least squares methods. *Journal of the American Statistical Association, 77,* 848–854.

Shadish, W. R. (1996). Meta-analysis and the exploration of causal mediating processes: A primer of examples, methods, and issues. *Psychological Methods, 1,* 47–65.

Shadish, W. R., & Baldwin, S. A. (2003). Meta-analysis of MFT interventions. *Journal of Marital and Family Therapy, 29,* 547–570.

Shadish, W. R., & Cook, T. D. (1999). Comment-design rules: More steps toward a complete theory of quasi-experimentation. *Statistical Science, 14,* 294–300.

Shadish, W. R., Cook, T. D., & Campbell, D. T. (2002). *Experimental and quasi-experimental designs for generalized causal inference.* Boston: Houghton Mifflin Company.

Shadish, W. R., Matt, G. E., Navarro, A. M., & Phillips, G. (2000). The effects of psychological therapies under clinically representative conditions: A meta-analysis. *Psychological Bulletin, 126,* 512–529.

Shadish, W. R., & Sweeney, R. B. (1991). Mediators and moderators in meta-analysis: There's a reason we don't let dodo birds tell us which psychotherapies should have prizes. *Journal of Consulting and Clinical Psychology, 59,* 883–893.

Shaffer, D., Philips, I., Garland, A., & Bacon, K. (1989). Prevention issues in youth suicide. In D. Shaffer, I. Philips, & N. B. Enzer (Eds.), *Prevention of mental disorders, alcohol, and other drug use in children and adolescents* (pp. 373–412). (Office for Substance Abuse Prevention Monograph 2, U.S. DHHS Publication No. (ADM) 90-1646). Washington, DC: U.S. Government Printing Office.

Sharma, S., Durand, R. M., & Gur-Arie, O. (1981). Identification and analysis of moderator variables. *Journal of Marketing Research, 18,* 291–300.

Sheets, V. L., & Braver, S. L. (1999). Organizational status and perceived sexual harassment: Detecting the mediators of a null effect. *Personality and Social Psychology Bulletin, 25,* 1159–1171.

Sherman, S. J., & Gorkin, L. (1980). Attitude bolstering when behavior is inconsistent with central attitudes. *Journal of Experimental Social Psychology, 16,* 388–403.

Shipley, B. (2000). *Cause and correlation in biology: A user's guide to path analysis, structural equations, and causal inference.* Cambridge, England: Cambridge.

Shrout, P. E., & Bolger, N. (2002). Mediation in experimental and nonexperimental studies: New procedures and recommendations. *Psychological Methods, 7,* 422–445.

Shultz, T. R. (1982). Rules of causal attribution. *Monographs of the Society for Research in Child Development, 47*(1, Serial No, 194).

Sidani, S., & Sechrest, L. (1999). Putting program theory into operation. *American Journal of Evaluation, 20,* 227–238.

Silver, A. A., & Hagin, R. A. (1989). Prevention of learning disorders. In D. Shaffer, I. Philips, & N. B. Enzer (Eds.), *Prevention of mental disorders, alcohol, and other drug use in children and adolescents* (pp. 413–442). (Office for Substance Abuse Prevention Monograph 2, DHHS Publication No. (ADM) 89-1646). Washington, DC: U.S. Government Printing Office.

Simon, H. A. (1954). Spurious correlation: A causal interpretation. *Journal of the American Statistical Association, 49,* 467–479.

Singer, J. D., & Willett, J. B. (2003). *Applied longitudinal data analysis: Modeling change and event occurrence.* London: Oxford University Press.

Skinner, B. F. (1961). A functional analysis of verbal behavior. In S. Saporta & J. R. Bastian (Eds.), *Psycholinguistics: A book of readings* (pp. 67–74). New York: Holt, Rinehart, and Winston.

Smith, B. W., & Freedy, J. R. (2000). Psychosocial resource loss as a mediator of the effects of flood exposure on psychological distress and physical symptoms. *Journal of Traumatic Stress, 13,* 349–357.

Smith, E. R. (1982). Beliefs, attributions, and evaluations: Nonhierarchical models of mediation in social cognition. *Journal of Personality and Social Psychology, 43,* 248–259.

Smith, H. F. (1957). Interpretation of adjusted treatment means and regressions in analysis of covariance. *Biometrics, 13,* 282–308.

Snedecor, G. W. (1946). *Statistical methods* (4th ed.). Ames: The Iowa State College Press.

Sobel, M. E. (1982). Asymptotic confidence intervals for indirect effects in structural equation models. *Sociological Methodology, 13,* 290–312.

Sobel, M. E. (1986). Some new results on indirect effects and their standard errors in covariance structure models. *Sociological Methodology, 16,* 159–186.

Sobel, M. E. (1987). Direct and indirect effects in linear structural equation models. *Sociological Methods & Research, 16,* 155–176.

Sobel, M. E. (1990). Effect analysis and causation in linear structural equation models. *Psychometrika, 55,* 495–515.

Sobel, M. E. (1998). Causal inference in statistical models of the process of socioeconomic achievement: A case study. *Sociological Methods and Research, 27,* 318–348.

Sobel, M. E. (in press). Identification of causal parameters in randomized studies with mediating variables. *Journal of Educational and Behavioral Statistics.*

Spencer, S. J., Zanna, M. P., & Fong, G. T. (2005). Establishing a causal chain: Why experiments are often more effective than mediational analyses in examining psychological processes. *Journal of Personality and Social Psychology, 89,* 845–851.

Spirtes, P., Glymour, C., & Scheines, R. (1993). *Causation, prediction, and search*. New York: Springer-Verlag

Springer, M. D. (1979). *The algebra of random variables*. New York: Wiley.

Springer, M. D., & Thompson, W. E. (1966). The distribution of products of independent random variables. *SIAM Journal on Applied Mathematics, 14*, 511–526.

SPSS, Inc. (1999). *SPSS base 9.0 user's guide*. Chicago: SPSS.

StatXact 4 for Windows [computer software] (1999). Cambridge, MA: Software Corp.

Stelzl, I. (1986). Changing a causal hypothesis without changing the fit: Some rules for generating equivalent path models. *Multivariate Behavioral Research, 21*, 309–331.

Stephenson, M. T., & Holbert, R. L. (2003). A Monte Carlo simulation of observable versus latent variable structural equation modeling techniques. *Communication Research, 30*, 332–354.

Stewart, J. (1999). *Calculus: Early Transcendentals* (4th ed.). New York: Brooks Cole.

Stolzenberg, R. M. (1980). The measurement and decomposition of causal effects in nonlinear and nonadditive models. *Sociological Methodology, 1*, 459–488.

Stolzenberg, R. M., & Relles, D. A. (1990). Theory testing in a world of constrained research design. *Sociological Methods & Research, 18*, 395–415.

Stone, A. A. (1992). Selected methodological concepts: Mediation and moderation, individual differences, aggregation strategies, and variability of replicates. In N. Schneiderman, P. McCabe, & A. Baum (Eds.) *Perspectives in behavioral medicine: Stress and disease processes* (pp. 55–71). Hillsdale, NJ: Lawrence Erlbaum Associates.

Stone, C. A., & Sobel, M. E. (1990). The robustness of estimates of total indirect effects in covariance structure models estimated by maximum likelihood. *Psychometrika, 55*, 337–352.

Stouffer, S. A., Suchman, E. A., DeVinney, L. C., Star, S. A., & Williams, R. M., Jr. (1949). *The American soldier: Adjustments during army life* (Vol. 1). Princeton, NJ: Princeton University Press.

Suppes, P. C. (1970). *A probabilistic theory of causality*. Amsterdam: North-Holland.

Susser, M. (1973). *Causal thinking in the health sciences: Concepts and strategies of epidemiology*. New York: Oxford University Press.

Susser, M. (1991). What is a cause and how do we know one? A grammar for pragmatic epidemiology. *American Journal of Epidemiology, 133*, 635–648.

Sussman, S. (Ed.) (2001), *Handbook of program development for health behavior research and practice*. Thousand Oaks, CA: Sage.

Swanson, J. M., & Chapman, L. (1994). Inside the black box: Theoretical and methodological issues in conducting evaluation research using a qualitative approach. In J. M. Morse (Ed.), *Critical issues in qualitative research methods* (pp. 66–93). Thousand Oaks, CA: Sage.

Taborga, M. P. (2000, May). *Effect size in mediation models*. Unpublished master's thesis, Arizona State University, Tempe.

Taborga, M. P., MacKinnon, D. P., & Krull, J. L. (1999, June). *A simulation study of effect size measures in mediation models*. Poster presented at the 7th annual meeting of the Society for Prevention Research, New Orleans, LA.

Tang, T. Z., & DeRubeis, R. J. (1999). Sudden gains and critical sessions in cognitive-behavioral therapy for depression. *Journal of Consulting and Clinical Psychology, 67*, 894–904.

Tatsuoka, M. M. (with Lohnes, P. R.) (1988). *Multivariate analysis: Techniques for educational and psychological research* (2nd ed.). New York: MacMillan.

Taylor, S. E., & Fiske, S. T. (1981). Getting inside the head: Methodologies for process analysis in attribution and social cognition. In J. H. Harvey, W. Ickes, & R. F. Kidd (Eds.), *New directions in attribution research* (Vol. 3, pp. 459–524). Hillsdale, NJ: Lawrence Erlbaum Associates.

Taylor, A. B., & MacKinnon, D. P. (2006). *Permutation tests for the mediated effect.* Unpublished manuscript.

Tein, J. Y., & MacKinnon, D. P. (2003). Estimating mediated effects with survival data. In H. Yanai, A. O. Rikkyo, K. Shigemasu, Y. Kano, & J. J. Meulman (Eds.) *New developments in psychometrics: Proceedings of the International Meeting of the Psychometric Society,* (pp. 405–412). Tokyo: Springer-Verlag.

Tein, J. Y., Sandler, I. N., MacKinnon, D. P., & Wolchik, S. A. (2004). How did it work? Who did it work for? Mediation in the context of a moderated prevention effect for children of divorce. *Journal of Consulting and Clinical Psychology, 72,* 617–624.

Tinklepaugh, O. L. (1928). An experimental study of representative factors in monkeys. *Comparative Psychology, 8,* 197–236.

Tisak J., & Meredith, W. (1990). Descriptive and associative developmental models. In A. von Eye (Ed.), *Statistical methods in longitudinal research* (Vol. 2, pp. 387–406). New York: Academic Press.

Tobler, N. S. (1986). Meta-analysis of 143 adolescent drug prevention programs: Quantitative outcome results of program participants compared to a control or comparison group. *Journal of Drug Issues, 16,* 537–567.

Tofighi, D., MacKinnon, D. P., & Yoon, M. (2006). *Covariance among regression coefficients in a single mediator model.* Unpublished manuscript.

Tolman, E. C. (1935). Psychology versus immediate experience. *Philosophy of Science, 2,* 356–380.

Tolman, E. C. (1938). The determiners of behavior at a choice point. *Psychological Review, 45,* 1–41.

Törnqvist, L., Vartia, P., & Vartia, Y. O. (1985). How should relative changes be measured? *American Statistician, 39,* 43–46.

Trochim, W. M. K. (1985). Pattern matching, validity, and conceptualization in program evaluation. *Evaluation Review, 9,* 575–604.

Turner, R. J., Wheaton, B., & Lloyd, D. A. (1995). The epidemiology of social stress. *American Sociological Review, 60,* 104–125.

U.S. Department of Health, Education, and Welfare. (1964). *Smoking and health: Report of the advisory committee to the Surgeon General of the public health service* (DHEW Publication No. PHS 1103). Washington, DC: U.S. Government Printing Office.

Vandenbroucke, J. P. (1988). Which John Snow should set the example for clinical epidemiology? *Journal of Clinical Epidemiology, 41,* 1215–1216.

Verhaeghen, P., & Salthouse, T. A. (1997). Meta-analyses of age-cognition relations in adulthood: Estimates of linear and nonlinear age effects and structural models. *Psychological Bulletin, 122,* 231–249.

Wall, M. M., & Amemiya, Y. (in press). Nonlinear structural equation modeling as a statistical method. In S. Y. Lee (Ed.), *Handbook of latent variable and related models* (pp. 321–344). Amsterdam: Elsevier.

Walsh, J. E. (1947). Concerning the effect of the intraclass correlation on certain significance tests. *Annals of Mathematical Statistics, 18*, 88–96.

Warner, B. D., & Rountree, P. W. (1997). Local social ties in a community and crime model: Questioning the systemic nature of informal social control. *Social Problems, 44*, 520–536.

Weed, D. L. (1998). Commentary: Beyond black box epidemiology. *American Journal of Public Health, 88*, 12–14.

Weersing, V. R., & Weisz, J. R. (2002). Mechanisms of action in youth psychotherapy. *Journal of Child Psychology and Psychiatry, 43*, 3–29.

Wegener, D. T., & Fabrigar, L. R. (2000). Analysis and design for nonexperimental data: Addressing causal and noncausal hypotheses. In H. T. Reis & C. M. Judd (Eds.), *Handbook of research methods in social and personality psychology* (pp. 412–450). New York: Cambridge University Press.

Weiner, B., Russell, D., & Lerman, D. (1979). The cognition-emotion process in achievement-related contexts. *Journal of Personality and Social Psychology, 37*, 1211–1220.

Weiss, C. H. (1997). How can theory-based evaluation make greater headway? *Evaluation Review, 21*, 501–524.

Weisz, J. R., & Kazdin, A. E. (2003). Concluding thoughts: Present and future of evidence-based psychotherapies for children and adolescents. In A. E. Kazdin & J. R. Weisz (Eds.), *Evidence based psychotherapies for children and adolescents* (pp. 439–452). New York: Guilford.

West, S. G., & Aiken, L. S. (1997). Towards understanding individual effects in multicomponent prevention programs: Design and analysis strategies. In K. Bryant, M. Windle, & S. West (Eds.), *The science of prevention: Methodological advances from alcohol and substance abuse research* (pp. 167–209). Washington, DC: American Psychological Association.

West, S. G., Aiken, L. S., & Todd, M. (1993). Probing the effects of individual components in multiple component prevention programs. *American Journal of Community Psychology, 21*, 571–605.

Wheelwright, P. (1951). *Aristotle*. New York: Odyssey.

Wiley, D. E. (1973). The identification problem for structural equation models with unmeasured variables. In A. S. Goldberger & O. D. Duncan (Eds.), *Structural equation models in the social sciences* (pp. 69–83). New York: Seminar Press.

Wilkinson, L., & the Task Force on Statistical Inference, APA Board of Scientific Affairs (1999). Statistical methods in psychology journals: Guidelines and explanations. *American Psychologist, 54*, 594–604.

Williams, J., & MacKinnon, D. P. (in press). Resampling and distribution of the product methods for testing indirect effects in complex models. *Structural Equation Modeling*.

Wineburg, S. S. (1987). The self-fulfillment of the self-fulfilling prophecy. *Educational Researcher, 16*, 28–37.

Winship, C., & Mare, R. D. (1983). Structural equations and path analysis for discrete data. *American Journal of Sociology, 89*, 54–110.

Witteman, J. C. M., D'Agostino, R. B., Stijnen, T., Kannel, W. B., Cobb, J. C., de Ridder, M. A. J., et al. (1998). G-estimation of causal effects: Isolated systolic hypertension and cardiovascular death in the Framingham Heart Study. *American Journal of Epidemiology, 148*, 390–401.

Wohlwill, J. F. (1973). *The study of behavior development.* New York: Academic Press.

Wolchik, S. A., West, S. G., Westover, S., Sandler, I. N., Martin, A., Lustig, J., et al. (1993). The children of divorce parenting intervention: Outcome evaluation of an empirically based program. *American Journal of Community Psychology, 21,* 293–331.

Wolfle, L. M. (1999). Sewall Wright on the method of path coefficients: An annotated bibliography. *Structural Equation Modeling, 6,* 280–291.

Woodworth, R. S. (1928). Dynamic psychology. In C. Murchison (Ed.), *Psychologies of 1925* (pp. 111–126). Worcester, MA: Clark University Press.

Word, C. O., Zanna, M. P., & Cooper, J. (1974). The nonverbal mediation of self-fulfilling prophecies in interracial interaction. *Journal of Experimental Social Psychology, 10,* 109–120.

Wright, S. (1920). The relative importance of heredity and environment in determining the piebald pattern of guinea-pigs. *Proceedings of the National Academy of Sciences, 6,* 320–332.

Wright, S. (1921). Correlation and causation. *Journal of Agricultural Research, 20,* 557–585.

Wright, S. (1923). The theory of path coefficients: A reply to Niles's criticism. *Genetics, 8,* 239–255.

Wright, S. (1934). The method of path coefficients. *Annals of Mathematical Statistics, 5,* 161–215.

Yung, Y. F., & Bentler, P. M. (1996). Bootstrapping techniques in analysis of mean and covariance structures. In G. A. Marcoulides & R. E. Schumacker (Eds.), *Advanced structural equation modeling: Issues and techniques* (pp. 195–226). Mahwah, NJ: Lawrence Erlbaum Associates.

Appendix A

Answers to Odd-Numbered Exercises

Chapter 1

1.1. There are many interesting aspects of mediation definitions in the OED. For example, the word *mediate* is from the Latin word *mediare*, to be in the middle.

1.3. Two examples of S–O–R models are the following (a) Pavlov's bell leads to conditioned hunger response that leads to eating. (b) Putting an animal in a maze leads the animal to remember prior rewarded maze actions that leads to behavior to complete the maze. Two examples of mediation in prevention are the following. (a) Tobacco prevention programs are designed to change social norms to be less tolerant of tobacco use and reduced tolerance for tobacco use is hypothesized to reduce smoking. (b) A health promotion program encourages team members to communicate about healthy eating and healthy eating reduces percent body fat.

1.5. Most models of human behavior are likely to be affected by more than one variable so it makes sense to consider models with many variables. The drawback of including several variables is the number of possible relations among the variables. One option is to hypothesize and to test the different types of effects described in this chapter such as mediator, moderator, and confounder variables in more complicated models.

1.7. a. confounder
   b. moderator
   c. mediator
   d. moderator

1.9. The Horst (1941) study is considered one of the first examples of suppression because the addition of a third variable, verbal ability, increased the relation between mechanical ability and pilot training success. Mechanical ability was related to success in pilot training during World War II. Verbal ability predicted the test of mechanical ability because increased verbal ability made it easier to read the test and increased test performance. Verbal ability had only a small relation with pilot training success. As a result, removing the relation of verbal ability from the test of mechanical ability actually increased the relation between mechanical ability and piloting success. Verbal ability can also be considered a confounder because including it changes the relation between mechanical ability and piloting success.

1.11. The simple X to Y relation was that suicide rates were higher for married persons compared to unmarried persons. When stratified by age, suicide rates were actually lower for married persons compared with unmarried persons for most age groups. Rosenberg (1968) calls age a distorter variable because including it in the analysis revealed that the correct interpretation was actually the reverse of the interpretation when the distorter variable was not included. The distorter variable was also a confounding variable because it changed the relation between two variables. In this case it reversed the sign of the relation.

Chapter 2

2.1. They criticized the typical way of assessing mediation because it failed to consider the relation of the mediator to the dependent variable. It is possible that there is a significant relation of the independent variable on the mediator and a significant relation of the independent variable on the dependent variable yet no or very little evidence for the relation of the mediator to the dependent variable.

2.3. Briefly, action theory would focus on the three mediators targeted. Smoking cessation programs targeted smoking, medication is used to lower cholesterol, and medication is used to lower blood pressure. Prior research, especially from the Framingham study found a substantial associations between smoking, cholesterol level, and blood pressure and cardiovascular disease

2.5. Mediation for explanation example: Physical abuse in early childhood is associated with violence later in life. Dodge, Bates, and Pettit (1990) found evidence that deviant social processing measures mediated the relation between early childhood physical abuse and later aggressive behavior. Mediation for design example: Middle school drug prevention programs target social norms, resistance skills, and communication skills because changing these mediating variables are hypothesized to reduce tobacco, alcohol, and marijuana use.

2.7. Surrogate endpoints are typically variables that are used instead of an outcome and as a result are more closely related to the ultimate outcome. Surrogate endpoints also tend to explain the entire relation between an independent variable and a dependent variable. A mediator is less clearly related to the dependent variable because it is not considered a surrogate for the dependent variable and often more than one mediator explains a relation between the independent variable and the dependent variable.

2.9. Surrogate endpoints tend to lie very close to the ultimate endpoint. In some mediation studies, a surrogate endpoint would actually be considered a useful dependent variable. For example, blood pressure may be considered in some cases as a surrogate for cardiovascular health, but it is also used as a dependent variable in other studies. Another study may attempt to change mediators to change blood pressure.

2.11. For school-based prevention, social learning theory provides a rationale for the modeling of resisting drugs and changing norms to be less tolerant of drug use. Some of the mediators targeted in drug prevention campaigns include knowledge, social norms, beliefs about positive and negative consequences of drug use, bonding with school, adults, and family, communication skills, and intentions to use drugs.

Chapter 3

3.1. a. $s_{ab} = \sqrt{(0.2^2)(0.01^2) + (0.4^2)(0.1^2)} = 0.0400$, $z' = 0.08 / 0.0400 = 1.998$

b. $s_{ab} = \sqrt{(0.22^2)(0.1^2) + (0.22^2)(0.1^2)} = 0.0311$, $z' = 0.0484 / 0.0311 = 1.556$

c. $s_{ab} = \sqrt{(0.2^2)(0.01^2) + (0.4^2)(0.2^2)} = 0.0800$, $z' = 0.08 / 0.0800 = 1.0$

d. $s_{ab} = \sqrt{(0.2^2)(0.4^2) + (0.4^2)(0.01^2)} = 0.0801$, $z' = 0.08 / 0.0801 = 1.0$

e. The significance levels of the individual coefficients are positively related to the significance level of the mediated effect, such that two individually significant coefficients are more likely to yield a significant mediated effect. In general, both coefficients must be statistically significant for the test of the mediated effect to be statistically significant. Note also that dividing the mediated effect by the standard error does not necessarily have a normal distribution. A test of significance based on the distribution of the product is more accurate.

3.3. The causal step method does not provide a direct test of significance for the mediated effect. Instead, one assesses mediation through the presence or absence of several model criteria in the steps. Calculating

the ratio of the mediated effect to its standard error not only provides a point estimate of the mediated effect, but also allows for sig-
nificance testing of the $\hat{a}\hat{b}$ or $\hat{c} - \hat{c}'$ quantity. Finally, the causal steps
method requires a significant overall effect of X on Y, which reduces
power of the mediation test and does not support the estimation
of models in which there may be a significant mediated effect but
nonzero overall effect (e.g., suppression or inconsistent mediation
models).

3.5. Donaldson, Graham, & Hansen (1994) evaluated the Adolescent
Alcohol Prevention Trial (AAPT), an intervention program designed
to prevent the onset of adolescent drug/alcohol use. Two psychological mediators, resistance skills training and social norms, were
hypothesized to link the program to desired outcomes. Donaldson
et al. implemented path analysis in an analysis of covariance design
to test for possible mediation effects. They examined the significance
of all component paths (i.e., direct and indirect) to provide evidence
for mediation.

Chapter 4

4.3. Component Quantities:

$N = 15$	$r_{XY} = .01576$	$r_{XM} = -.90500$
$r_{YM} = .40843$	$s_Y = .13601$	$s_X = 0.09865$
$s_M = .32515$		
$\hat{a} = -2.98297$	$\hat{b} = .97701$	$\hat{c} = .02173$
$\hat{c}' = 2.93612$	$r_{YM.X} = 0.9937$	

Note that these data were simulated with $a = -3$, $b = 1$ and $c' = 3$ for
an inconsistent mediation model.

Calculations:

$$\text{Regression coefficient for } \hat{c}' = \frac{.0158 - (-.9050)(.4084)(.1360)}{1 - (-.9050)^2(.0986)} = 2.9361$$

$$\text{Regression coefficient for } \hat{b} = \frac{.4084 - (-.9050)(.0158)(.1360)}{1 - (-.9050)^2(.3252)} = .9770$$

$$\text{Proportion Mediated} = \frac{(-2.9830)(.9770)}{.02173} = -134.118$$

Ratio of mediated effect to direct effect: $\dfrac{(-2.9830)(.9770)}{2.9361} = -.9926$

Ratio of X on Y to X on M: $\dfrac{.0217}{-2.9830} = -.9926$

R^2 *Multiple*: $\dfrac{(0.4084^2 + .0158^2) - (2(0.4084)(0.0158)(-.9050)}{1 - (-.905)^2} = 0.9875$

R^2 #1: $0.4084^2 - (0.9875 - (.0158^2) = -.8204$

R^2 #2: $(-.9050^2)(0.9937^2) = -.8088$

R^2 #3: $\dfrac{(-.9050^2)(.9937^2)}{.9875} = -.8242$

4.5. The proportion mediated equals −825.425 and the ratio of mediated to direct effect equals 0.73547. A negative value for the proportion mediated and a value outside the range of ±1 is not sensible. This illustrates the problem with the proportion mediated measure. The ratio mediated makes more sense here but is often very unstable even at large sample sizes.

4.7. a. See Equation 4.30; b. See Equation 6.23, where $a = \gamma$, $b = \beta_1$, and $d = \beta_2$.

4.9. The function for the difference between c and c' for standardized variables equals $r_{XY} - ((r_{XY} - r_{MY}r_{XM})/(1 - r_{XM}^2))$. The partial derivatives with respect to r_{XY}, r_{XM}, and r_{MY} equal $r_{XM}/(1 - r_{XM}^2)$, $(-2r_{XM}r_{XY} + r_{MY} + r_{XM}^2 r_{MY})/(1 - r_{XM}^2)^2$, and $-((r_{XM}^2)/(1 - r_{XM}^2))$, respectively. As described in the chapter, the multivariate delta method can be used to obtain the asymptotic variance by pre- and post-multiplying the vector of partial derivatives by the covariance matrix among r_{XY}, r_{XM} and r_{MY}.

4.11. Here are some of the steps in the derivation:

$\mathrm{Cov}(c, c') = t/s\,(X_2{}^\mathsf{T}X_2)(X_1{}^\mathsf{T}X_1)\sigma^2 y - t/s(X_2{}^\mathsf{T}X_1)(X_1{}^\mathsf{T}X_2)\sigma^2 y$

$\mathrm{Cov}(c, c') = [[(X_2{}^\mathsf{T}X_2)(X_1{}^\mathsf{T}X_1) - (X_2{}^\mathsf{T}X_1)^2]\sigma^2 y]/[(X_1{}^\mathsf{T}X_2)s]$

$\mathrm{Cov}(c, c') = s\sigma^2 y/[s(X_1{}^\mathsf{T}X_1)]$

$\mathrm{Cov}(c, c') = \sigma^2 y/(X_1{}^\mathsf{T}X_1)$

Chapter 5

5.1. a. $\hat{a}_1\hat{b}_1 = (0.3441)(-0.4830) = -0.1662003$

$\hat{a}_2\hat{b}_2 = (0.0542)(0.3365) = 0.0182383$

$s_{\hat{a}_1\hat{b}_1} = \sqrt{(0.3441^2)(0.0647^2) + (-0.4830^2)(0.0471^2)} = 0.031831$

$s_{\hat{a}_2\hat{b}_2} = \sqrt{(0.0542^2)(0.0562^2) + (0.3365^2)(0.0129^2)} = 0.0053023$

$$\frac{\hat{a}_1\hat{b}_1}{s_{\hat{a}_1\hat{b}_1}} = \frac{-0.1662003}{0.031831} = -5.22141$$

$$\frac{\hat{a}_2\hat{b}_2}{s_{\hat{a}_2\hat{b}_2}} = \frac{0.0182383}{0.005302956} = 3.43927$$

b. Assess $X \rightarrow Y: \dfrac{\hat{c}}{s_{\hat{c}}} = \dfrac{-0.0014}{0.0603} = 0.02322$, ns

Assess $X \rightarrow M1: \dfrac{\hat{a}_1}{s_{\hat{a}_1}} = \dfrac{0.3441}{0.0471} = 7.30573$, $p < 0.05$

Assess $M1 \rightarrow Y: \dfrac{\hat{b}_1}{s_{\hat{b}_1}} = \dfrac{-0.4830}{0.0647} = 7.46522$, $p < 0.05$

Assess $X \rightarrow M2: \dfrac{\hat{a}_2}{s_{\hat{a}_2}} = \dfrac{0.0542}{0.0129} = 4.20155$, $p < 0.05$

Assess $M2 \rightarrow Y: \dfrac{\hat{b}_2}{s_{\hat{b}_2}} = \dfrac{0.3365}{0.0562} = 5.9875$, $p < 0.05$

Assess $\hat{c}$ vs. $\hat{c}'$: $0.2332 > 0.0044$

c. 95% CI for $\hat{a}_1\hat{b}_1$: $= -0.1662003 \pm 1.96(0.031831)$

$$LCL = -0.228589$$
$$UCL = -0.10381$$

95% CI for $\hat{a}_2\hat{b}_2$: $= 0.0182383 \pm 1.96(0.0053023)$

$$LCL = .007845$$
$$UCL = 0.02863$$

d. Because the overall effect of X on Y is nonsignificant, the causal steps method finds that there is no mediation. This contrasts with the finding in part A of 5.1, in which the point estimates divided by their respective standard errors show significant mediated effects. Given that zero is not included in the 95% confidence intervals, and significant mediated effects based on the product of coefficients computation method, there is significant mediation of the prevention program on subsequent alcohol use by both social norms and resistance skills. A follow-up study may investigate possible moderation effects to determine whether the program worked differentially on subjects given particular characteristics. Studies to manipulate more specific aspects of the norms and skills manipulation may be useful.

5.3. a. $\hat{a}_1\hat{b}_1 = (0.237149)(0.281868) = 0.06684$

$\hat{a}_2\hat{b}_2 = (0.131117)(0.059703) = 0.00783$

$\hat{a}_3\hat{b}_3 = (0.242897)(0.335794) = 0.08156$

$\hat{a}_4\hat{b}_4 = (0.243409)(0.114041) = 0.02776$

Total mediated effect:

$$\sum_{\hat{a}_1\hat{b}_1}^{\hat{a}_4\hat{b}_4} = 0.06684 + 0.00783 + 0.08156 + 0.02776 = 0.18399$$

b. $\hat{a}_1\hat{b}_1 = (0.237149)(0.281868) = 0.06684$

$$s_{\hat{a}_1\hat{b}_1} = \sqrt{(0.237149^2)(0.053233^2) + (0.281868^2)(0.046217^2)} = 0.018140$$

$$\frac{\hat{a}_1\hat{b}_1}{s_{\hat{a}_1\hat{b}}} = \frac{0.06684}{0.018140} = 3.68459$$

$$= 0.06684 \pm 1.96(0.018140)$$
95% Confidence Limits: $= 0.06684 \pm 0.03555$
$$LCL = 0.03129$$
$$UCL = 0.10239$$

$$\hat{a}_2\hat{b}_2 = (0.131117)(0.059703) = 0.00783$$

$$s_{\hat{a}_2\hat{b}_2} = \sqrt{(0.131117^2)(0.054959^2) + (0.059703^2)(0.044780^2)} = 0.007686$$

$$\frac{\hat{a}_2\hat{b}_2}{s_{\hat{a}_2\hat{b}_2}} = \frac{0.00783}{0.007686019} = 1.01873$$

$$= 0.00783 \pm 1.96(0.007686)$$
95% Confidence Limits: $= 0.00783 \pm 0.01506$
$$LCL = -0.000723$$
$$UCL = 0.02289$$

$$\hat{a}_3\hat{b}_3 = (0.242897)(0.335794) = 0.08156$$

$$s_{\hat{a}_3\hat{b}_3} = \sqrt{(0.242897^2)(0.054272^2) + (0.335794^2)(0.045270^2)} = 0.020121$$

$$\frac{\hat{a}_3\hat{b}_3}{s_{\hat{a}_3\hat{b}_3}} = \frac{0.08156}{0.020121} = 4.05345$$

$$= 0.08156 \pm 1.96(0.020121)$$
95% CI for $\hat{a}\hat{b}_2$: $= 0.08156 \pm 0.03944$
$$LCL = 0.04212$$
$$UCL = 0.121$$

$$\hat{a}_4\hat{b}_4 = (0.243409)(0.114041) = 0.02776$$

$$s_{\hat{a}_4\hat{b}_4} = \sqrt{(0.243409^2)(0.053507^2) + (0.114041^2)(0.045899^2)} = 0.014037$$

$$\frac{\hat{a}_4\hat{b}_4}{s_{\hat{a}_4\hat{b}_4}} = \frac{0.02776}{0.014037} = 1.97769$$

$$= 0.02776 \pm 1.96(0.014037)$$

95% CI for $\hat{a}\hat{b}_2$: $\quad = 0.02776 \pm 0.02751$

$$LCL = 0.00025$$

$$UCL = 0.05527$$

c. $\dfrac{a_1b_1 - a_2b_2}{s_{a_1b_1-a_2b_2}} = \dfrac{0.05902}{0.01181} = 4.9985, \, p < 0.05$

$$\left(\begin{aligned}
s_{a_1b_1-a_2b_2} &= \sqrt{s^2_{s_{a_1b_1}} + s^2_{s_{a_2b_2}} - 2a_1a_2s_{b_1b_2}} \\
&= \sqrt{0.018140^2 + 0.007686^2 - 2(0.237149)(0.131117)(0.0040)} \\
&= \sqrt{0.000329 + 0.000059 - 0.000249} \\
&= \sqrt{0.000139} \\
&= 0.01181
\end{aligned} \right)$$

Chapter 6

6.1.

$$
\begin{bmatrix} M_1 \\ M_2 \\ Y \end{bmatrix} = \begin{bmatrix} 0 & 0 & 0 \\ 0 & 0 & 0 \\ b_1 & b_2 & 0 \end{bmatrix} \begin{bmatrix} M_1 \\ M_2 \\ Y \end{bmatrix} + \begin{bmatrix} a_1 \\ a_2 \\ c' \end{bmatrix} \begin{bmatrix} X \end{bmatrix} + \begin{bmatrix} e_1 \\ e_2 \\ e_3 \end{bmatrix}
$$

$$
= \begin{bmatrix} 0 & 0 & 0 \\ 0 & 0 & 0 \\ -0.4830 & 0.3365 & 0 \end{bmatrix} \begin{bmatrix} M_1 \\ M_2 \\ Y \end{bmatrix} + \begin{bmatrix} 0.3441 \\ 0.0542 \\ 0.0044 \end{bmatrix} \begin{bmatrix} X \end{bmatrix} + \begin{bmatrix} e_1 \\ e_2 \\ e_3 \end{bmatrix}
$$

6.3.a. Selected CALIS output

The CALIS Procedure

Covariance Structure Analysis: Maximum Likelihood Estimation

Observations	40	Model Terms	1
Variables	4	Model Matrices	4
Informations	10	Parameters	9

Manifest Variable Equations with Estimates

m1 =	0.8401*x	+ 1.0000 e1
Std Err	0.1559 a1	
t Value	5.3883	
m2 =	0.2219*x	+ 1.0000 e2
Std Err	0.1441 a2	
t Value	1.5396	
y =	0.5690*m1	+ 0.5297*m2 + 0.1122*x + 1.0000 e3
Std Err	0.1507 b1	0.1630 b2 0.1992 c
t Value	3.7769	3.2502 0.5631

Variances of Exogenous Variables

Variable	Parameter	Standard Estimate	Error	t Value
x		84.84872		
e1	ee1	80.44700	18.21766	4.42
e2	ee2	68.74247	15.56710	4.42
e3	ee3	64.94416	14.70696	4.42

Covariances Among Exogenous Variables

Var1	Var2	Parameter	Standard Estimate	Error	t Value
e1	e2	cm1m2	−22.06700	12.42111	−1.78

6.3. b. Yes, the estimates from SAS Proc CALIS are the same, within rounding error, as the estimates from EQS and LISREL.

6.5. Due to measurement error, it is unlikely that any of these constructs are perfectly reliable, which affects the validity of these constructs. One way to account for measurement error is to use latent variables with multiple indicators. Three indicators of father's occupation are income, size of company, and job title. Three indicators of father's education are highest degree attained, number of years of school, and grade point average. Three indicators of respondent's occupation are income, size of company, and job title. Three indicators of respondent's education are highest degree attained, number of years of school, and grade point average. It is more difficult to specify three indicators for respondent's number of siblings or income.

6.7. MODEL INDIRECT:

OCC1962 ind FATHOCC;
OCC1962 ind FATHEDUC;
OCC1962 ind NUMSIB;

INC1961 ind FATHEDUC;
INC1961 ind FATHOCC;
INC1961 ind NUMSIB;
INC1961 ind EDUC;

—OR—

MODEL INDIRECT:

OCC1962 ind EDUC FATHOCC;
OCC1962 ind EDUC FATHEDUC;
OCC1962 ind EDUC NUMSIB;

INC1961 ind EDUC FATHEDUC;
INC1961 ind EDUC FATHOCC;
INC1961 ind EDUC NUMSIB;
INC1961 ind OCC1962 FATHEDUC;
INC1961 ind OCC1962 FATHOCC;

INC1961 ind OCC1962 NUMSIB;
INC1961 ind EDUC OCC1962 FATHEDUC;
INC1961 ind EDUC OCC1962 FATHOCC;
INC1961 ind EDUC OCC1962 NUMSIB;

INC1961 ind EDUC;

Chapter 7

7.1.

$$
\Lambda_x = \begin{bmatrix} \lambda_{x1} \\ \lambda_{x2} \\ \lambda_{x3} \\ \lambda_{x4} \end{bmatrix} \quad
\Theta_\delta = \begin{bmatrix} \delta_{11} & 0 & 0 & 0 \\ 0 & \delta_{22} & 0 & 0 \\ 0 & 0 & \delta_{33} & 0 \\ 0 & 0 & 0 & \delta_{44} \end{bmatrix}
$$

$$
\Lambda_y = \begin{bmatrix} \lambda_{y11} & 0 \\ \lambda_{y21} & 0 \\ \lambda_{y31} & 0 \\ \lambda_{y41} & 0 \\ 0 & \lambda_{y52} \\ 0 & \lambda_{y62} \\ 0 & \lambda_{y72} \\ 0 & \lambda_{y82} \end{bmatrix} \quad
\Theta_\varepsilon = \begin{bmatrix} \varepsilon_{11} & 0 & 0 & 0 & 0 & 0 & 0 & 0 \\ 0 & \varepsilon_{22} & 0 & 0 & 0 & 0 & 0 & 0 \\ 0 & 0 & \varepsilon_{33} & 0 & 0 & 0 & 0 & 0 \\ 0 & 0 & 0 & \varepsilon_{44} & 0 & 0 & 0 & 0 \\ 0 & 0 & 0 & 0 & \varepsilon_{55} & 0 & 0 & 0 \\ 0 & 0 & 0 & 0 & 0 & \varepsilon_{66} & 0 & 0 \\ 0 & 0 & 0 & 0 & 0 & 0 & \varepsilon_{77} & 0 \\ 0 & 0 & 0 & 0 & 0 & 0 & 0 & \varepsilon_{88} \end{bmatrix}
$$

$$
\Gamma = \begin{bmatrix} \gamma_1 \\ \gamma_2 \end{bmatrix} \quad
B = \begin{bmatrix} 0 & 0 \\ \beta_{21} & 0 \end{bmatrix} \quad
\Psi = \begin{bmatrix} \psi_{11} & 0 \\ 0 & \psi_{22} \end{bmatrix} \quad
\Phi = \begin{bmatrix} \phi_{11} \end{bmatrix}
$$

```
EQS:
/TITLE
      Three Factor Latent Variable Model
/SPECIFICATIONS
VARIABLES=12; CASES=100;
MATRIX=CORRELATION; ANALYSIS=COVARIANCE;
METHOD=ML;
/LABELS
       V1=X1;   V2=X2;   V3=X3;    V4=X4;
       V5=M1;   V6=M2;   V7=M3;    V8=M4;
       V9=Y1;   V10=Y2;  V11=Y3;  V12=Y4;
       F1=X;    F2=M;    F3=Y;
```

```
/EQUATIONS
        V1   = 1 F1  + E1;
        V2   = *F1  + E2;
        V3   = *F1  + E3;
        V4   = *F1  + E3;
        V5   = 1 F2  + E5;
        V6   = *F2  + E6;
        V7   = *F2  + E7;
        V8   = *F2  + E8;
        V9   = 1 F3  + E9;
        V10  = *F3  + E10;
        V11  = *F3  + E11;
        V12  = *F3  + E12;
        F2   = *F1  + D2;
        F3   = *F1  + *F2 + D3;
/VARIANCES
        F1 = *;
        D2 TO D3 = *;
        E1 TO E12 = *;
/END
LISREL:
THREE FACTOR MODEL
DA NI=12 NO=100
LA
X1 x2 x3 x4 m1 m2 m3 m4 y1 y2 y3 y4
SE
4 5 6 7 8 9 1 2 3
MO NX=4 NK=1 NY=8 NE=2 PS=SY,FIGA=FU,FIPH=FU,FITE=DI,
FR LX=FU,FILY=FU,FIBE=FU,FI
FR LX(2)LX(3)LX(4)
FR LY(2,1) LY(3,1) LY(4,1)
FR LY(6,2) LY(7,2) LY(8,2)
VA 1 LX(1) LY(1,1) LY(4,2)
FR BE(2,1)
FR GA(1) GA(2)
FR PS(1,1) PS(2,2)
FR PH(1,1)
OU MI RS EF MR SS SC


MPLUS:
TITLE: Three Factor Three Indicator Model Chapter 7
Example 1;
```

```
DATA:
  FILE IS "C:\chapt7 _ exp1";
  TYPE IS CORRELATION STD;
  NGROUPS = 1;
  NOBSERVATIONS = 100;

VARIABLE:
  NAMES ARE x1 x2 x3 x4 m1 m2 m3 m4 y1 y2 y3 y4;
  USEVARIABLES ARE x1 x2 x3 x4 m1 m2 m3 m4 y1 y2 y3 y4;

ANALYSIS:
  TYPE IS GENERAL;
  ESTIMATOR IS ML;
  ITERATIONS = 1000;
  CONVERGENCE = 0.00005;

Model:
  x by x1@1 x2 x3 x4;
  m by m1@1 m2 m3 m4;
  y by y1@1 y2 y3 y4;
  y on x m;
  m on x;

OUTPUT:   SAMPSTAT STANDARDIZED;
```

7.3. The additional indirect effect matrices for multiple indicator models represent the indirect effects of the η variables on the Y variables and the indirect effects of the ξ variables on the Y variables.

7.5. THREE FACTOR MODEL
Number of Iterations = 7
LISREL Estimates (Maximum Likelihood)

LAMBDA-Y

	ETA 1	ETA 2
coach1	1.00	—
coach2	1.75	—
	(0.25)	
	6.96	
coach3	1.48	—
	(0.21)	
	6.94	

severe1	—	1.00
severe2	—	1.18
		(0.08)
		15.30
severe3	—	1.27
		(0.08)
		15.44

LAMBDA-X

	KSI 1
intent1	1.00
intent2	1.47
	(0.07)
	21.41
intent3	1.50
	(0.07)
	20.97

BETA

	ETA 1	ETA 2
ETA 1	—	—
ETA 2	−0.38	—
		(0.09)
		−4.31

GAMMA

	KSI 1
ETA 1	−0.06
	(0.04)
	−1.62
ETA 2	0.30
	(0.05)
	5.54

Covariance Matrix of ETA and KSI

	ETA 1	ETA 2	KSI 1
ETA 1	0.47		
ETA 2	−0.20	0.97	
KSI 1	−0.05	0.26	0.80

PHI

KSI 1
0.80
(0.08)
9.93

PSI

Note: This matrix is diagonal.

ETA 1	ETA 2
0.47	0.82
(0.12)	(0.10)
3.78	8.24

Squared Multiple Correlations for Structural Equations

ETA 1	ETA 2
0.01	0.16

Squared Multiple Correlations for Reduced Form

ETA 1	ETA 2
0.01	0.09

Reduced Form

	KSI 1
ETA 1	−0.06
	(0.04)
	−1.62
ETA 2	0.32
	(0.06)
	5.84

THETA-EPS

coach1	coach2	coach3	severe1	severe2	severe3
3.26	0.91	0.63	1.10	0.86	0.53
(0.21)	(0.16)	(0.12)	(0.08)	(0.08)	(0.08)
15.81	5.65	5.49	13.57	10.64	6.78

Squared Multiple Correlations for Y - Variables

coach1	coach2	coach3	severe1	severe2	severe3
0.13	0.61	0.62	0.47	0.61	0.75

THETA-DELTA

intent1	intent2	intent3
0.63	0.22	0.56
(0.04)	(0.05)	(0.06)
14.47	4.76	9.73

Squared Multiple Correlations for X - Variables

intent1	intent2	intent3
0.56	0.89	0.76

Goodness of Fit Statistics
Degrees of Freedom = 24
Minimum Fit Function Chi-Square = 29.11 (P = 0.22)
Normal Theory Weighted Least Squares Chi-Square = 28.44
  (P = 0.24)
Root Mean Square Residual (RMR) = 0.073
Standardized RMR = 0.030
Goodness of Fit Index (GFI) = 0.99

Note that all the fit indices are the same as the model without variables reversed. Perceived severity does not appear to mediate the effect of intentions on coach tolerance because the $\hat{a}$ path from intentions to severity is not statistically significant. These results may simply reflect that intentions are not significantly related to perceived severity, not any mediation relation. Longitudinal data may shed light on the relation among these variables. Experimental manipulation of the variables such as in a prevention program to manipulate coach tolerance to change intentions may also help clarify the ordering of the variables. In addition, the sequence of variables is not consistent with theory for how the variables are related.

7.7. The higher the reliability of X1, the closer the observed partial correlation is to the true partial correlation.

Chapter 8

8.1.   a. The values in Tables 8.1 are correct.
       b. .90.
8.3.   In the typical parallel process latent growth curve model, the relation
       of the slope in the X variable is related to the slope in the M variable,
       which is related to the slope in the Y variable. These relations are
       essentially correlations among slopes, which does not clearly reflect
       a time ordering. It is possible to estimate latent growth models such
       that the slope in variables does reflect time ordering such as when
       the slope in the X for the first three waves is related to the slope in
       M for the next three waves, and the slope in M is related to the slope
       in Y for the last three waves. The latent difference score explicitly
       models change between waves in a way that change in earlier waves
       can be related to change in later waves.
8.5.   It is interesting to conceive of the Collins et al. person-centered
       approach with continuous variables. One option is to specify a test
       for each condition but with continuous data. Another option is to
       dichotomize continuous measures to form binary variables suitable
       for analysis with the Collins et al. method. Many different cut points
       could be used and mediation investigated for each of the cut points.
       These analyses may reveal important thresholds with continuous
       data.

Chapter 9

9.1.   The correlation would be zero.
9.3.   a. Individual attitudes about drug use affect individual intentions
          to use drugs, which then affects an individual's actual drug use,
          where the Level 1 variable is individuals.
       b. An intervention given to sports teams to improve nutrition
          increases team cohesion, which then increases the number of
          games won by the teams, where the Level 2 variable is teams
          and the Level 1 variable is individuals.
       c. Perceived classmate intelligence affects an individual's percep-
          tion of his or her own intelligence, which affects individual
          achievement, where the Level 2 variable is classrooms and the
          Level 1 variable is students.
       d. Budgetary differences at schools affect classroom size, which
          affects student learning, where the Level 3 variable is schools,
          the Level 2 variable is classrooms, and the Level 1 variable is
          students.

e. Differences in the amount of resources a state allocates to mental health issues affects how close an individual lives to a mental health care facility, which affects the likelihood of seeking help for depression, which affects the number of times an individual attempts suicide, where the Level 3 variable is states, a Level 2 variable could be counties, and the Level 1 variable is individual.

Chapter 10

10.1. A mediator is a third variable that explains the mechanism by which two other variables are related, thus answering "how" or "why" there is a relation between the other variables. For example, drug resistance skills for refusing drug offers may mediate the relation between a program that taught those skills and a drug use outcome. A moderator is a third variable that defines the conditions (e.g., levels of a variable) under which a given relation between other variables is true. For example, increased achievement may decrease depression, but this effect may only hold for subjects with low initial achievement (Merrill, 1994). Mediated moderation is used to explain the source of an overall moderated treatment effect of X on Y, where mediation (i.e., XZ→M→Y) is responsible for the overall moderated relation. For example, the influence of a cognitive prime on game behavior may be moderated by one's social value orientation. The reason for this moderation could be the result of forming expectations of one's partner's behavior in a game, given the social value orientation (Muller et al., 2005). Moderated mediation is used to describe when a mediated relation of X→M→Y differs across the levels of another variable. For example, intentions to use drugs may mediate the relation between a prevention program and drug use, but this effect may only be present for subjects who were risk takers; a program's effect on intentions to use drugs may affect those subjects who are risk takers.

10.3. It is reasonable to expect both mediation and moderation effects in prevention research for example. There should be a quantifiable mechanism by which a program is intended to achieve success (i.e., a mediator of the program), although that mechanism may not hold true for all recipients (i.e., moderation). How much or how little one should tailor a prevention/intervention based on program efficacy in certain subgroups is a compound decision.

10.5. There are several ways that a measure of work completed could be used in the analysis. Fit persons may just be able to complete more tasks. The number of tasks completed could be a measure of energy expenditure which ought to be related to water consumed thereby reducing unexplained variability in water consumed. It is also possible that self-reported thirst may be related to tasks completed. Temperature may be related to tasks completed which then affects thirst and water consumed; the rationale being that tasks are more easily completed in cooler temperatures.

Chapter 11

11.1. The product of coefficients and difference in coefficients methods of computing mediation are not equivalent in logistic and probit regression because the residual variances associated with the mediation regression equations are fixed, to set the metric of the latent outcome. Thus, any change in model coefficients is dependent on the error term, and the scale of the dependent variables differs across equations.

11.3. a. $Y^* = -0.6409 + 0.2771X$

$(se_{\hat{c}} = 0.1118)$

$Y^* = -1.4507 + 0.139X + 0.4406M$

$(se_{\hat{c}} = 0.1213, se_b = 0.1244)$

$M = 1.78228 + 0.33748X$

$(se_{\hat{a}} = 0.06067)$

b. $\hat{c} - \hat{c}' = 0.2771 - 0.139 = 0.1381$

$\hat{a}\hat{b} = (0.33748)(0.4406) = 0.1487$

c. $s_{\hat{a}\hat{b}} = \sqrt{(0.33748^2)(0.1244^2) + (0.4406^2)(0.06067^2)} = 0.04977$

$s_{\hat{c}-\hat{c}'} = \sqrt{0.1118^2 + 0.1213^2 - (2)(0.0125)} = 0.047042$

$\dfrac{\hat{c} - \hat{c}'}{s_{\hat{c}-\hat{c}'}} = \dfrac{0.1381}{0.047042} = 2.9374$

$\dfrac{\hat{a}\hat{b}}{s_{\hat{a}\hat{b}}} = \dfrac{0.1487}{0.04977} = 2.9877$

95% Confidence Limits $(c - c')$: $= 0.1381 \pm 1.96(0.047042)$

$= 0.1381 \pm 0.0922$

$LCL = 0.0459$

$UCL = 0.2303$

$$= 0.1487 \pm 1.96(0.04977)$$

95% Confidence Limits (ab): $= 0.1487 \pm 0.0975$

$$LCL = 0.0512$$
$$UCL = 0.2462$$

Although the mediated effect estimates across the $\hat{a}\hat{b}$ and $\hat{c} - \hat{c}'$ methods differ in the 10ths decimal place, results associated with significance tests and confidence limits are consistent.

d. Proportion Mediated $= \dfrac{(0.33748)(0.4406)}{0.2771} = 0.5366$

$$= 0.5366 \pm 1.96(0.2632)$$

95% CI for the proportion mediated: $= 0.5366 \pm 0.5159$

$$LCL = -0.0174$$
$$UCL = 1.0142$$

e. The unstandardized difference estimate was .1381 and the product estimate was .1489. By using the standardization in Equation 11.6, the value of the difference method was .1479, which is now much closer to the product estimate standardization with Equations 11.4 and 11.5 yields a product and difference estimate of .078 and .077, respectively.

Chapter 12

12.1. $(8!)^2 = 1{,}625{,}702{,}400$ unique data sets with eight subjects and three observations.

12.3. The bootstrap may yield more accurate confidence intervals for the mediated effect because it does not require a normal distribution for the mediated effect.

12.5. The definition of bootstrap is to rely only on one's own efforts and resources, as in pulling one's self up by the bootstraps. Bootstrap resampling is so named because the method relies only on the data in your sample, not on any other data or data distributions.

The jackknife is so called because a jackknife is a very useful tool to have handy, just as the jackknife method of estimating variance is a very useful tool to have handy.

Chapter 13

13.1. A statistical simulation was conducted using the simulation program described in chapter 4 for a sample size of 100 and 500 replications for 16 different values of a, b, c', and three values of d (0, .2, and 0.5). Overall, there were more Type I errors for the b coefficient, which is not surprising because d is added to the b coefficient in the population model. Regarding detection of mediation effects, there was no increase in Type I error rates when b was equal to zero, but the power to detect the mediated effect was greater for nonzero values of d.

13.5. There are four variables in the two mediator models discussed in chapter 4. Each of the variables, X, M1, M2, and Y may be in all possible positions in the model. Path relations and correlations may be reversed and still have equivalent models. It is also important to note that there are six possible two-way interactions, four three-way interactions, and one four-way interactions that may be necessary to accurately represent the data.

Chapter 14

14.1. The dummy codes listed correspond to the difference between the control and cognitive (C1) and between control and psychoanalytic (C2).

Group	C1	C2
Control	0	0
Cognitive	1	0
Psychoanalytic	0	1

14.3. This statement is true in that mediation ideas and theory are not strictly quantitative. However, it is somewhat inaccurate because in testing mediation ideas and theory, it is helpful to obtain quantitative information on theory to assess effects.

14.5. The stage of the research would dictate the design. Let's say that I start with studies of conceptual and action theory to understand what actions can be taken to change a mediator and also the extent to which the mediator is related to the dependent variables. Once a reasonable strategy to change the mediators is determined, a randomized study would be planned to compare different theories about how the dependent variable comes about. After the results of this study are obtained, several follow-up experimental studies would be conducted, such as blockage or enhancement designs. Ideally qualitative studies would be conducted along with replication studies consisting of extensions of the mediation theory to other contexts.

Appendix B

Notation

Chapter 1

X	Independent variable
M	Mediating variable
Y	Dependent variable
Z	Third variable

Chapter 3

c	Coefficient relating X to Y
a	Coefficient relating X to M
b	Coefficient relating M to Y adjusted for X
c'	Coefficient relating X to Y adjusted for M
$b_{unadjusted}$	Coefficient relating M to Y not adjusted for X

Hats above coefficients represent estimates or estimators, for example, $\hat{a}$, $\hat{b}$, $\hat{c}$, $\hat{c}'$, and $\hat{a}\hat{b}$, $\hat{c}-\hat{c}$

LCL	Lower confidence limit
UCL	Upper confidence limit
i	intercept
e	residual
MSE	Mean Square Error
N	Sample Size
z	value on the standard normal distribution
t	value on the t distribution
s_{first}	standard error of $\hat{a}\hat{b}$ based on first derivatives
s_{second}	standard error of $\hat{a}\hat{b}$ based on first and second derivatives
$s_{unbiased}$	unbiased standard error of $\hat{a}\hat{b}$

Chapter 4

r_{XY}	correlation between X and Y
r_{XM}	correlation between X and M
r_{MY}	correlation between M and Y
$r_{XY.M}$	correlation between X and Y partialled for M
$r_{XM.Y}$	correlation between X and M partialled for Y

$r_{MY.X}$	correlation between M and Y partialled for X
$R^2_{Y,XM}$	correlation squared between Y and both X and M
$E(X)$	Expectation of X
$Cov[X,Y]$	Covariance of X and Y
θ	parameter
Σ_θ	covariance matrix among parameters
s_X	standard deviation of X
c'_s	standardized $\hat{c}'$ coefficient
$\sigma^2_{e_2}$	population residual variance for Equation 3.2
$\hat{\sigma}^2_{e_2}$	sample estimate of residual variance for Equation 3.2
σ	standard error if subscript has a hat and standard deviation of an estimator if there is not a hat on the subscript
$s_{\hat{a}}$	standard error of $\hat{a}$
$\sigma_{\hat{a}T}$	theoretical or true standard error of $\hat{a}$
$\sigma_{\hat{a}}$	standard deviation of estimated $\hat{a}$ across replications in the Monte Carlo study
$\bar{s}_{\hat{a}}$	average standard error of $\hat{a}$ across replications in the Monte Carlo study

Chapters 6 and 7

RMSEA	Root mean square error of approximation
B	Beta matrix of coefficients relating dependent variables
β	Beta, elements in the B matrix
Γ	Gamma matrix of coefficients relating independent (exogenous) to dependent (endogenous) variables
γ	Gamma, the elements in the Γ matrix
Λ_y	Lambda Y is the matrix of coefficients relating indicators of Y to latent measures
λ_y	Lambda y, elements of Λ_y
Λ_x	Lambda X is the matrix of coefficients relating indicators of X to latent measures
λ_x	Lambda x, elements of Λ_x
Φ	Phi, covariance matrix among independent (exogenous) latent variables
ϕ	Phi, elements of Φ
Ψ	Psi, covariance matrix among dependent (endogenous) latent variables
ψ	Psi elements of Ψ
Θ_δ	Theta delta, matrix of errors in X variables
θ_δ	Theta delta, elements of θ_δ matrix
Θ_ε	Theta epsilon, matrix of errors in Y variables
θ_ε	Theta epsilon, elements of θ_ε matrix

η	Eta, latent dependent variables
ξ	Ksi, latent independent variables
ζ	Zeta, residual variance for latent dependent variables
p	Number of observed dependent or Y variables
q	Number of observed independent or X variables
m	Number of latent independent η variables
n	Number of latent dependent ξ variables
$V_{\Lambda y}$	Selection matrix for partial derivatives for Λ_y
V_B	Selection matrix for partial derivatives for B
V_Γ	Selection matrix for partial derivatives for Γ
$T_{\eta\eta}$	Total effects of latent dependent variables on latent dependent variables.
$I_{\eta\eta}$	Indirect effects of latent dependent variables on latent dependent variables.
$T_{\eta\xi}$	Total effects of latent independent variables on latent dependent variables
$I_{\eta\xi}$	Indirect effects of latent independent variables on latent dependent variables.
$I_{y\eta}$	Indirect effects of latent dependent variables on Y
$I_{\eta\xi}$	Indirect effects of latent independent variables on Y
se	standard error
sd	standard deviation

Chapter 8

τx	intercepts for X variables
τy	intercepts for Y variables
κ	intercepts for latent independent (exogenous) variables
α	intercepts for latent dependent (endogenous) variables
I_{Xi}	intercept for X
S_1	stability coefficient
I_{Mi}	LGC intercept for the M variable
S_{Mi}	LGC slope for the M variable
I_{MOi}	LGC intercept for the prediction of I_{Mi}
S_{MOi}	LGC intercept for the prediction of S_{Mi}
ΔM_2	Latent difference between wave 2 and wave 1 for the M variable
M_t	Mediator stage at time t
nM_t	Not in Mediator at time t

Chapter 9

ICC	Intraclass correlation
β_{0j}	Group level intercept for j groups in the multilevel model

e_{ij}	Individual error associated with the ith individual in the jth group in the multilevel model
γ_{00}	Overall mean of the groups in the regression models where group mean is the dependent variable in the multilevel model
u_{0j}	Random deviation of the predicted group-level mean from the observed group-level mean in the multilevel model
τ_{00}	Var (u_{0j}) Variation between group means in the multilevel model
σ^2	variance of the residuals at the individual level in the multilevel model
u_{1j}	Random error of the a coefficient at the group level in the multilevel random effects model
u_{2j}	Random error of the b coefficient at the group level in the multilevel random effects model
u_{3j}	Random error of the c' coefficient at the group level in the multilevel random effects model

Chapter 11

Y^*	Continuous latent variable underling a categorical variable
$\hat{c}_{corrected}$	$\hat{c}$ coefficient corrected to be in the same metric as $\hat{c}'$
$\hat{\sigma}^2_{Equation\ 11.3}$	Estimated residual variance in Equation 11.3

Chapter 13

RCM	Rubin's causal model
ACE	Average causal effect
FACE	Prima facie causal effect
C-FACE	Covariate adjusted prima facie causal effect
ITT	Intention to treat
TOT	Treatment effect among treated
ICC	Intraclass correlation
LATE	Local average treatment effect
SUTVA	Stable unit treatment value assumption
ALICE	Additive linear and constant effects
M'	Predicted value of M
U	set of units
u	Individual unit
K	Set of conditions
t	Treatment or encouragement to study
c	Control or no encouragements to study
X(u)	Unit in a condition
M(u,x)	Mediator score for unit u in condition x

Y(u,x,m)	Dependent variable score for unit u in condition x and a value of m
Y(u,t,m)	Score for unit u if u is encouraged to study and studies m hours
Y(u,c,m)	Score for unit u if u is not encouraged to study and studies m hours
Y(u,c, M(c))	Score for unit u if u is not encouraged to study, and a mediator score in the control group
Y(u,t, M(t))	Score for unit u if u is encouraged to study, and a mediator score in the treatment group
p	Constant number of hours that encouragement increases each student's amount of study; the causal effect of t on M
$f + pB_c$	Constant linear improvement in test scores due to encouragement to study; the causal effect of t on Y
f	Constant amount that encouragement increases the test scores of a student who always studies m hours; the causal effect of encouragement on test scores for a student who always studies m hours
B_c	Constant amount that studying 1 more hour increases a student's test score
g	Average value of test scores for students when they are not encouraged to study and they do not study for all students who would study an amount m when they are not encouraged to study
d	Slope relating the more a student studies when not encouraged, the higher he or she would score on the test without studying and without encouragement

Author Index

Bursten, B. E., 4
Burzykowski, T., 384
Buyse, M., 33*t*, 83, 91, 304, 384

C

Campbell, D. T., 4, 196, 350, 352, 355, 356, 370, 371, 377
Campbell, N. A., 4
Carmack, C., 35
Castellino, D. R., 216
Castro, F. G., 382
Catalano, R. F., 41
Catellier, D. J., 238
Chamberlain, P., 29
Chapman, L., 390
Chassin, L., 30, 382
Chen, H. T., 39, 41
Cheng, T., 90, 91, 110
Cheong, J., 211, 212, 213
Chernick, M. R., 334
Choi, S., 32, 33*t*, 35
Clarke, G. N., 38, 68, 241, 271, 330
Cliff, N., 15
Clogg, C. C., 69, 90, 91, 110
Cobb, J. C., 230, 364
Cochran, W. G., 16, 31
Cohen, J., 53, 54, 70, 80, 84, 128, 191
Cohen, P., 53, 54, 70, 128
Cole, D. A., 200, 201, 202
Collins, L. M., 9, 230, 231, 235, 236, 396, 405
Conger, A. J., 7
Cook, T. D., 350, 352, 355, 356, 370, 371, 377, 378, 383, 384, 386
Cooper, H., 378, 383, 384, 386
Cooper, J., 378
Cordray, D. S., 378, 383, 384, 386
Cornwell, L. W., 95, 96
Cox, G. M., 31
Coyle, S. L., 36
Crabtree, B. F., 388
Craig, C. C., 95, 96
Crocker, L., 174
Cronbach, L. J., 197, 370, 388
Cudeck, R., 193
Cuijpers, P., 37
Cummings, G., 364
Curran, P. J., 30, 209, 223, 289, 295, 383

D

D'Agostino, R. B., 230, 364
Darlington, R. B., 65, 175
Darwin, C., 327
Davenport, J. M., 239
Davis, J. A., 110
Davis, M. A., 37
Dawber, T. R., 299
Day, N. E., 32, 33*t*
de Leeuw, J., 240, 244
DeMets, D. L., 32, 33*t*, 34
de Ridder, M. A. J., 230, 364
DeRubeis, R., J., 29, 65
DeVinney, L. C., 17
Diaconis, P., 390
DiClemente, C. C., 37
Dodge, K. A., 216, 436
Donaldson, S. I., 35, 38, 438
Dosman, D., 364
Downer, A., 37
Dryfoos, J. G., 36
Dudley, H., 328
Duffy, S. W., 32, 33*t*
Duncan, B., 17, 18, 30, 136, 149, 151, 209, 365
Duncan, O. D., 149, 151
Duncan, S. C., 209
Duncan, T. E., 209
Dunn, A. L., 36
Durand, R. M., 10, 276
Dusenbury, L., 38
Duval, R. D., 326
Dworkin, S. L., 388
Dwyer, J. H., 19, 34, 37, 38, 60, 73, 82, 85, 90, 91, 94, 100, 196, 197, 209, 223, 230, 240, 302, 304, 306, 307, 373

E

Earls, F., 241, 272, 274
Echt, D. S., 33
Eddy, J. M., 29
Eden, T., 327
Edgington, E. S., 326, 330, 334
Efron, B., 326, 333, 334, 354, 355
Ehrhardt, A. A., 388
Eisenberg, L., 79
Elliot, D. L., 38, 68, 241, 271, 330
Eng, A., 38
Escobar, L. A., 96

Subject Index